THE DUCT TAPE DIET

A frustrated dieter's way of taking fat off...
A registered dietitian's way of keeping it off

By Leonard Malysz and
Theresa Malysz, RD

Drivetime Publishing, Rochester, Michigan

Library of Congress

Publisher's Cataloging-in-Publication
(Provided by Quality Books, Inc.)

Malysz, Leonard
The duct tape diet : a frustrated dieter's way of taking fat off--a registered dietitian's way of keeping it off / by Leonard Malysz and Theresa Malysz.
p. cm.
Includes bibliographical references and index.
LCCN 2003095368
ISBN 0-9643610-0-0

1. Reducing diets. I. Malysz, Theresa. II. Title.

RM222.2.M319 2004 613.2'5
QBI03-200655

The information provided by the authors is intended for educational and entertainment purposes, and not as a substitute for advice and/or treatment obtained from a consultation with your physician. Please see a qualified health professional if you suspect you are unwell. Your reading of this book indicates your acknowledgement of and agreement with this disclaimer.

Edited by: Renea Schultz
Cover Design: AnneMarie Malysz

Published by Drivetime Publishing
P.O. Box 80246, Rochester, Michigan 48308-0246 U.S.A.

Printed in the United States of America

Acknowledgments

Many thanks are due to those who've contributed to this effort in countless ways and helped us bring this book to completion. The task was more than we expected.

Our peer review group included Betty Kriegel, MS, RD; and Debbie Socks, RD, CDE; both of whom spent many hours reading our manuscript to ensure the accuracy of the content and the appropriateness of the material. Another reading was done by Nancy McLuckie, an avid reader of diet books, who gave us valuable feedback regarding our approach and style.

Our editor, proofreader and daughter, Renea Schultz, struggled through a medical emergency to fulfill her responsibilities to this project. We are indebted to her for this personal commitment of time and talent above and beyond the call of duty.

Graphic designer and daughter-in-law AnneMarie Malysz brought a wealth of knowledge and creativity to our book cover and website design, which we believe are unique and most appealing. Her contributions are greatly appreciated.

We also want to acknowledge the support of Theresa's transplant team management, especially Dr. Henry Oh, Director of Transplant Surgery; and Transplant Specialist Nancy Satmary, RN; both of whom graciously lent their names to our back cover testimonials.

The support from colleagues, family and friends has taken us through some challenging phases of our journey to bring this dream to reality. For that, we are truly grateful.

INTRODUCTION

Can a weight–loss diet actually be fun? Can we laugh at ourselves when the emotional need to binge on "diet villains" is thwarted by a thin, gray strip? Can you decide what foods to allow on your diet and still lose weight? The answer to all three questions is a resounding YES!

And it's all here in *The Duct Tape Diet* (DTD). Born out of a frustrated dieter's "battle of the binge," the DTD is an approach that allows us to be fallible human beings. Regardless of age, gender, apple shape or pear – the decision as to what constitutes a diet villain and whether it deserves to do hard time in duct tape jail is yours alone to make. Solitary confinement or weekly visits is the issue that makes it a Phase I accelerated weight-loss stage or Phase II maintenance for life.

What it all boils down to is making a lifestyle change – where you judge the merits of continuing down the road you're on – or taking another way that gets you to a smaller you without the pain of "a diet." This journey involved me – Len Malysz (pronounced may – liss). Yours truly lost 35 pounds on that road – and had fun doing it. The fun was knowing my destination, enjoying the scenery, smelling the flowers along the way and not missing anything I might have thought was vital to my former way of life.

You've heard of "no pain, no gain" as it relates to building muscle and strength. Well, the DTD offers "no pain, no insane diet game" in the pursuit of weight loss. This means you can take off the pounds you want without feeling hungry and without resorting to an extreme diet that loads you up with unhealthy foods or deprives you of necessary nutrients.

The DTD encourages you to enjoy the real deal when it comes to treats like ice cream rather than those pale imitations. It also makes it possible for you to eat six or more times a day, and insists that you never skip a meal.

Sounds too good to be true? If I hadn't gone through it, I'd think so too. But this diet is unique in that it puts you in control of what goes into your mouth and gives you the freedom to decide what those foods should be. It employs one of the oldest methods known to human kind – the strip of something around your finger or wrist – that reminds you of a promise you made – to yourself. This promise is affirmed through the judicial use of duct tape against your diet villains – those insidious goodies that lurk around the house as if waiting to pounce when your defenses are weakened by moods, events or powerful cravings.

The DTD was born of my personal journey through the theoretical, emotional, psychological, pharmacological and – finally – professional turns in my personal weight-loss saga. I've got a closet full of heavy/skinny-size clothes. My book shelves are bulging with nearly every fad diet published in the last 30 years. My computer hard drive is loaded with files from countless websites featuring diets and weight control subject matter.

Spouse and co-author of this book – Theresa Malysz, RD – contributed a huge chunk of knowledge and strategies gained from over ten years working as a clinical dietitian in a variety of settings. She made it clear that the mainstream of nutritional science might know something about weight loss that doesn't get headline attention in the popular press.

I learned a lot about why some of the old maxims like "an apple a day keeps the doctor away" have significant scientific and nutritional validation. I've achieved an appreciation for the great gift of life bestowed upon us all and realized that we have a duty to be responsible caretakers of the bodies we inhabit.

Perhaps the most stunning revelation is that obesity takes the lives of up to 300,000 annually. It currently condemns about a third of the total U.S. population to a life of poor health and limited opportunities. The trend is unfortunately on the rise over the past several decades – and many of the fad diets are only contributing to this worsening situation. From my standpoint, the problem rides the wave of misinformation crashing through the popular culture – and the purposeful over-complication of what is one of the simplest things in the world – healthy eating.

Our intention with the DTD is to establish a baseline of simple, easy-to-understand strategies for gradual weight loss instead of the risky fad-diet approaches that may do more harm than good. It makes no sense for you to risk your health in pursuit of something that could backfire and bring you to the brink of disaster.

I promise you one thing in this book – a painless strategy for weight loss that can change your life and allow you to reach your ideal weight without feeling hungry or exercising yourself to exhaustion. You'll get nothing but straight talk here – and some entertaining writing along the way. At least we hope it is – because the goal here is to have fun while learning the way to a healthy lifestyle. What could be easier or more enticing?

So in keeping with our straight talk promise, let's bring up a major expectation of most diet books – recipes. Many readers usually skip through these books looking for those secret recipes that are supposed to melt the fat away. Sorry to disappoint, but this is not a cookbook, it is a weight-loss book based on healthy eating strategies.

We are focusing on getting you thinner rather than padding our efforts here with recipes that fewer of you would have the time or inclination to prepare in the first place. Therefore, we do not include recipes other than those that illustrate a strategy – such as our stove-top "kettle popcorn" using canola oil and popcorn seasoning to prepare a healthy snack.

But we do know that many of you who thumb through these pages are searching for ways to get past the frustrations of yo-yo dieting and wishing to start a new life in a thinner and healthier body. That – friends – is what we're here for.

Our hope is that whoever reads these pages is motivated to take action today regarding an overweight or obese condition, and realize that lifestyle modification does not have to be an all or nothing proposition. Think about how Michaelangelo started with a slab of marble. He never took drastic action with a sledge hammer and bashed away with potentially catastrophic consequences. He chipped a little here, a little there, and over time created a figure of great beauty.

That's what you can do in terms of changing the way you have thus far molded your body. Small efforts here and there over time add up to lifestyle changes that can help you bring out that beautiful body and keep it for the rest of your life.

The important thing is to make a commitment to do something about it and start on that day-by-day, step-by-step walk toward your ideal weight. It didn't just take six weeks to acquire your excess weight – so you can't expect to lose it that quickly. Realize that your body needs enough time to lose those unwanted pounds so it can find that set point where it wants to stabilize. Otherwise, you're gambling with your health and subjecting yourself to unnecessary risk.

This is an opportunity for us to embark on an important quest, perhaps the most important ever. It's an event that could very well change your life – for the better.

Every journey begins by taking that first step. Let's join together and walk this path toward a new life – and a healthier lifestyle.

Table of Contents

INTRODUCTION 5

CHAPTER 1~BIRTH OF THE DUCT TAPE DIET 11

CHAPTER 2~TAKING CONTROL 17

CHAPTER 3~WARNING – CARBS/CALORIES, ETC. 25

CHAPTER 4~RISKS OF QUICK WEIGHT LOSS 35

CHAPTER 5~LADIES – START YOUR ENGINES 43

CHAPTER 6~THE BUZZ ON SUGAR 65

CHAPTER 7~ROAD TO OBESITY 71

CHAPTER 8~FOOD LABEL LITERACY 79

CHAPTER 9~THROWING WEIGHT AROUND 85

CHAPTER 10~WEIGHT-LOSS STRATEGIES 91

CHAPTER 11~MIND OVER FATTER 107

CHAPTER 12~FOOD FIGHT 115

CHAPTER 13~MEALS AWAY 121

CHAPTER 14~MANDATORY EXERCISE? 129

CHAPTER 15~PUTTING IT ALL TOGETHER 133

APPENDIX A~ADDITIONAL READING, MEASURE EQUIVALENTS 139

APPENDIX B~ABBREVIATIONS IN USDA NUTRIENT DATABASE FOR STANDARD REFERENCE RELEASE 15 143

APPENDIX C~USDA NUTRIENT DATABASE FOR STANDARD REFERENCE RELEASE 15 .. 147

INDEX 327

Chapter 1
BIRTH OF THE DUCT TAPE DIET

Take control of your diet villains with the "tool kit on a roll."

You'll have to trust us on this, but the idea of The Duct Tape Diet (hereafter known as the DTD) was born about three weeks before the federal government's endorsement of duct tape as a citizen's best defense against evil doers on U.S. soil.

The whole idea of using this most unlikely diet enhancer came about because Len was fussing about the issue of carbohydrates making him fat. So in an effort to bring you the full measure of what drove him to take immediate action on that fateful night, the telling of it shifts to a first-person narrative. This is a technique we'll employ throughout the book, so please take note of it and enjoy the fun.

DIET VILLAINS GET MUMMIFIED

I was tossing and turning my way through a sleepless night brought about by a binge of carbohydrates in the form of 10 cups of oil-popped popcorn (55-cal./cup x 10 = 550 calories) and 8-ounces of red wine (85-cal./4 oz. x 2 = 170 calories) – and doing this math in my mind over and over again.

"Good grief – that's a total of 720 calories! What was I thinking?" This kept going through my brain like a hammer once used in those old headache commercials.

And what made it all the worse – I was working on a diet book at the time. Not this book, but one that focused on the role of insulin reacting to high levels of metabolized carbohydrates that turn to sugar in the bloodstream. So all of this was vividly recycling through my insulin-ravaged brain cells.

Not only did I ingest a whopping amount of calories just before bedtime (one of the worst times to stuff your face), but I violated some basic theories concerning the role of insulin contributing to the formation of fat from excessive amounts of carbs in the diet.

Finally, I couldn't stand it another second – and bounded out of bed on a mission.

"Where are you going?" my wife mumbled from her disturbed slumber.

"I'm going crazy with guilt over all the calories I just put into my body," I bleated, while stumbling into every piece of furniture on the way to my bathrobe.

"Nothing you can do about it now," she said with a yawn.

"Maybe not, but at least I can keep from doing it again," I bellowed.

"Don't you dare throw out any food, just leave it alone," she cautioned, now with a edge creeping into her voice.

"All right, then I'm going to make it as hard to get at as I can," and away I went.

What I had in mind is what food packagers do all the time – defeat the purpose of the purchase. In other words – make it impossible to get at the contents.

"Press here to open" means "lose a fingernail."

"Tear along this line" translates into "watch it tear everywhere <u>but</u> the dotted line."

Fully charged for my mission, crazed on carbs and stubbing my toes in a darkened room, I make my way to solving every dieter's problem; that is – holding those "diet villains" at bay even when they're in the house. To some, these take the form of chips, ice cream and candy. In my case, they've already been identified, if not vilified.

It's the middle of the night and I'm storming through the basement, searching for something to solve the problem once and for all. What I'm looking for has got to have the tenacity of super glue on your fingertips and the bulletproof quality of the plastic that holds beverage six-packs together.

It's always the last thing you consider – but gadzooks – I finally discovered it – quite by accident. As I stumbled into the boxes stacked chin-high – the one that crashed to earth first was the one we never opened.

It hid all my skinny clothes – bought when I slimmed down on that fad diet – and too good and expensive to throw out. But keeping the box from busting wide open was a strip of what would be the answer to my temporary insanity – duct tape.

This was not the kind originally developed to seal ammunition boxes during WWII, and evolved to sealing duct work in forced air systems with the adhesive strength of Post-it™ notes. No, my duct tape was the kind that you had to really work at to peel off the roll. And if you ever stripped some off and accidentally let the two sticky sides meet – might as well throw it away and start over because it just won't let go.

It turned out to be exactly what I needed to seal (wine connoisseurs, please avert your eyes) the twist-off cap on the gallon jug that serves as everyday table wine at our house. (It's hidden whenever guests come over.)

In my frenzy, I peeled off a 12-inch strip and brought it around and over the cap, making sure the sticky sides met. Then I lost control and started wrapping half the bottle, just to make it look less appealing.

Next was the open bottle of popcorn kernals (45 ounces/with 50% more – free). I neglected the other 12 bottles of the stuff we had squirreled away just in case the food company stopped offering the 50% more free deal. Those were factory sealed and – therefore – not a threat, but that open bottle was unlocked and loaded, so it got wrapped like an Egyptian mummy.

By now, the wife is out of bed and taking this all in. Did I mention that she's a registered dietitian? How about the part where she works with a hospital transplant team? Did I leave out that she's responsible for helping overweight patients lose weight before they can qualify for a new kidney or pancreas? And that she helps them keep the weight off after the transplant?

Well, at this point, she's talking about how after years in the profession, nothing like this scene has ever been described in any of her professional conferences or nutrition literature. Sure, there are some bizarre stories out there regarding people and their food, but this was one for the books. A man striking out against his caloric tormentors?

Okay, perhaps this concept is a little wacky, but it gets the idea across real fast to anyone in the house who really needs the message and isn't as motivated as you. Wait a second! Who am I kidding? It's for me – and you – for those times when the weight-loss motivation goes to that unceremonial burial ground. You know the place. It's where New Year's resolutions can be found in shallow graves, long forgotten and moldering away.

So – was duct tape the answer? Most of the time, it was enough to be confronted by this guardian of the goodies. It made no sound, but said plenty about why it was there in the first place. Like a nagging reminder of promises made, it drove off all but the most determined popcorn and wine junkie. And yes, there were those occasions when desire overcame resolve, but unless I was armed with a utility knife and pliers, there was just no way to get past the duct tape chastity belt.

This is how it went with my personal diet villains. Yours could be temptations of a different, more caloric variety. They might include ice cream, donuts, chips, chocolate, pizza, cheese puffs, cup cakes – you name it.

Just keep in mind that even though these &#@%$* little demons might win now and then – you can do something about it. When I jumped out of bed that night, I needed to put my tormentors in their place – bound and gagged – or something like that. Sure, you could throw these temptations out in the trash, but when you mummify them in duct tape – those multiple layers of gray vinyl and cloth are the ultimate revenge.

So there it is, boiled down. The essence of *The Duct Tape Diet* is that certain foods are real villains to your quest for a thinner body – and need to be avoided while you're trying to lose weight. In my world, they deserve their fate.

Chapter 2
TAKING CONTROL

Never let your demons get the upper hand – or allow them in your house unless bound and gagged.

Yours truly and wife have discussed this book from a number of different perspectives, and we always end up on the same basic theme – taking control of one's future through action.

The need to do so was overwhelming the night of my struggle over the popcorn and wine calories. There was this compelling need to take some kind of direct action. I felt that my diet villains were in control – and either they were going to run my life or I was going to regain the upper hand.

I had to find a way to confine these little monsters and demonstrate to myself that I could chart the course of my food intake, and not allow the temptations of these so-called comfort foods to take over and control my destiny.

It seemed that whenever I encountered a weak moment in my life, these "friends" would make things a little easier to cope. During the eating process, I felt comforted as the feelings of depression or tension would fade into the background. But as soon as the last morsel was consumed, they all came back – only this time they were holding hands with another, uglier relative – self loathing.

It's that moment where you realize how many calories you've ingested, and how much that puts you behind in your quest to lose excess weight. You begin questioning your resolve and listing all the many other qualities lacking in your makeup. Before long, you could be on the road that many travel in American society today – obesity. And more people are finding themselves in this category than ever before.

EXCUSES, EXCUSES

Theresa has heard nearly every excuse for keeping diet villains around the house from her patients at the transplant center. These include:

- The kids want it
- For when guests drop over
- I have money-off coupons
- To celebrate a small victory
- It's wasteful to throw food away
- It was on sale
- Everything else tastes like sawdust

If you have "reasons" why you can't take action against your diet villains, then you're not really serious about losing weight. It's basically that simple. Somewhere, somehow you need to find the motivation to do what has to be done.

One of the most effective techniques for getting the motivation engine started and running is a photograph that catches you as others see you. An obese woman interviewed on TV got her motor kick started when she was photographed with an infant on her lap. The stark comparison between herself and the child was so overwhelming that she became relentless in maintaining her resolve to lose 150 pounds – and did it.

A photograph taken of me at a family function accentuated my "nice round face" that my mother thought was so becoming – and served as the final straw in my motivation to get thin and find some cheek bones.

Another technique is putting a magnetized mirror on the refrigerator that flashes your image back as you open the door. If you visit our website – www.ducttapediet.com – you'll find a number of helpful items that could be the catalyst for your personal march toward a smaller-size you.

THE ORIGINAL IS ALWAYS BETTER

We've been evaluating the just-released clear version of duct tape, and find it to be much like the second, third and fourth iterations of hit movies – not always up to the standards set by the original.

For the purposes of the DTD, what I need is to hide the diet villains away and make them look like a bad day at the duct tape repair shop. That bag of chips needs to be mummified in good, old-fashioned duct tape gray. If I can still see the packaging in all its glory with just a few layers of clear tape, the allure is hardly dented at all.

Let's see if we can really nail this point. Okay – try this. Depending on your orientation, think of your favorite male or female movie star wearing nothing but crystal-clear plastic rather than opaque gray. Get the picture?

The objective is to be turned away by the sight of your favorite goodie all wrapped up and ready for the trunk of someone's car. It's that level of disgust that we're trying to achieve with this process. So when you want to make your villains pay the price for making your life miserable, use the good stuff – and show them no mercy.

A SIMPLE K.I.S.S. (Keep It Simple & Successful)

Before launching into this book project, we made a promise to ourselves that above all else, this effort would produce something uncomplicated, easy to understand and fun to read.

As stated earlier, the DTD was born out of frustration. Basically, I was unable to control periodic binges of calorie-dense snacks. But beyond that, it was frustration with the whole, complicated world created by the fad diet industry. It seems the emphasis is on obscuring the relatively simple concept of healthy eating, which leads to long-term weight loss.

In a former life, I had to edit the writings of rocket scientists (true story) and make it understandable to federal government employees who decided whether to award the contract. With that background, I have trouble grappling with the language and theories in many fad diet books today.

I'm looking at the back cover of one book at this moment and it cites a complex formula to adjust proteins, carbs and fats to fit your own unique biochemistry. Sorry, but unless you're a biochemist, how in the world are you going to deal with this subject matter – and jump through all the required hoops to weight loss?

We believe that you have better things to do with your life than deciphering fad diet mumbo-jumbo and doctoral thesis concepts that require Ph.D.-level comprehension skills. This is why we chose the title and approach you see unfolding in these pages. For those who appreciate our efforts, welcome. For others, we invite you to plow through everything else out there – and look forward to seeing you back here afterwards.

WHY STUDIES ARE NOT QUOTED

If you came to this book expecting to find it chock full of studies supporting various conclusions, I'm afraid you'll be disappointed. Why? I'll try to be as charitable as possible. A wise person once said: "statistics don't lie, but many lies can be supported by statistics." I think the same may be said about many research findings. It's almost a cliché that research studies hyped by the media are often totally contradicted by subsequent studies, most of which are health or diet related.

A classic example is the great oat bran crusade of the late 1980s. This high-fiber food source was hailed as the magic bullet after several studies found it to be a significant factor in lowering cholesterol and facilitating other health-related benefits. One year later, another study threw cold water on the original findings and sent oat bran sales into a tailspin. Therefore, if we cited a number of current studies to support a breakthrough finding, we'd be vulnerable to another oat bran scenario and – quite possibly – out of date before the printer's ink was dry.

The major purpose of the DTD is to offer weight-control information based on Theresa's professional experience with patients who successfully lost weight in a clinical environment at a major big-city medical center.

Our view is that if this book was targeted to the medical/nutritional community, we would most certainly focus on the latest research to underscore any breakthrough methodology being proposed. But since we're actually targeting the community of people who are much like those she's consulted over the years, we need to emphasize the practical, how-to aspects of permanent weight loss that have proven successful for so many.

FAT OR THIN? IT'S YOUR CHOICE

You obviously want to get your life in order and embark on a new course regarding your weight and overall health. Otherwise, you wouldn't be this far into the book. That's a choice you've made – and a wise one – if I may be so bold.

Choices are critical to how we live our lives. Even though you may not have control over certain aspects of your life – job related and otherwise – you do have control over what goes into your mouth and how often.

If everyone around you is overweight, you can choose not to be. If everyone in your office snacks on donuts in the morning, pizza at lunch and chips throughout the day, you can choose not to. You are the most important person in this whole process – and sometimes just coming to that realization is all it takes to start you on the road to a new life.

Basically, that's what this book is all about. It's ludicrous to suggest that anyone give up, overnight, the eating habits developed over a lifetime. But if you really want a new life, it's imperative that you work on those tough guys who contribute the most trouble in your diet game plan.

Some people are playing doctor with herbal supplements that can aggravate an existing condition or interfere with medically prescribed drugs intended to alleviate a problem. If your source of information is someone at the health food store, you're getting advise from an individual trying to sell you something – a motive not always in your best interest. Medical training is another issue you should consider when following a course of action.

Some of you might have a prejudice against doctors or other health care professionals, but all I can offer is my own experience. My mother and older brother both suffered from high blood pressure, but despite a long history of debilitating headaches, mine was always normal. One day, I came down with a bad cold and went to see Dr. Bill (William P. Bowman, MD). The nurse took my blood pressure and looked puzzled. Then she took a second reading from my other arm, this time with a look of concern.

Long story short, my blood pressure was so high the good doctor gave me something for it immediately and prescribed some tests that indicated I'd had it for a while. A thickened wall in one of my heart valves was evidence of that. Since then, I've been on daily medication, my blood pressure is under control, the headaches mysteriously disappeared – and my heart valve is almost back to normal. This was one bad cold I was very glad to get.

Theresa indicates that undetected high blood pressure led many of her patients to lose normal kidney function, resulting in the need for a kidney transplant. For those who might be willing to take that chance, consider that transplant recipients have a long road of anti-rejection medications and possible failure of the transplanted kidney sometime in the future. Modern medicine is a miracle of our times, but it doesn't take the place of preventive action on our part. Hypertension is the technical name, but the more common term "silent killer" nails it exactly.

If you do nothing else in response to what you read here, please get your blood pressure checked at least twice a year. If there's hypertension in your family's history, purchase an electronic blood pressure monitor and check your blood pressure weekly, if not daily. For an investment of around $35 you can keep track of something that may rob you of a healthy future.

Chapter 3
WARNING – CARBS/CALORIES, ETC.

Avoid the "white carbs" – bread, pasta, potatoes, rice – and embrace whole grain versions for the fiber and slower absorption.

I'm all for using duct tape like that yellow police line tape at crime scenes – across the whole pantry where many carbs and calories make their home. It's plainly a warning. You might even want to write the words "Caution – Do Not Enter" with a black marking pen.

I hear you. Some out there think this is a bit extreme, but if it keeps you from diving into the villains, well, mission accomplished. Presidential nominee Barry Goldwater once said: "Extremism in the defense of liberty is no vice." By posting the caution tape, however, we're interested in liberating you from excess body fat, as well as the related health problems almost certainly in your future if nothing is done about it.

Warnings of this nature have roots in other cultures. Some voodoo practitioners use the entrails of chickens. The mob sends out dead fish or a horse's head. We use duct tape to ward off the diet villains.

And we all know the vile deeds these villains commit, because we see the results in the mirror every day. If we're not careful, that image can take on the proportions of Jackie Gleason's moon face in the opening credits of the old *Honeymooner's* television series.

It's the face we see reflected in department store windows, hoping distorted glass is the reason why we hate that image. It appears in those fitting-room mirrors that add another 10-to-15 pounds. It haunts us with subtle reminders of holiday parties, Mardi Gras celebrations, St. Patrick's day binges and spring break bashes where we threw caution to the wind. Who knew then that – ounce for ounce – booze has about the same caloric punch as sugar syrup?

FOCUS ON THE "WHITE CARBS"

The media is full of anecdotal evidence on weight loss from those who've shared their stories. A common theme throughout many of these reports is the elimination of "everything white" from their diet, including bread, pasta, potatoes, cereal and rice. We're referring to an offshoot of several high-protein, low-carb diets that underscore the high glycemic values of these foods, which means they quickly metabolize into glucose.

This theory holds that a spike in blood sugar causes a response of insulin that spells big trouble for those of us concerned about weight. Excess insulin levels are said to cause fat accumulation. We maintain a neutral position on this theory until more research confirms it one way or another, but my experience in losing 35 pounds in 21 weeks seems to support it.

Here's what happened. I duct taped all the refined flour, pasta, white rice, cereal and potatoes. Then, to keep carbohydrates in my diet, I switched to 100% whole wheat bread, whole wheat pasta, brown rice, bran cereal and yams.

This accomplished a number of things. The whole grains slowed down the absorption of carbs into the bloodstream, which kept the insulin levels from spiking. They accomplished this by introducing both soluble and insoluble fiber into my system. The soluble fiber helps me feel full, while the other (also known as roughage) helps with regularity.

Dietary fiber is somewhat of a magic bullet in the arena of weight loss and long-term health. Research findings indicate a strong correlation between fiber in the diet and reduced risk of type 2 diabetes, heart disease, and several types of cancer. It also accounts for improved health of the gastrointestinal tract, where the formation of pouches can lead to diverticulitis – an inflamation of this area and possible further complications that are too indelicate for these pages. In short – eat more fiber.

HOW TO INCREASE YOUR INTAKE OF WHOLE GRAIN FOODS

Choose foods that name one of the following ingredients *first* on the label's ingredient list:

- brown rice
- oatmeal
- whole oats
- bulgur (cracked wheat)
- popcorn
- whole rye
- graham flour
- pearl barley
- whole wheat flour
- whole grains

Try some of these whole grain foods: whole wheat bread, whole grain ready-to-eat cereal, *whole wheat crackers, oatmeal, whole wheat pasta, whole barley in soup and tabouli salad.

* No hydrogenated oils in ingredients.
NOTE: "Wheat flour," "enriched flour," and "degerminated corn meal" are not whole grains.

But I also drank eight glasses of water each day, reduced my portion sizes to coincide with the serving sizes the USDA Food Pyramid recommends, focused on eliminating fatty and sweet foods, enjoyed alcohol only on special occasions, and rarely ate in restaurants. I reinstituted my 30-minute per day on the cross-country skiing machine and walked the dog about two miles every day.

So, was it the elimination of white carbs that helped me lose weight? I maintain that it was a factor, particularly from the fiber that came from substituting whole wheat bread and brown rice – all of which helped keep my cholesterol and blood pressure in the best range I've seen in years.

Please forgive the "I" references that follow, but they make a point. To this day I avoid anything with refined white flour, white rice, white potatoes, bagels, rice- or corn-based cereal. It's fixed in my mind that these foods lead me to a place I used to occupy – where excess weight dwells – and I do not want to reside there ever again. It's my non-alcoholic version of staying on the wagon.

I enjoy the comments from family and friends who remark on my smaller size, and I feel better about it. My self-esteem is at an all-time high – and I feel much younger than my age. There's nothing about my former size that I want to revisit. My clothes fit better, my wife likes the way I look, my doctor tells me he's happy with all the test results, and my dog enjoys our daily walks.

The bottom line to this new me is that I finally realized the key to weight loss and lifelong weight maintenance – calories.

THE REAL DEAL – CALORIES

Wait a second! Now you're talking about calories; what happened to carbs?

High glycemic and simple carbs are important in terms of their hunger-inducing effect – all related to their role in elevating blood sugar, stimulating the release of insulin and theoretically promoting the storage of fat.

But, if you recall, the original catalyst for the DTD was a sleepless night caused by worry over a high-calorie binge. The reason for all that angst was that I acquired a bit of knowledge through extensive research to do a book on weight loss.

I had also struggled to lose about 30 pounds and was trying to get through the "wall" – where you hit a point on the scale and make no progress on the downside for a while. Some refer to this as the "set point," which didn't really apply in my case.

But when the weight loss progress abates, your mind starts working on you with questions:

> "Why are you torturing yourself?
> Since it's not working, why not enjoy life?
> Don't you deserve it?
> After all, didn't you lose a lot already?"

These questions start chipping away at your resolve and you begin thinking "What the heck, one 4-ounce glass of wine can't hurt." But that amount goes down so well it leads to another 4-ounces, which then stimulates your appetite for something salty.

So out comes the 5-quart pot. In goes the popping corn with some canola oil – and 10 cups later, you've got 550 calories plus 170 in the wine. Nobody needs to take 720 extra calories to bed, because that's when metabolism slows down and fat can accumulate.

But your other self chimes in to justify it by pointing out the benefits of red wine for the heart. And don't forget the canola oil is monounsaturated, and popcorn is great dietary fiber, and ... well, you get the picture.

So the story goes for many of us, but for me – when the head hits the pillow – all these justifications get trumped by the calorie drum that keeps beating out the same tune. And the chorus of carbohydrates chime in for good measure. It goes something like this:

> "Let's see – 4 grams of carbs per cup of popped popcorn times 10 equals 40 plus 2 grams of carbs per 4-ounce glass of wine equals 4, totaling 44 grams of carbs. Don't you realize what all these calories are doing to the diet just before bedtime?"

At 720 calories and 44 grams of carbs, I could've had half a small cheese pizza. The difference, however, is that my popcorn and wine had no saturated fat, which can't be said of the pizza.

So it does make a difference in what you eat, even though the calories are the same. But any way you slice it, you're hard pressed to make a good case for taking on significant calories just before bedtime or any other time when the goal is to take off some excess weight.

Truth is, when all is said and done, it's calories that determine whether you're going to gain or lose weight. Since a calorie – or kilocalorie, as it's called in the scientific community – is a measurement of energy, it counts in terms of what goes in (food energy content) and what goes out (energy used by the body).

YOUR CALORIC REQUIREMENTS

Before you start eliminating calories to meet your weight-loss goals, it's really important to determine how many calories you need to keep the body functioning properly on a daily basis.

The official word from the U.S. Food and Drug Administration is in the Daily Values guide, which states that:

> "a 2,000-calorie level is about right for moderately active women, teenage girls and sedentary men, and 2,500 calories is the right target level for many men, teenage boys and active women. Many older adults, children, and sedentary women need fewer than 2,000 calories a day and may want to select target levels based on 1,600 calories a day. Some active men and teenage boys and very active women may want to select target levels based on 2,800 calories per day."

This is the FDA's range of calorie requirements. Your's may be lower or higher depending on activity level.

With as many variables as there are people, it's always a good idea to consult your doctor or dietitian before moving forward on any weight-loss plan. A registered dietitian will want to do an analysis of your specific situation before you go on any diet. Without that, it would be like a doctor trying to diagnose your medical complaint at a cocktail party without taking basic readings of weight, blood pressure, pulse rate, etc.

An RD would want to know these vital statistics, as well as any pre-existing medical conditions, such as kidney problems, heart disease, blood sugar medications and medical history involving you and your ancestors. Otherwise, you're out there on your own, self-medicating with a powerful drug – food. And make no mistake, you can drastically alter your body's chemistry by engaging in some fad diet that restricts certain nutrients necessary for good health. A registered dietitian can help you determine your specific calorie needs.

YOUR PROTEIN REQUIREMENTS

Aside from determining your basic calorie needs, there's another nutrient that's key to achieving your weight-loss goals – protein.

We can't stress enough how important it is to get an adequate supply of "complete" proteins, which are defined as having all nine amino acids involved in supporting the body's growth and maintenance. If your diet lacks any of the nine, your body starts losing muscle cells and other tissues that need rebuilding on a daily basis.

As we note elsewhere in these pages, muscle is vital to building a highly tuned calorie burning machine that metabolizes all those carbohydrates and other nutrients you consume every day.

In addition, these essential amino acids play an important part in pushing the right buttons in the brain regarding hunger sensation so that you feel full on smaller amounts of food. They also help stave off food cravings and influence feelings of alertness, depression, energy and well being. Therefore, it's important to not only ensure you're getting enough protein every day, but that your getting complete proteins.

Okay, so you're sold on the idea. But then the question is: which foods provide the complete proteins and which do not? Animal products, such as cheese, milk, meat, fish, poultry and eggs have all nine essential amino acids, while most vegetable proteins are incomplete. However, soy protein and many varieties of nuts are complete proteins.

The good news is that you can eat foods with incomplete proteins and combine them with others to get all nine essential amino acids. For example, corn lacks certain amino acids that beans have in abundance, so the two eaten together complete the protein. Most of you have been unconsciously achieving this result by combining your pasta with meat or cheese, corn tortilla with beans and your morning cereal with milk.

It's important to note that – despite being incomplete proteins – vegetables are rich sources of antioxidants – the body's best defense against free-radicals, which are responsible for many diseases. All you need is about 9% of your total calories from protein. Currently, many Americans get double that amount, with some thinking that by overindulging in protein, more muscle will be formed. Alas, that's not a proven theory.

The downside of protein overconsumption is that it puts an added strain on the kidneys, and it can cause the body to excrete calcium in the urine.

One final downside, the body is unable to store the extra dose of amino acids, so they're either excreted, burned off through exercise or stored as fat. So – if your goal is to lose weight – it's a good idea to moderate your intake of protein.

THE SOY ALTERNATIVE

The soybean is not only a complete protein – but as a vegetable – it takes on a chameleon-like role in various products as a meat-protein substitute. This unique food source assumes several disguises that nearly duplicate the original.

One of our favorite foods is a soy burger grilled on a non-stick surface, seasoned with barbecue sauce, heaped with sautéed onions (in teaspoon of olive oil) and served on a whole wheat bun. Topped with lettuce and tomato, deli mustard and low-fat mayonnaise – it's a delicious alternative to a beef burger.

Another favorite is spaghetti sauce made of one 15-oz can each of stewed tomatoes, pasta-ready tomato sauce and diced tomatoes spiced with Italian seasonings; a 4-oz can of chopped mushrooms (drained) and a 6-oz. can of Italian-style tomato paste – plus 2 cups diced onions (sautéed), a clove of finely chopped garlic and 1 cup of port wine – all simmered together with 12-oz. of soy-based recipe crumbles instead of ground beef. Every now and then, I try real meat instead of the soy product, and find it nearly impossible to tell the difference. By the way, this sauce is always used over whole wheat pasta at our dinner table.

Soy butter was a surprise discovery in the store one day. It's made of soy milk – an extract of the soy bean. I tried it, liked the taste and have used it ever since instead of the 50-50 canola oil/butter mix that was my previous favorite. For each tablespoon, soy butter has 35 calories, no saturated fat, 2 grams of monounsaturated fat and 1 gram of polyunsaturated fat.

Compare this with butter, which has 7.6 grams of saturated fat, 3.5 of monounsaturated fat, 0.5 of polyunsaturated fat and 100 calories per tablespoon. Bottom line – 75% less fat and calories per serving for soy butter. Some are turned off by its light beige color, but to my taste buds, it's the only difference.

Here's one more favorite – soy cheese. It looks, tastes, melts, and has all the texture of dairy cheese. We have it during those celebratory wine and cheese moments out on the patio.

Please note that there is a controversy about soy products having some side effects. Your family doctor should be consulted if your own level of soy protein is excessive.

OTHER ALTERNATIVES

- A long time ago, we substituted ground turkey for ground beef in most of our meals, and found it to be a good trade.

- When it comes to pizza, consider ordering a Greek pizza, which is meatless, but oh-so delicious. Ask them to use low-fat cheese, if possible.

- Salads are a great place to try some crabmeat substitute – made of fish processed to taste like the more tasty and costly crustacean.

- Try making your own salad croutons out of whole wheat pita, flavored with garlic cooking spray and Italian seasonings, and baked in a toaster oven until crisp.

Chapter 4
RISKS OF QUICK WEIGHT LOSS

If you expect to lose excess weight in a hurry, you can also expect potentially serious health consequences.

We run into people all the time who would never bet on a horse race, put money on a stock market tip or buy a car without first reading *Consumer Reports,* but think nothing of plunging into a risky diet plan because they heard someone lost weight on it.

If there's only one thing you get out of this book, we hope it's this: DON'T PLAY ROULETTE WITH YOUR HEALTH!

There are no quick, easy solutions that come from a supplement, diet pill or fad diet without risking your overall health. You didn't put the weight on overnight, and you can't expect to lose it quickly either – unless you're prepared to suffer the ocassionally serious consequences that could stay with you for a lifetime.

The human body is a fabulous creation that's developed a self-preservation mechanism evolving over thousands of years to maintain the human species during floods, famines and other interruptions to the availability of food. Then, along comes some proponent of a particular weight-loss theory that supposedly does away with all this and it's – well – a breathtaking example of arrogance.

We believe that the only sensible, healthy way to lose weight is to slowly reverse the process of weight gain with foods that fulfill your need for nutrients, fiber and satisfaction with less of the calories, saturated fat and simple carbohydrates that got you there in the first place.

We also encourage at least 30 minutes of daily exercise – be it walking the dog, taking the stairs instead of the elevator, biking or using a treadmill. It all works to rev up your metabolism, build muscle and keep your calorie burning machine in good operating condition. However, you should consult your doctor before embarking on any exercise program.

WHY FAD DIETS ULTIMATELY DON'T WORK

The truth is, most fad diets do produce quick weight loss. If you don't mind the maladies that often accompany the "emergency" weight loss for your high school reunion, then you've found your answer – temporarily, that is.

When you eventually leave that diet behind – look out – because the body's natural tendency to recover quick weight loss will kick in and you'll probably gain it all back and then some. The reason is that your fad diet threw the body's equilibrium off balance and starved it of essential nutrients, such as carbohydrates, which are necessary to feed the muscles and brain.

If you follow any diet that limits carbohydrates, the body has no choice but to get its energy from fat or muscle, which can lead to dehydration. Since the body is around 70% water, most of the weight loss on a low-carb diet can be attributed to water lost through dehydration.

Some diets that include unlimited amounts of fat – particularly saturated fat found in meat and dairy products – can lead to an increased risk of heart disease. It's particularly insidious because saturated fat induces the liver to produce cholesterol – a process that's more responsible for higher levels of blood cholesterol than what you might consume in cholesterol-rich foods. Saturated fat stimulates production of LDL (bad) cholesterol, which is primarily responsible for clogging arteries.

All of this is why you need to consult a health-care professional before embarking on any weight-loss program. Otherwise, you're embarking on a risky sea voyage without a lifeline.

INSULIN

To keep the blood sugar level in check, the pancreas secretes insulin – a powerful hormone that provides the pathway for glucose to enter the cells and feed the muscles. Since carbs turn to glucose rather quickly, those with an active lifestyle need to stoke up on muscle fuel, and carbs are the way to go.

However, when you examine the lifestyles of most adults and children in the U.S. – "active" does not describe the typical day of office workers, truck drivers, students, store clerks or Game Boy® jockeys. What does describe the American workday is a sedentary lifestyle, one that can't burn all that fuel, which then ends up being stored as fat.

The other major issue with carbs is they bring the old cliché about Chinese food to a new level of understanding because soon after eating a high-carb meal, you actually do feel hungry. That's because when blood sugar levels are high, you feel full. But when insulin rushes in to bring them back down, you often feel hungry again. And it's that cycle of frequent hunger that causes many people to eat more often and in greater quantities than they otherwise might.

Many in the diet book community argue that these high levels of insulin eventually cause the body's cells to be less sensitive to that hormone's effects, resulting in less glucose absorbed as energy and more processed into body fat. This insulin resistance syndrome is blamed for much of the obesity we see today and is becoming more of an issue with the skyrocketing number of type 2 diabetes cases occurring in the U.S. But this theory seems to have the cart before the horse, because obesity is more likely the cause of insulin resistance rather than the result.

Obesity tends to make folks less active and, therefore, less likely to burn excess fat. It also brings them down emotionally to the point where food becomes a tranquilizer – a way of easing the pain caused by self-loathing and society's intolerance. So they indulge themselves in the only way that brings them any solace – more food. Stated a bit more precisely – more of the wrong foods.

In summary, by eating too many high-glycemic carbohydrates that quickly metabolize into glucose, you get a yo-yo effect of high blood sugar levels and insulin responses, which – in turn – promote more hunger. Cells can become resistant to the frequent hits from insulin and the result may be blood sugar levels that no longer respond. Diagnosis – symptoms of insulin resistance.

The current emphasis on high glycemic foods as a major contributor to the problems of excess weight or obesity is something that merits further research. However, if we examine how the glycemic index (GI) of foods is determined, it'll help explain why this issue isn't as clear cut as some might conclude.

The method most frequently cited in the literature is the rather laborious task of asking a subject to ingest a single food item – such as white rice. Shortly thereafter, researchers take a series of blood samples from the individual to determine the blood sugar level and how quickly that specific food enters the bloodstream as glucose, which would then trigger a release of insulin.

Published results have indicated a considerable difference between GIs for the same foods. Variables that account for these differences raise questions as to the validity of the theory promoting the concept of the GI influencing weight gain on a consistent basis. For example, some people metabolize foods more quickly than others, while others have an insulin response that's faster.

Then there's the issue of glycemic load (GL), which factors in the amount of a specific food with its glycemic index to determine the overall effect that particular food has on the bloodstream. If we look at carrots, for example, the GI is rather high. But most of us would seldom make a meal out of carrots or eat more than a single serving of this food at one time, so the GL falls into the medium-to-low end of the spectrum. Unless you suffer from diabetes – that means the glycemic effects of such foods are relatively innocuous – and all the recent hype over glycemic index as a key factor in America's overweight crisis is in need of some serious re-examination.

WHO NEEDS CARBS? YOU DO!

We have some questions for the high-protein, low-carbohydrate fad diet community.

Why does the diet restrict fruits and vegetables – foods rich in antioxidants, fiber and essential nutrients?

If carbs make you fat, why are most Asians – who eat rice at nearly every meal – usually rail thin?

If carbs need to be restricted to induce weight loss, why are they so essential to brain and muscle function?

We have many more such questions but to use an analogy from the auto industry: a high-protein, low-carb diet would be like trying to improve the performance of your vehicle by draining the engine oil and crimping the fuel line. You may be able to drive it for a while, but you're flirting with a major breakdown down the road.

Responsible diet gurus ought to preach an awareness of the type of carbohydrates that cause an insulin spike and all that this entails. They should then recommend a switch from refined grains and white rice to whole grains and brown rice; and from simple sugars to complex carbohydrates that take time to break down.

We'd also like to hear them explain that Food Guide Pyramid recommendations of 6-11 servings from grains, cereal, rice and pasta translate to about 150 to 300 calories per meal. They should also educate their readers that a recommended serving size is ½ cup – not all that will fit into a pasta, rice or cereal bowl.

And finally, most of us seldom eat rice, pasta or cereal by itself without a protein like meat, cheese or milk. Among the fad diet crowd, it should be common knowledge that protein helps to slow the otherwise speedy metabolization process responsible for the dreaded spike in blood sugar levels. Unfortunately, this information rarely finds its way into their books.

One thing more. We are also waiting for solid evidence that excess insulin makes you fat. It does make you hungry by lowering your blood sugar, and that explains why refined grains are a problem. Hunger resulting from eating foods made of white flour, such as many crackers and breads, often leads to overeating.

The lack of sufficient fiber in refined grains also contributes to the hunger problem by leaving you less full than you do when you eat whole grains. It's just that simple. It's hunger that's the problem, not carbohydrates per se. That's why fruits, consisting almost totally of carbohydrates and fiber, keep you well satisfied.

If you lead an active lifestyle and engage in strenuous workouts everyday, your daily intake of 6-11 servings of whole-grain-based foods should not be a problem. In fact, your muscles love carbs because,when metabolized into glucose, carbs are what muscles use as fuel. The problem is that active muscles burn through this fuel quickly – just like a jet fighter – and require frequent trips to the tanker to keep the body flying high and fast.

Carbs can be simple – like white sugar, which is void of many other nutrients – or complex, such as pasta, which combines protein and fat, along with vitamins and trace elements the body requires. Simple carbs such as fruit juices, honey, candy, syrup, and fructose-sweetened drinks metabolize quickly. Complex carbs that fall into the "white carb" category – such as rice, bread, potatoes, cereal, and bagels – can also raise blood sugar levels, which is why we recommend they be replaced by whole grain versions. The fiber in whole grain carbohydrates acts to slow down metabolism, which keeps insulin levels from spiking.

We're proposing that you get off the fad diet merry-go-round and do something that works for the long run – a healthy eating weight-loss program that doesn't deprive you of the foods you crave, but replaces unwise food choices and moderates how much you eat.

It all comes down to portion sizes and fewer calories. But here's the good news. You should actually eat more frequently than the standard three meals a day and stoke up on foods that are filling but light on calories. We're talking vegetables and fruits here – the crunchy kind. In fact – you could find it really difficult to remain overweight if you filled up on fruits and veggies throughout the day. It worked for us – and it can do the same for you.

Chapter 5
LADIES – START YOUR ENGINES

It's the absence of love handles that makes the heart grow fonder.

Those who believe the DTD is somehow directed at men are half right. Men's health is a major issue today because more women realize the need to keep their men healthy, vigorous and living longer. As Mae West once said, "It's not the men in my life that counts, it's the life in my men."

We believe the one factor causing the most trouble for men's health in North America is their diet. It's usually why they carry excess weight around their midsection – the most dangerous place on the body for fat to accumulate – and why they often end up with type 2 diabetes.

But ladies, you have your own champion right here in the DTD. She's co-author Theresa Malysz, as mentioned elsewhere, a registered dietitian who's part of a transplant team at a major city hospital. She provides weight-loss counseling for many women and men who must lose weight as part of their eligibility criterion to qualify for a kidney or pancreas transplant. Her recommendations are based on American Dietetic Association guidelines, which in my case resulted in the loss of 35 pounds in 21 weeks. And I've kept those pounds off for more than a year. I now eat throughout the day, never feel hungry and have more energy and stamina than I can ever remember.

Much of what we cover in these pages is directed at weight reduction strategies that are most effective for both genders. Specifically, you can follow this healthy diet regimen and achieve a gradual one-to-two-pound-per-week weight loss leading to your ideal weight. The ultimate goal would be a lifestyle of better food choices and exercise that helps maintain the lower weight and improved health.

Now that you have a basic idea of what we provide here, let's cover what we don't endorse. If you're interested in a crash diet that promises you'll fit into that size "too small" in time for your high-school reunion next month, please look for that elsewhere. Those diets are potentially dangerous and don't prepare you to keep the weight off. Some do make that claim, but require you to buy their products. The only products we recommend are the good foods available at your local market.

WHAT'S THIS GUY THING?

Regarding the male and female appeals of the material in the DTD, it's no secret that most diet books are purchased by women – often with the intention of learning the diet so it can be applied to the weight problems of both people in the relationship.

However, it's well known in nutrition circles that many men turn up their noses at anything smacking of a feminine approach to weight loss. They've already made up their minds that "women's diet books" recommend salads at every meal, with dry toast and a chaser of herbal tea.

This is why the DTD book cover and title were thought to have a better chance at winning over the stubborn male in your life. If he sees you reading it and applying some of the recommendations within these pages, there's a better chance for success at slowly working in the changes in the food that's bought and put on the table. We also have some time-saving ideas for two-earner families. These strategies can save a considerable amount of money, as well, (men love that) and help the two of you look better, feel better and maybe even love better (see Meals Away).

The other appeal is that as a woman, you're concerned about your man. We recently had a phone conversation with a woman in her 30s whose husband of the same age is overweight and diagnosed with high cholesterol. He neglects to take the prescribed medication to keep it in check and doubts whether the expensive weight control program at the local hospital is something he wants to get into at this point.

Here's the inside story of what men go through at this critical point in their lives. Guys in their 30s are typically still trying to cope with the reality of no longer being in their 20s. They're also faced with mountains to climb in their careers, and the job thing is – forgive me, but you ladies probably know this already – often tops in their list of priorities.

They love you and the kids, but that's in a different compartment of their lives. They don't have the time or the inclination to worry about something like cholesterol or healthy eating. To them, all of this sounds like something older men have to deal with, and the whole concept of taking daily medication is not on their radar screen.

They'll work out at the gym, but only if they look good enough to be seen there. Otherwise, they'll hide behind their business suits or work clothes and put weight control on the back burner. Ladies, any of this sound familiar?

Guys – if you're reading – I've been there and then some. You strap on your emotional body armor every day to cope with a situation at work that often requires jousting with your peers or pulls you down like quick sand. There are some good work places out there, but if things were that good, you probably wouldn't have a weight problem.

The last thing on your agenda is daily medication that reminds you of advancing age or implies a weakness that you won't recognize under threat of death. And – in your world – all that extra weight is just winter fat that will come off in the summer with golf and outside activities. If it's later in the year, that beer belly from those summer barbecues will come off with hunting season and winter sports.

If some of this rings a bell, what you need is to get a grip on the reality of your situation. Chances are the promotions are going to those guys who look the part of a trim, up-and-coming leader. Whether you wear a white or blue collar to work, the more weight you carry, the less able you are to perform or look as good as someone of equal ability, but in a trimmer package.

I have personally witnessed a situation where a corporate vice president was seen enthusiastically feeding his large body from a food buffet at a company sponsored event. It occurred to me at the time that this didn't look good – and not more than three months later, he was forced to retire in his mid-50s. Was this cause and effect? Who knows, but it happened – and the executive who filled his job was a picture of ideal weight.

Many companies are scrutinizing their executives and workers for excessive weight, which is often perceived as a sign of unresolved emotional turmoil compensated by overeating. It's a common perception that those who excel in business are those who exhibit healthy eating habits, as well as superior work habits.

Regarding the concept of taking daily medication, it's really an indicator of a man's character and a married man's dedication to wife and family. The man who takes care of himself is like an athlete who knows the value of a healthy body. He thereby ensures that his loved ones benefit from his hard work, and that no one is burdened by the personal care required in the event of a preventable stroke or heart attack. To me, such a circumstance would be the ultimate humiliation for someone who prides himself on taking care of business or being the man of the family. Enough said.

Despite the deficiencies of the male gender cited thus far, Theresa has seen men in her weight-loss sessions take charge and employ inventive measures that enhance their progress toward a healthier lifestyle. In one case, a man used a spread-sheet computer program to track his daily food records and employed the search feature to identify problem foods that popped up too frequently. Give us guys some way to combine a gadget with weight-loss and it's a match made in heaven.

HE SAID/SHE SAID

You may have already detected a hint of disagreement between the co-author and me. As a health-care professional and DTD technical advisor, she has a definite point of view that deserves its moment in the sun. I can faintly hear the full-throated cheering from some of you, as well as the understanding silence from others who can empathize with my situation.

It so happens that Theresa does not give an inch on certain issues relating to her field of expertise, although she has to accommodate the occasional nugget of information I've been able to uncover, much like the hog that roots out a truffle now and then.

In an effort to highlight our differences and lend some perky dialog to these pages, we created a feature known as "HE SAID/SHE SAID," which appears throughout the book as a sidebar. It's designed to showcase how the person at the receiving end of diet information views the nutrition landscape (that's the HE SAID) followed by the professional take on how the perception might be off track (SHE SAID).

Read on to the next subject – Behavior Change – and see how this feature might be enlightening, as well as entertaining.

BEHAVIOR CHANGE

This morning, I again measured out my 1/2 cup of raisin bran cereal for breakfast and doused it with 1/2 cup of skim milk. After losing my excess weight, you'd think I wouldn't need to be that regimented. Truth is, I'm the last person in the world to whom the term "regimented" would apply.

What this behavior does represent is a new habit to replace an old one. I used to fill the biggest cereal bowl in the house with as large a helping of corn flakes as it could hold. And then – of course – milk was filled to the brim. In those days, we would only have 1% milk in the house, since Theresa was gradually moving the family in the direction of skim milk.

As human beings, we are creatures of habit – and eating habits are one of the most difficult behaviors to change. Our food preferences and eating habits evolved over many years, and most were established early in our childhoods. But as my new breakfast cereal habit illustrates, it's never too late to teach an old dog new tricks.

One of the most effective catalysts for behavior change is a medical event. I've had several and – believe me – there's nothing like an EMS ride to the emergency room to get your attention. In many cases, these events were diet related, so they accelerated changes in my eating habits that Theresa had been trying to steer me into for years. As I wrote earlier, eating habits are tough to change.

Hopefully, you can benefit from my experience. Take a long, hard look at your eating habits. Do they include eating your meals in front of the television or while driving? Neither is a good idea, because the objective is to enjoy your food, not feed on something that hardly registers as a meal.

Here's the problem. The habit turns into a cue for eating whenever you're watching TV or driving. It's like going to the movies and bingeing on theater popcorn and candy bars. This is something you wouldn't ordinarily do, but the defenses drop when you're in that environment.

The fact is, you go to the movies infrequently, but you probably watch TV and drive every day. This is why it's so important to identify those eating habits and food choices that put you in jeopardy of eating – not because you're hungry – but because you're doing something associated with eating.

For example, I used to finish my dinner and immediately grab a bag of pretzels to sit and watch TV. Was I hungry? No – it was a habit – much like a cigarette with coffee in the bad old days.

HE SAID: I actually had to give up eating pretzels to break myself of that habit. I'm convinced that pretzels are one of those "diet villain" carbohydrates. To this day, I don't eat pretzels because they represent a problem for me that I don't want to revisit.

SHE SAID: His "diet villain" approach is a psychological ploy that works for him and may work for others. However, foods aren't heroes or villains. It's possible to incorporate all foods into one's diet, but with moderation. When people binge on a particular food or eat it out of habit rather than satisfaction, that's when things can get out of hand.

So what do I do instead of snacking on these foods that I no longer consider friendly? Theresa cuts up several varieties of fruit – pears, peaches, apples, grapes, etc – and that's our dessert. No sugar, no cream, nothing added. And I consider it a huge treat.

ENOUGH'S AS GOOD AS A FEAST

A bargain hunter by nature, I used to scan the advertisement sections of the Sunday newspaper in search of money-saving coupons and all-you-can-eat restaurants. In those days, the goal was to ingest the maximum amount of food with little regard for its quality and let the restaurant owner worry about making a decent profit.

It took me some time to understand that our role in life is not to consume as much as possible at the least cost, but to enjoy the quality of nature's bounty in limited quantities. I was struck with this thought years ago when – of all things – the Mary Poppins character from the Disney movie captured my attention with the line: "Enough's as good as a feast."

That got me to thinking – was it really smart to continually ingest "man-sized" portions resulting in a midsection that felt like an inflated balloon?

It all led to a serious examination of my eating habits, which were based on generations of men whose daily activities involved hard labor – plowing the fields, assembling cars or building houses. The closest I ever came to that level of physical labor was working in a paper box factory while attending college.

It became obvious that my daily food intake was appropriate for a level of metabolism from another era. Instead of metabolizing my food at the rate of a younger man working his muscles on the job, I now spend my days in front of a computer keyboard, writing promotional material and books.

HE SAID: Thus began a journey of re-evaluating the age-old question: "Do I live to eat or eat to live?" The answer led to a whole, new relationship with food – one that focused on quality, not quantity. If I now step outside my healthy eating regimen, it's for a taste of the real thing instead of a pale substitute.

SHE SAID: A good rule to follow – particularly with snacks – is to measure out a serving amount into a small bowl, put away the larger source container and eat slowly to enjoy the taste. If you try to eat out of the original container, you'll end up eating more than you should, even if you adopt the "eat to live" philosophy.

If you think about it for a moment, it's usually the first few bites of food that are particularly enjoyable, while the remainder is more or less filling the fuel tank. This is why fine dining is made up of several courses – each with portions that by "super sized" standards might be considered small. These portions are just enough to capture the essence of the food's appeal without the bulk that would erode your enjoyment of succeeding courses.

The bottom line to this chapter is that you'll find satisfaction in smaller portions if you allow the fuel gauge in your brain to catch up to the fuel level in your stomach. It takes about 20 minutes for this action to happen, so if you keep shoveling in more food during this period, you're just overfilling the tank. If you were doing the same thing at the gas station, it would be spilling out the filler tube. However, since the stomach is a flexible tank, it stretches to accommodate the excess.

Now you know why the fast eaters, which include many of us guys, can be seen popping antacids to help relieve that "overstuffed" feeling. Obese people also tend to be fast eaters, going in for second and third helpings before their brains register anything from the first one. If you're one of those who fits the profile of a fast eater but haven't yet reached the obesity threshold, just keep doing what you're doing and you'll get there before you realize what's happening.

EAT ONLY WHEN HUNGRY

Why do most people drop everything at noon and have lunch? It's because the entire North American culture is built around the idea that the body needs to be fueled at that point of the day. And by no means are we talking about a small meal. Many folks really stoke up and consume a good portion of their total caloric intake for the day during this hour. And don't ever tinker with this lunch routine.

For example, my dad was great for helping us do things around a new home we bought years ago, but when the noon whistle blew, it was time to eat, no matter if we were pouring concrete or planting a tree. For us, it didn't matter if the big and little hands of the clock were together, but in his world, it was all that mattered at that moment. In fact, there was one occasion when we didn't have lunch set up for this magic hour, and it caused him thereafter to brown-bag it – complete with a raw onion for his sandwich.

This story illustrates how some of us never leave the rigid schedules originally created when nearly ninety percent of the population lived and worked on farms. Then it was customary for the wife to bring a massive lunch out to where the family was working in the north forty. She made the trip so they wouldn't lose all the time it took to get back to the main house, eat and then travel back to the fields. Today, we're all pretty much tied to this noon-hour ritual regardless of how hungry we might be.

Those who travel to the United States from third-world countries are awestruck by the nonstop 24/7 availability of food here. In fact, the concept of hunger in America is so uncommon that a number of sources we uncovered for this book had to actually describe the symptoms:

- gnawing feeling in the stomach
- headache
- lack of concentration
- light-headedness
- irritability
- growling of the stomach

Some people confuse a time to eat with hunger or, more precisely, with a sharpened appetite. Many nutritional experts advise us to eat only when hungry to avoid eating from habit, boredom or stress – all of which do nothing but add pounds rather than satisfy the body's signal that it's time to refuel.

This is why we recommend eating small meals more frequently throughout the day – to keep hunger from making us overeat or over-medicate. Food should not be used as a narcotic to dull the feelings of loneliness, depression or nervousness.

We also believe it's important to eat while sitting down at a table and taking time to enjoy the meal. Food can and should be a joyous occasion, not something to stuff in your mouth as you're rushing through the house or on the way to work.

It all adds up to building new eating habits designed to eliminate the consumption of food for reasons other than to sustain your energy level.

The typical American morning promoted in television commercials is where mom, dad and the kids are all rushing to meet their schedules. They're either eating on the run or standing up as they wolf down their breakfast.

Compare this with another era – *The Nelsons* or *Leave It To Beaver*. Ever notice how much calmer Ozzie Nelson or Ward Cleaver appeared as they sat down with their families for a sane breakfast? Is there a connection here or just nostalgia?

Of course Harriet Nelson and June Cleaver were stay-at-home moms, so that probably accounts for much of yesteryear's morning sanity. However, it just seems that we're chasing our tails these days when it comes to meal time, and the national trend has been toward expanding waistlines.

MARRIED TO A DIETITIAN

If you think being married to a registered dietitian is tough on a husband, understand that this is just a perception, not the reality. (Yes, I know how to dodge a bullet).

Not until later in life did Theresa earn her BS degree, complete her internship and establish her registered dietitian credentials. But she did learn a lot about nutrition through the years leading up to it. Thankfully, her knowledge was sourced from well-documented peer-reviewed studies rather than flavor-of-the-month theories that made the circuit from headline to trash can.

My role was that of a guinea pig, so to speak, for the experiment of how to change behavior or – more succinctly – how to alter eating habits developed over forty years of life.

Typically male – with a penchant for pancake breakfasts, salami sandwich lunches, and meat-and-potatoes dinners – I was a formidable example of set-in-cement attitudes toward food.

If she asked me about substituting my everyday food with healthier and lower calorie alternatives, my reaction was predictably negative. So, every now and then, she would secretly slip one of these ringers into the recipe and wait for any complaints. If nothing was said, she would try another alternative and continue this process until I noticed something was amiss. By then, the concept of substituting a better food choice was established, and the war was lost.

Over the years, Theresa gradually introduced a lot of new approaches and alternatives to our meals that made the entire family healthier and kept our weights from going over the edge. Our kids picked up these healthier eating habits, which carried them into controlled-weight adulthood. These include:

- fried foods banished from the kitchen
- steamed vegetables instead of canned
- ground turkey replacing hamburger
- nonstick sprays instead of oil
- fruit salads replacing traditional sugary desserts
- reduced fat milk and dairy products over whole milk
- zero calorie soft drinks instead of sugar sweetened
- tub margarine replacing stick margarine

The diet that evolved became the DTD, with the following additional refinements.

- more fish than beef
- zero calorie spray buttery flavor over butter
- soy products mimicking the original meats
- lite beer replacing regular
- brown rice instead of white rice
- 100% whole wheat replacing white bread
- yams in place of white potatoes

- whole wheat pasta replacing refined flour pasta
- bran cereal over corn flakes
- whole scrambled eggs replaced by egg substitutes
- veggie butter over margarine
- veggie crumbles instead of Italian sausage in spaghetti sauce
- veggie cheese replacing some dairy cheese products
- whole grain crackers minus trans fats over all others
- canola oil and some olive oil over all oils

ENJOY EATING

The one thing driving many people away from doing anything about their unhealthy diets is that the alternatives aren't very exciting compared to the tasty, high-fat, high-calorie foods they're used to. We believe it takes some creativity in meal planning and preparation to get over that mental turn-off.

HE SAID: For example, seafood is naturally low in saturated fat, which is good – and often higher in omega 3 fatty acids – which are beneficial in many ways. But if you just look at caloric content, a 4-oz. portion of most white/pale colored fish that's baked, broiled or steamed comes in at about 90 calories with 1 gram of omega 3 fatty acids. Compare that with an average for cooked beef at 344 calories per 4-oz portion, with 6 grams of saturated fat.

SHE SAID: Many people think that ordering a fish sandwich or fried fish is a better alternative when eating out, but are probably unaware of the high fat and calorie content in the fish breading that's part of the deep frying process – translating into 50 calories or more than a comparable hamburger. This holds true even if the fish is battered and fried at home. Try baking, broiling or grilling fish coated with olive oil with smoky seasoning or preferred spices that add flavor and mask objectionable fish aroma without adding significant calories.

Many folks look at the price per pound of seafood and compare that with inexpensive cuts of beef and pork. The difference often stops them cold in their pursuit of making better food choices.

But if they consider it from the standpoint of – let's say – horse meat versus beef – the price differential would most likely be a non-issue.

DIET VILLAINS – BOUND AND GAGGED

They can hide, but they can't run. I'm talking about those villains in your diet that seem to call out to you because you know they're there. The DTD solution? Leave them bound and gagged with an impenetrable layer of duct tape that silences the calls targeted at your weakest moments.

I don't care if the potato chips are stashed in a hat box, on the top shelf, way in the back corner of your closet. You know they're there. And when the craving for chips hits, you home in on them like a cruise missile. If you were six-months into a weight-loss regimen and close to achieving your ideal weight, maybe it wouldn't be so bad to have just a handful. But chances are that it wouldn't be over until the entire bag was consumed.

Face it. You can't afford to let this event knock you off course and possibly be the catalyst that puts you back where you started – self-defeated and miserable. So, armed with your duct tape, remove every item: candy, alcohol, chips, or whatever your worst villains might be. Throw them into an old box and start wrapping it with duct tape. Round and round it goes and where it stops, nobody knows. Don't worry about using too much, because this is going to be a fortress of vinyl, cloth and adhesive. Mark it "Caution – Keep Out."

Now, you know yourself best. You've probably been down this road before. If even this level of deterrent can't keep you from attacking the box with a knife or box cutter, then it's probably better to just throw these diet villains into the trash. But do it with coffee grounds, egg shells and peelings mixed in so you won't be tempted to retrieve the goodies before the trash collectors arrive.

Believe me, these cravings can drive a person to the most extreme examples of bizarre behavior. Let me refer you to the *Seinfeld* character – George Costanza – who once retrieved an eclair from the trash – one that had a bite out of it – and was caught by his girlfriend's mother in the act of eating it. But Len, you might say, this is a fictitious character. Okay, but I've worked in offices where I saw ... never mind.

On a serious note, in some cases one might need the guidance of a clinical psychologist who can help diagnose emotional issues that are intertwined with excess weight. This professional can also deal with issues that some young women face, where they see themselves as overweight even though they're actually underweight. In cases like this, the body has very little left to lose and the lack of sufficient caloric intake causes it to begin sacrificing vital organs. Since the heart is primarily a muscle, it can be one of the first to go.

HE SAID: If you identify all the villains in your diet and replace them with low-fat, low-calorie alternatives, the only way you're not going to lose weight is if you ingest more of the replacement food. This is where so many who went through the low-fat/non-fat era went off the deep end – and couldn't understand why.

SHE SAID: If activity levels remain constant, the human body responds to reduced intake of calories by burning its stores of energy. But the kind of weight you lose is important. Stores of energy can be fat – or it can be muscle. That's why it's critical that you lose weight slowly – about one to two pounds per week, unless you're obese, in which case you should be under the weight-loss guidance of a physician or RD.

If you participate in some fad diets that promise quick weight loss you could be endangering your health in any number of ways. But one of the greatest dangers is that you might be losing muscle instead of fat, particularly if you're not exercising. Muscles and muscle tone are essential to weight control because they feed on carbohydrates and function as an effective calorie burning machine.

THE DUCT TAPE DIET

It's instructive to note that the DTD evolved over a number of years where Theresa kept nudging me in the direction she knew I needed to go regarding my high blood pressure and overweight condition. Since I was the "patient" in this weight-loss regimen, the client/patient privilege has been waived so we can share the experience and explore the outright stubbornness of this sometimes noncompliant patient.

She gradually introduced lower-fat dairy products starting with 2% milk instead of whole milk, then 1%, ½ %, and finally skim. Instead of a three-egg omelet, I would get one egg and two-egg whites. Rather than white bread, she would buy a variety of semi-whole-grain breads before finding a 100% whole wheat that I liked. Hard stick margarines were abandoned long ago in favor of reduced-fat tub margarine. All sweetened drinks were replaced with water or diet soda. Juices were limited to ½ cup servings. More fruits and vegetables were introduced until we achieved the Food Pyramid numbers – a milestone in helping the pounds melt away. Her approach was much like cooking a frog. If thrown in hot water, he'll jump out. But by gradually raising the heat ...

I admit to the rather common state of inertia among members of my gender and age group that grew up on meals that "stick to your ribs." What actually stuck was our tendency to eat as if we were still working on the farm instead of the office. To give you an idea of how I ate then compared to now, we offer the following comparison:

THEN	NOW
Breakfast	
8 oz. of orange juice	one orange, quartered
2 bacon strips & 2 eggs, fried	one poached egg & soy sausage
white bread toast	1 slice 100% whole wheat toast
gobs of margarine & jam	1 tsp. soy butter
4-5 cups of coffee, black	2 cups of coffee, black

THEN	NOW
Snack	
bagel & coffee	6 oz. nonfat yogurt
Lunch	
Salami sandwich, white bread	½ turkey sandwich on rye
hydrogenated margarine	1 tsp. soy butter
2 tbs. Italian dressing	1 tbs. deli mustard
bag of salted pretzels	1-oz. low-fat string cheese
glass of 2% milk	12-oz. diet soda
Snack	
2 chocolate-chip cookies	1 medium apple
	1-oz. mixed nuts
Dinner	
4 slices pepperoni pizza	3-oz. grilled tuna steak
2 12-oz. cans regular beer	1 cup brown rice
	2 cups broccoli/cauliflower
	12-oz. diet soda
	½ cup mixed fruit
Snack	
8-12 pretzel sticks	4 whole grain crackers
	½ cup bing cherries

SNACKING

If anyone thinks this writer doesn't consume a lot of food in the course of a day, consider the foregoing "then and now" comparison, where I'm continually amazed at the results.

As you can see, I nibble throughout the day, but it's what I put in my mouth and how much of it goes in that may be different from what you're doing. What I haven't listed are the sprigs of steamed cauliflower and broccoli that don't even have to be accounted for because they're so low in calories and high in volume. They have the effect of filling up my stomach with lots of low-cal vegetation – kind of like delicious, nutritious packing material. They're so effective, it's rare for me to have any sensation of hunger, unless I forget to eat. Yes, it does happen, but the stomach reminds me.

Note: snacking is a major element of this weight-loss regimen. A healthy snack item evens out the daily intake of food and removes the mid-morning and mid-day hunger attacks that could lead to trouble unless you're prepared. If you stick to fresh fruits and vegetables as your snacks of choice, eliminate sweet and alcoholic beverages and avoid fast food, I don't see how it's possible for you to NOT lose weight.

Assuming you don't immediately jump on the broccoli and cauliflower bandwagon, we've put together a short list of snacks that really can get you through the day without blowing your weight-loss goals:

100 Calories (or less)
- ½ cup ice milk or sherbet
- 6-oz. nonfat yogurt with fruit
- 1 thin slice whole wheat bread with fat-free cheese single
- ½ cup 1% low-fat cottage cheese with 1/3 cup sliced fruit
- 2 cups fresh strawberries
- 1 cup unsweetened applesauce
- 2-oz. roasted chicken breast
- 15 almonds or 30 pistachios
- 1 cup sliced pear
- 1 large orange
- 1 extra large peach
- 1 medium apple
- 2 medium plums

Remember, your best friends are fruits and vegetables. Keep them out in plain sight and make sure you get at least 2-4 servings every day. If you could manage a combined nine servings, you're well on your way to a slimmer, healthier future. And it's not that difficult if you slice some tomatoes on your sandwich, spoon some salsa into your pita, add some black beans to your salad, etc.

By the way, it's not will power that keeps me from making a meal out of the mixed nuts or cheese spread on crackers, it's that my stomach is used to small quantities of food on a more frequent basis. And we don't allow some of the food villains to take up residence; they might otherwise be tempting me into big trouble.

Here's how we keep some sense of sanity regarding potential problem scenarios. My birthday is coming up and – breaking tradition – I've requested that we celebrate at a restaurant instead of having ice cream and cake at our place. The reason? I know at an at-home celebration that whatever's left over will stay in the house, since the grown-up kids won't take any with them. And throughout the days that follow, these goodies will beckon to me. Since I come from the school of: "somewhere in the world people are starving, therefore you can't throw out good food," it's a problem. And if these leftovers make it through the day without being eaten, guess what will be dessert for two or three days. So, it's best to cut all this off at the pass and do the birthday thing at some other venue besides our home. You've got to be true to yourself and work around your weaknesses as well as your strengths.

LATE NIGHT SNACKS

Late night snacking is a problem that many of us have to deal with in our own way. The issue is not as benign as some might think. Many experts believe that eating before bed is the worst time of all to be snacking.

If you recall, this book started with the story of my evening snacking crisis. Late night bingeing on popcorn and wine haunted me with the thought of all those calories and carbs – and prompted me to duct tape off the remaining supply. That event represented a catharsis, in which I took a long, hard look at the totality of my weight-loss efforts. I decided at that point to take the concept of lifestyle change seriously and embark on a healthy, blood-pressure sensitive regimen.

HE SAID: Those six meals a day we've recommended can often be three regular meals and three snacks. But that doesn't mean candy bars and chips between breakfast, lunch and dinner. In my case, I steam up enough cauliflower and broccoli the previous evening for snacking throughout the day. It's a favorite food now, and I just can't seem to get enough of what used to be on my "ugh" list.

SHE SAID: I would never argue against his passion for these highly nutritious veggies, but the danger of having any foods so often is that you end up hating them. Remember the key to healthy eating – many foods eaten together in moderation. There's an interesting story about how an all-day popcorn eating binge caused someone to make a visit to the emergency room and undergo a rather embarassing procedure – but we won't mention any names.

The theory is that everyone's metabolism slows down as bedtime draws near, so whatever passes your lips has a better chance of landing on your hips (or where ever you least want it).

Some authoritative sources, however, categorize this concept as a myth. It seems that research studies on both sides of the issue are inconclusive. But my hunch is that late night snacking is probably not a good idea if you're trying to lose weight.

You haven't asked the question, but I'm answering it anyway. My 35-pound weight loss occurred while snacking on fresh fruit somewhere between 8 and 9 p.m.

BLOWN THE DIET

Those of you who've traveled this path before may have experienced the typical dieter's approach to a weight-loss regimen. We're speaking here of the many juncture points throughout the process of getting you from fat to thin.

First, you decide to do something and seize on the latest fad diet. It has to be good – you surmise – because everyone's talking about it. Then comes the pre-diet stage where you binge on every goodie on your villains list because – come Monday morning – you start the new diet.

For the next two weeks or so, you're wrapped up in that strong phase of strict adherence to the regimen, followed by the wobbly stage where you crave those foods you've been denying yourself.

Then, one day, an event sets you back on your heels. It could be a romantic breakup, a job-related upheaval, a financial reversal, or some other kind of emotional crisis. It has the effect of erupting into a psychological need for comfort food – that soothing friend that's always been there during those difficult times in your life.

Now you treat yourself to one of these off-limits food temptations, but instead of just a brief fling at goody junction, you stay the whole night. The morning after, you can't look at yourself in the mirror because you've blown the diet and you're back to square one. Now you have to start all over to crank up your motivation and get back on the weight-loss track. That can take from a few weeks, to months, or years.

If any of this sounds familiar – we understand – and welcome you to the DTD safe house. There's no one here so pure that he or she can cast the first stone.

In fact, we set forth the circumstances of our genesis at the outset of the book. You can't admit to the need for duct taping your diet villains and then take a superior position in terms of what the rest of the world needs to do regarding weight loss. Never forget this – we are marching with you toward that same battleground where the fight to keep the pounds from gaining is an everyday struggle. And we expect to win – one day at a time.

Chapter 6
THE BUZZ ON SUGAR

Zap the sweet drinks – 150 calories per 12 ounces of regular soda is why nutritionists call it "liquid candy."

My mother came to these shores from the old country, where sugar was a treat. Therefore, anything resembling a special food would get the sugar hit. Whenever it was strawberry season, she'd marinate them in sugar, then added more in the serving dish.

Growing up this way, I expected the same from Theresa and she obliged; that is, until her education caught up with the reality of how sugar represents empty calories. Thereafter, she prepared marvelous fruit salads in their natural state. Today, I would never think of adding sugar to my strawberries or any other food. It's not a good idea for anyone who's trying to fight the good fight against an expanding waistline.

HE SAID: But then there's always the helpful advice from those who should really know better. I came across an article about "healthy eating," and the food writer suggested slicing strawberries and adding sugar, cream and perhaps some bits of chocolate, all in the name of a healthy dessert. To me, this is one foot on that slippery slope of inviting your diet villains back for a brief visit. Ask a recovering alcoholic if having just a taste of booze now and then is a good way of staying sober. It's the same for those of us trying to stay on the food wagon. So, beware of the sugar hustlers.

SHE SAID: This strict approach may work for some people, but it doesn't have to be that rigid for everyone. If an individual has conquered a weight problem, it isn't necessary to permanently give up a favorite food. In fact, those who achieve a healthy lifestyle have changed their relationship with food in fundamental ways, and need to know that they can experience those occasional treats again without the fear of falling back into old habits. We each have to know our limits, but nobody wants to be locked in a food prison with no possibility of parole. It might be reason enough to attempt an escape.

Buried in the government mandated food labels is the awful truth about what really goes into many of these lower-fat products. When fat is reduced or removed from food, it takes flavor with it. Consequently, a large number of processed foods are often fortified with – surprise, surprise – sugar.

When we speak of reducing sugar in our diets, it means extracting yourself from the clutches of what has become an intrinsic part of everything we eat or drink. Government statistics reveal that the average American consumes more than 158 pounds of the sweet stuff every year.

That's not hard to understand when you consider that a 12-ounce can of regular soda, for example, contains the equivalent of 10 teaspoons of sugar. Most nutrition experts cite this amount as the upper daily limit for a healthy diet.

YIKES! YOU DRINK HOW MANY?

This is going to shock some people, but I know of individuals who drink six-to-seven 12-oz. cans of sweetened soft drinks a day. At 150 calories per can, that's nearly 1,000 calories daily or the equivalent of about 2 pounds of body fat per week. Unless these calories are offset by reduced food intake and exercise, we're talking about 100 pounds of needless, unhealthy and potentially dangerous body fat accumulated over one year.

Known as liquid candy in the nutritional community, sugared drinks are a primary source of calories for many overweight people. In nearly every case, these are empty calories, with little or no nutritional value. They're also stealth calories, because they seldom register as food in your stomach or brain compared with the solid food that requires chewing, another fullness signal for the brain.

Therefore, it's understandable that most folks with weight problems rarely ever consider drinks when they document their food intake.

And it isn't just soft drinks. Some folks think fruit juice is really good for you, which it is, but like anything else, in moderation. One half-cup (4 ounces) of orange juice in the morning represents the equivalent of one fruit. Since the nutrients in fruit juice are formidable, you can increase the portion if you account for it in your total servings of fruits for the day or the total number of calories in your weight-loss plan.

For example, an eight-ounce glass of orange juice contains more than a day's requirement of vitamin C, 20% of the daily need of folic acid, 10% of potassium and thiamin, and at least 5% of vitamins A and B, magnesium and copper. However, it contains very little fiber and doesn't fill you up very much. A large orange, on the other hand, does fill you up and contains a decent amount of fiber. Both contribute about 100 calories, but the juice hits your bloodstream with a thunderclap of sugar, which is why people with diabetes sometimes need it to stabilize their blood sugar. Because of its soluble fiber, the juice of an orange enters the bloodstream more slowly and has less impact on your insulin level.

Now for the problem drinkers. There are a few gentle souls out there who think orange juice is so good for them that they consume up to three 16-ounce glasses of it every day. That amounts to 48-ounces – the equivalent of 12 fruits per day. At 110 calories per 8-ounce serving, that's 660 calories, with a huge blast of natural sugar into the bloodstream, causing insulin to spike with all its associated effects. Not good.

However, there is one advantage orange juice has over the orange – it can be fortified with calcium. Pay careful attention to the carton, because you can buy it with or without calcium, so make sure it's been fortified. Many adults, particularly women, just don't get enough calcium, and orange juice is a convenient method of increasing one's intake. Just make sure you're getting 100% juice and not a sugar flavored drink with just a smidgen of juice. The government is now forcing these drinks to start labeling the amount of real juice in a typical serving, which I saw superimposed over one of their commercials the other day. It turned out to be 5% real juice, so be sure to check it out for yourself.

One last thing about juice. Just because the label may include the word "unsweetened," the amount of natural sugar in the juice is significant. Fructose is the natural form of fruit juice sugar, and there's about 110 calories in 8-ounces of orange juice, 160 in grape juice and 180 in prune juice. They may all be artificially unsweetened, but naturally they pack a wallop in natural sugar content. Consequently, you really need to watch sugar content.

We started this chapter by citing those who drink 6 to 7 sweetened sodas a day. If these folks would just switch to 0-calorie soda, they could potentially lose 15 to 20 pounds in ten weeks without breaking a sweat. That's what some fad diets promise and seldom deliver over the long run, which in this case would amount to nearly 100 lb. in a year.

Theresa often hears concerns from obese patients at the transplant center about the supposed dangers of artificial sweeteners. Yet these same people think nothing about the dangers of drinking huge amounts of sweetened soda every day that account for a large part of their excess weight.

It's a devastating toll these pounds take on the obese person's heart, pancreas, kidneys and other vital organs. Consider also how the pressure from all this weight can lead to problems with knees and hip joints, making life miserable to say the least. Obesity is also socially ostracizing, often keeping those who suffer its effects from full participation in our society.

So, comparing the downsides of obesity with the decades-old controversy swirling around artificial sweeteners, it seems like a no-brainer decision to trade sweet drinks for the no-cal variety. However, just to play it safe and give yourself some peace of mind, keep your intake to a minimum. It's those lab rats that were fed megadoses of the stuff per day that had problems.

OTHER HIGH-OCTANE DRINKS

We haven't even considered alcoholic drinks, which can be just as weighty as anything else in your diet. Someone drinking a six-pack of beer is getting from 660 to 1,200 calories, depending on whether it's light, ice or heavy lager.

Most experts advise against more than two drinks per day, but as long as you compensate for these extra calories by eating less for that day, there's nothing wrong with an occasional high-octane drink. On the other hand, it's difficult to see how anyone on a 2,000 calorie diet could get through the day on what's left after all that beer.

For anyone wondering what actually counts as "a drink:

- 12 ounces of regular beer (149 calories)
- 5 ounces of wine (100 calories)
- 1.5 ounces of 80-proof distilled spirits (100 calories)

There's growing evidence that a glass or two of red wine every day is beneficial for most people, but unless you already consume alcohol on a regular basis, it's not advisable to start now. And the wine should be table wine instead of heavier port or sweet desert wines.

Use the following table to track your alcohol intake for the various types of drinks you might consume over a week, month and year.

*For example, if you're consuming two 4-oz. glasses of red wine every night @ 80 calories/4 oz., that amounts to 160 calories per day, or 1,120 per week, or 4,480 calories per month. Over a year's time, that's 53,760 calories. If you divide that amount by 3500 calories, the result is over 15 pounds of excess fat that you might gain if these calories were not compensated by additional exercise or reduced calories elsewhere in your diet.

Alcohol Calorie Calculator

Beverage	**Serving Amount (ounces)**	**Average (calories)**	**Average Drinks Per Week**	**Monthly Subtotal Calories**
Beer				
Regular	12	149		
Light	12	110		
Distilled (80 proof)				
Gin, rum, vodka, whisky, tequila	1.0	65		
Brandy, cognac	1.0	65		
Liqueurs (Drambuie, Cointreau, Kahlua)	1.5	188		
Wine				
Red	4	80	14 (see example)*	4,480*
Dry white	4	75		
Sweet	4	105		
Sherry	2	75		
Port	2	90		
Champagne	4	84		
Vermouth, sweet	3	140		
Vermouth, dry	3	105		
Cocktails				
Martini	3.5	140		
Manhattan	3.5	164		
Daiquiri	4	122		
Whiskey sour	3	122		
Margarita cocktail	4	168		
Coolers	6	150		
Monthly Total				4,480* Calories
Yearly Total				53,760* Calories

Chapter 7
ROAD TO OBESITY

If you control portions and serving sizes, you're on your way to a simple, effective weight-loss program – of your own design.

Much has been written lately about the connection between carbs and obesity. According to a study by the federal Centers for Disease Control and Prevention, more than 31% of the U.S. population is considered obese (defined as a body-mass index of 30 or above), and many point fingers at excessive carbohydrate intake as the principal cause.

By the way, researchers believe the percentage of obesity is even higher because people tend to underestimate their own weight, and this data was self-reported during telephone interviews with 195,000 respondents. Self-deception is rampant in the human species – as demonstrated by those who don shorts, bathing suits and stretch pants over bodies that definitely aren't flattered by these choices of wearing apparel.

The reason so many diet books focus on carbs is that the obesity problem started to get out of hand just about when the USDA released its Food Guide Pyramid. This is where the foundation for a healthy diet begins with a base of between 6 and 11 servings a day of what dietitians call the starches – bread, cereal, rice, pasta and potatoes. The problems associated with this recommendation are many, but let's sift out the major ones.

When the Food Guide Pyramid indicates 6-to-11 servings, most folks go for the high end of the range, and assume a serving is what fits onto a standard dinner plate. Wrong! And those taking pot shots at the Pyramid seem to be excusing the misapprehension of the public regarding food-group serving recommedations and portion sizes, which are considered by most in the nutrition community as totally out of control.

USDA Food Guide Pyramid

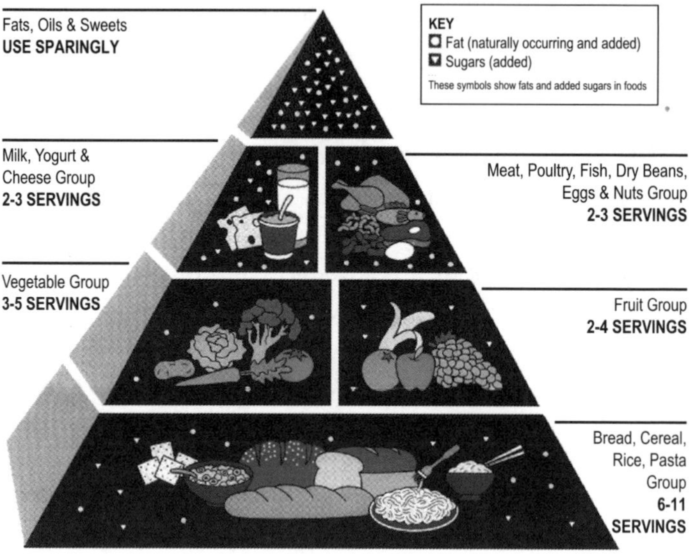

http://www.cnpp.usda.gov/pyramid.html

Let's face it – the vast majority of Americans have no idea what a serving of a specific food looks like.

For example, spaghetti servings are often viewed as the amount that fills one of those fancy pasta bowls. If that's what you think, stand by for a shock. The official USDA serving size is one-half cup of cooked pasta.

For those of you who don't cook and are unfamiliar with what that looks like, may I invite you to any store selling kitchen do-dads, even supermarkets have them, and look at a set of measuring cups. Take a look at that 1/2 cup size and try not to let your jaw drop. This gives you some idea of where the problem might be residing. Fill your bowl, and you've got maybe 6, 8 or 10 servings.

Now, how about some marinara sauce for your pasta? Okay, but you'll need to move down to the 1/3 cup measure for a serving size. I'm sorry, but this doesn't get any better. For a side dish, look at the 1/4 cup measure for an official serving of cottage cheese.

Enough of this fun. Leave the cups and consider the serving size of meat, poultry and fish. It's 2-3 ounces, but to get an idea of what that looks like, compare it to a deck of cards or an audio cassette. In fact, as an alternative to weighing and measuring your food, the USDA cites a whole list of everyday items that will lead you in the right direction.

Measure	**Approximate size**
2 tbs.	Ping-Pong ball
1/3 cup	level handful
1/2 cup	half tennis ball
1 cup	tennis ball
1 oz.	thumb
3 oz.	deck of cards

Keep in mind that the number of servings of any group in the Pyramid is a range instead of a fixed number. That's for a very good reason. We're all different in terms of our energy needs, which are determined by size, age, gender and activity level.

That's why when I asked my live-in registered dietitian about servings and portions, she couldn't give me a one-size-fits-all answer. Unfortunately, she married someone who always wants the simple, quick-fix solution. My apology for grilling her about this included the face-saving comment: "Opposites attract, honey. That's why we've been together so long."

So here's the real lowdown.

- Serving sizes recommended by the Food Guide Pyramid are how the USDA factors the amounts of all food group recommendations in some sort of equivalent measure.

For example, one slice of bread was the baseline for determining the starch group.

- Serving size in the Nutrition Facts food label is related to the amount customarily eaten at one time, determined by national surveys, and by how they match nutritional content of similar foods in a group.

- Serving sizes for food exchanges between various food groups are critical for those with diabetes and are consequently stricter than those found in most government and weight-loss charts. Fruit juice, for example, is 1/3 cup for prune and grape juice, while most other juices are 1/2 cup equaling one fruit. Otherwise, the most widely recommended serving size is 3/4 cup for most juices. If you have diabetes, you must consult with your physician or registered dietitian to ensure the accuracy of your serving sizes to achieve proper exchanges between basic food groups.

- Portion size is basically what you decide it is. If you decide that your spaghetti dinner will have 2 cups of pasta, just know that this counts as 4 of the 6-to-11 servings from the starch food group that forms the base of the pyramid.

The number of servings of each group that you can have (since there is a range) depends on how many calories your gender, age, height, and activity level are determined to be right for you. This is where a registered dietitian/nutritionist can help you calculate the number of calories you need. Otherwise, just follow the USFDA recommendations cited in Chapter 3.

WHAT COUNTS AS A SERVING?

Bread, Cereal, Rice, and Pasta Group (Grains Group)–whole grain and refined

- 1 slice of bread
- About 1 cup of ready-to-eat cereal
- 1/2 cup of cooked cereal, rice, or pasta

Vegetable Group
- 1 cup of raw leafy vegetables
- 1/2 cup of other vegetables cooked or 1 cup raw
- 3/4 cup of vegetable juice

Fruit Group
- 1 medium apple, banana, orange, pear
- 1/2 cup of chopped, cooked, or canned fruit
- 3/4 cup of fruit juice

Milk, Yogurt, and Cheese Group (Milk Group)*
- 1 cup of milk** or yogurt**
- 1 1/2 oz. of natural cheese** (such as Cheddar)
- 2 oz. of processed cheese** (such as American)

Meat, Poultry, Fish, Dry Beans, Eggs, and Nuts Group (Meat and Beans Group)
- 2-3 oz. of cooked lean meat, poultry, or fish
- 1/2 cup of cooked dry beans# or tofu counts as 1 oz. of lean meat
- 2 1/2-oz. soyburger or 1 egg counts as 1 oz. of lean meat
- 2 tbs. of peanut butter or 1/3 cup of nuts counts as 1 oz. of meat

NOTE: Many of the serving sizes given above are smaller than those on the Nutrition Facts Label. For example, 1 serving of cooked cereal, rice, or pasta is 1 cup for the label but only 1/2 cup for the Food Guide Pyramid.

* This includes lactose-free and lactose-reduced milk products. One cup of soy-based beverage with added calcium is an option for those who prefer a non-dairy source of calcium.

** Choose fat-free or reduced-fat dairy products most often

Dry beans, peas, and lentils can be counted as servings in either the meat and beans group or the vegetable group. As a vegetable, 1/2 cup of cooked, dry beans counts as 1 serving. As a meat substitute, 1 cup of cooked, dry beans counts as 1 serving (2 oz. of meat).

Adapted from U.S. Department of Agriculture, Center for Nutrition Policy and Promotion. The Food Guide Pyramid, Home and Garden Bulletin Number 252.

FOOD GUIDE SERVINGS CAN LIMIT CALORIES

The shouting about the USDA's Food Guide Pyramid being responsible for making people fat is a fallacy. Consider the following 2,000 calorie plan based on those recommendations.

Typical eating plan based on 2,000 calories a day

Food Group	Daily Servings	Serving Size	Examples and Notes
Grains and grain products	7-8	• 1 slice bread • ½ cup dry cereal • ½ cup cooked rice, pasta, or cereal	whole wheat bread, English muffin, pita bread, bagel, cereals, grits, oatmeal
Vegetables	4-5	• 1 cup raw leafy vegetable • ½ cup cooked vegetable • 6 oz. vegetable juice	tomatoes, potatoes, carrots, peas, squash, broccoli, turnip greens, collards, kale, spinach, artichokes, beans, sweet potatoes
Fruits	4-5	• 6 oz. fruit juice • 1 medium fruit • ¼ cup dried fruit • ½ cup fresh, frozen, or canned fruit	apricots, bananas, dates, grapes, oranges, orange juice, grapefruit, grapefruit juice, melons, mangoes, peaches, pineapples, prunes, raisins, strawberries, tangerines
Low-fat or nonfat dairy	2-3	• 8 oz. milk • 1 cup yogurt • 1½ oz. cheese	skim or 1% milk, skim or low-fat buttermilk, nonfat or low-fat yogurt, part skim mozzarella cheese, nonfat cheese
Meats, poultry, and fish	2	• 3 oz. cooked meats, poultry, or fish	lean meats (trimmed of visible fat), broiled, roasted or baked poultry with skin removed
Nuts, seeds, and legumes	4-5 per week	• 1½ oz. or 1/3 cup nuts • ½ oz. or 2 tbs. seeds • ½ cup cooked legumes	almonds, filberts, mixed nuts, peanuts, walnuts, sunflower seeds, kidney beans, lentils

Source: The DASH Eating Plan. U.S. DEPARTMENT OF HEALTH AND HUMAN SERVICES/National Institutes of Health/National Heart, Lung, and Blood Institute.

www.nhlbi.nih.gov/health/public/heart/hbp/dash/new_dash.pdf

PORTION AS A MARKETING TOOL

It's no surprise that folks are confused about portion size, because the trend in American culture is to expect more for your money, and many in the food business have locked onto that mindset. A growing number have figured out that by offering super-sized portions, they're attracting a significant segment of the public motivated in that direction.

With competition being what it is, restaurants and other food outlets are looking for signature items on the menu to increase market share. Instead of investing heavily in creating something new and different, they focus on portion size as an easy way to gain an advantage.

Notice we're not addressing the quality of the food, only the amount. Since food cost is only about 30% of the total cost involved in bringing a menu item to your table, it represents an inexpensive way of attracting the typical American consumer.

If you find yourself motivated by the super-sized menu items or the all-you-can-eat restaurants, you might want to consider whether it makes sense to continue down this road, or to choose a lifestyle that concentrates on enjoying the finer things in life, in moderation. This is the real key to life-long weight control.

LOW-FAT MANIA

The low-fat approach adopted by the processed food industry in the early 90s was a response to the publicity generated by the Food Guide Pyramid. Note that dietary fat occupies the smallest unit (use sparingly) of the daily number of servings recommended for a healthy diet.

Upon the release of the pyramid, the media jumped on the bandwagon and created a frenzy over the low-fat approach to weight loss.

All this publicity jump-started nearly every food producer on the planet to rush a low-fat or nonfat version of their product to market. Their packaging bristled with labels that screamed the low-fat message. In 1996-97, the zenith of this movement, some 38 percent of new product launches had low-fat claims. Since then, the hype has diminished considerably to where the percentage of new product launches in this category are close to single digits.

HE SAID: This low-fat tsunami gave the food industry a golden opportunity to tap into America's delusion that you could eat all you wanted of something as long as the label contained the words "low fat" or "nonfat." They ultimately found to their dismay that nonfat often translated into more calories per serving as food manufacturers boosted sugar content to retain the flavor lost when fat was removed. Sugar – after all – is totally nonfat.

SHE SAID: There's a little-known caveat regarding how a food can be labeled nonfat if it tests out to have 0.5 grams or less of fat per serving. The problem arises when shoppers buy a basket full of these products and consume multiple servings on the mistaken belief that nonfat translates into "nonfattening." Consider that if you ingest 4 servings of something containing 0.5 grams per serving, you've just consumed 2 grams of fat.

Remember, fat free does not mean calorie free. That's the insidious part of the whole nonfat processed food tango. And it's another reason to take a crash course on reading food labels.

Chapter 8
FOOD LABEL LITERACY

Read the label – low-fat versions can have a higher calorie content after food manufacturers replace fat with sugar.

Yes, food labelese is a language all its own, and you need to become literate in reading it, if not speaking it conversationally. And we're lucky, because the government offers language courses right off the Internet. What follows is exactly that, with some editing, but let me warn you, it can make your eyes glaze over the more you get into it. So here's a "Quick Start" version from yours truly, using the label on the following page as an example.

- Serving size is not necessarily what the USDA Food Pyramid or dietitians recommend
- Calories tell the real story, but focus on how many are from fat (30% in this case), and beware of saturated fat, hydrogenated/partially hydrogenated oil (see Food Fight)
- Pay close attention to % Daily Values of sodium, total carbohydrates, dietary fiber
- Watch the sugars, keep them as low as possible
- Shop for foods that have high nutritional values, low fat and low sodium
- Females and older males should look for higher % calcium

CHECK THE FOOD LABEL BEFORE YOU BUY

Food labels have several parts, including the front panel, Nutrition Facts and ingredient list. The front panel often tells you if nutrients have been added. For example, "iodized salt" lets you know that iodine has been added, and "enriched pasta" (or "enriched" grain of any type) means that thiamin, riboflavin, niacin, iron and folic acid have been added. Now we're entering the area where things gets a bit heavy, so hang on.

The ingredient list tells you what's in the food, including any nutrients, fats or sugars that have been added. The ingredients are listed in descending order by weight.

Use the Nutrition Facts to see if the food is a good source of a nutrient or to compare similar foods. For example, which brand of frozen dinner is lower in saturated fat, or which kind of breakfast cereal contains more folic acid? Look at the % Daily Value (%DV) column to see whether a food is high or low in nutrients. If you want to limit a nutrient (such as fat, saturated fat, cholesterol, sodium), try to choose foods with a lower %DV.

Nutrition Facts

Serving Size ½ cup (114G)
Servings Per Container

Amount Per Serving	
Calories 90	**Calories from Fat 30**
	% Daily Value
Total Fat 3g	5%
Saturated Fat 0g	0%
Cholesterol 0mg	0%
Sodium 300mg	13%
Total Carbohydrate 13g	4%
Dietary Fiber 3g	12%
Sugars 3g	
Protein 3g	
Vitamin A 80% •	Vitamin C 60%
Calcium 4% •	Iron 4%

*Percent Daily Values are based on a 2,000 calorie diet. Your daily values may be higher or lower depending on your needs:

	Calories:	2,000	2,500
Total Fat	Less than	65g	80g
Saturated Fat	Less than	20g	25g
Cholesterol	Less than	300mg	300mg
Sodium	Less than	2,400mg	2,400mg
Total Carbohydrate		300g	375g
Dietary Fiber		25g	30g

Calories per gram:
Fat 9 • Carbohydrate 4 • Protein 4

If you want to consume more of a nutrient (such as calcium, fiber, other vitamins and minerals), try to choose foods with a higher %DV. As a guide, foods with 5%DV or less contribute a small amount of that nutrient to your eating pattern, while those with 20% or more contribute a large amount. Remember, Nutrition Facts serving sizes may differ from those used in the Food Guide Pyramid. For example, 2 ounces of dry macaroni yields about 1 cup cooked or two (1/2 cup) Pyramid servings.

Source: www.fda.gov/opacom/backgrounders/foodlabel/newlabel.html

NUTRIENT CONTENT CLAIMS

Food Label regulations also spell out what terms may be used to describe the level of a nutrient in a food and how they can be used. The FDA's website lists the following core terms:

Free. This term means that a product contains no amount of, or only trivial or "physiologically inconsequential" amounts of, one or more of these components: fat, saturated fat, cholesterol, sodium, sugars, and calories. For example, "calorie-free" means fewer than 5 calories per serving, and "sugar-free" and "fat-free" both mean less than 0.5 g per serving. Synonyms for "free" include "without," "no" and "zero." A synonym for fat-free milk is "skim".

Low. This term can be used on foods that can be eaten frequently without exceeding dietary guidelines for one or more of fat, saturated fat, cholesterol, sodium and calories.

Here's how these descriptors are defined:

low-fat: 3 g or less per serving

low-saturated fat: 1 g or less per serving

low-sodium: 140 mg or less per serving

very low sodium: 35 mg or less per serving

low-cholesterol: 20 mg or less and 2 g or less of saturated fat per serving

low-calorie: 40 calories or less per serving.
Synonyms for low include "little," "few," "low source of" and "contains a small amount of."

Lean and extra lean: These terms can be used to describe the fat content of meat, poultry, seafood and game meats.

lean: less than 10 g fat, 4.5 g or less saturated fat, and less than 95 mg cholesterol per serving and per 100 g.

extra lean: less than 5 g fat, less than 2 g saturated fat, and less than 95 mg cholesterol per serving and per 100 g.

High. This term can be used if the food contains 20 % or more of the Daily Value for a particular nutrient in a serving.

Good source. This term means that one serving of a food contains 10-to-19 % of the Daily Value for a particular nutrient.

Reduced. This term means that a nutritionally altered product contains at least 25 % less of a nutrient or of calories than the regular, or reference, product. However, a reduced claim can't be made on a product if its reference food already meets the requirement for a "low" claim.

Less. This term means that a food, whether altered or not, contains 25 % less of a nutrient or of calories than the reference food. For example, pretzels that have 25 % less fat than potato chips could carry a "less" claim. "Fewer" is an acceptable synonym.

Light. This descriptor can mean two things:

First, that a nutritionally altered product contains one-third fewer calories or half the fat of the reference food. If the food derives 50 % or more of its calories from fat, the reduction must be 50 % of the fat.

Second, that the sodium content of a low-calorie, low-fat food has been reduced by 50 %. In addition, "light in sodium" may be used on food in which the sodium content has been reduced by at least 50 %.

The term "light" still can be used to describe such properties as texture and color, as long as the label explains the intent; for example, "light brown sugar" and "light and fluffy."

More. This term means that a serving of food, whether altered or not, contains a nutrient that is at least 10 % of the Daily Value more than the reference food. The 10 % of Daily Value also applies to "fortified," "enriched" and "added" "extra and plus" claims, but in those cases, the food must be altered.

Healthy. A "healthy" food must be low in fat and saturated fat and contain limited amounts of cholesterol and sodium. In addition, if it' s a single-item food, it must provide at least 10 % of one or more of vitamins A or C, iron, calcium, protein, or fiber. Exempt from this "10 %" rule are certain raw, canned and frozen fruits and vegetables and certain cereal-grain products. These foods can be labeled "healthy," if they do not contain ingredients that change the nutritional profile and, in the case of enriched grain products, conform to standards of identity, which call for certain required ingredients. If it's a meal-type product, such as frozen entrees and multi-course frozen dinners, it must provide 10 % of two or three of these vitamins or minerals or of protein or fiber, in addition to meeting the other criteria. The sodium content cannot exceed 360 mg per serving for individual foods and 480 mg per serving for meal-type products.

OTHER DEFINTIONS

The regulations also address other claims. Among them:

% fat free: A product bearing this claim must be a low-fat or a fat-free product. In addition, the claim must accurately reflect the amount of fat present in 100 g of the food. Thus, if a food contains 2.5 g fat per 50 g, the claim must be "95 % fat free."

Implied: These types of claims are prohibited when they wrongfully imply that a food contains or does not contain a meaningful level of a nutrient. For example, a product claiming to be made with an ingredient known to be a source of fiber (such as "made with oat bran") is not allowed unless the product contains enough of that ingredient (for example, oat bran) to meet the definition for "good source" of fiber. As another example, a claim that a product contains "no tropical oils" is allowed, but only on foods that are "low" in saturated fat because consumers have come to equate tropical oils with high saturated fat.

Meals and main dishes: Claims that a meal or main dish is "free" of a nutrient, such as sodium or cholesterol, must meet the same requirements as those for individual foods. Other claims can be used under special circumstances. For example, "low-calorie" means the meal or main dish contains 120 calories or less per 100 g. "Low-sodium" means the food has 140 mg or less per 100 g. "Low-cholesterol" means the food contains 20 mg cholesterol or less per 100 g and no more than 2 g saturated fat. "Light" means the meal or main dish is low-fat or low-calorie.

Standardized foods: Any nutrient content claim, such as "reduced fat," "low calorie," and "light," may be used in conjunction with a standardized term if the new product has been specifically formulated to meet FDA's criteria for that claim, if the product is not nutritionally inferior to the traditional standardized food and the new product complies with certain compositional requirements set by FDA. A new product bearing a claim also must have performance characteristics similar to the referenced traditional standardized food. If the product doesn't, and the differences materially limit the product's use, its label must state the differences (for example, not recommended for baking) to inform consumers.

Chapter 9
THROWING WEIGHT AROUND

Skin that chicken – remove skin and breading to avoid most fat, calories and white-flour carbs.

The daily caloric intake recommendation from the U.S. Food and Drug Administration is what the USDA's Food Guide Pyramid is based on. So, like it or not, the federal government plays a major role in how Americans eat.

By now it's clear that you have minimum requirements for calories and vital nutrients, but the government's guidelines seem to allow for a lot of leeway. And your energy needs may fluctuate with the kind of lifestyle you lead at various points on the calendar.

Spring kicks off the year with gym memberships, yard work and weekend marathons. Summer may be full of morning runs, water aerobics or company softball games. Fall is leaf raking season, touch football, bicycling through the country or walks in the woods. Winter is slower paced and full of holiday parties, so it may be why New Year's resolutions are usually focused on losing weight. Hence, gym memberships in the spring.

Also, work schedules have a busy season, sometimes keeping you at the workplace hours longer than off-peak times. This cuts into your activity regimen, forces unhealthy meal decisions and creates stressful situations that often get resolved with food. So, not only are you challenged to maintain your caloric burn rate, you may also be stoking the furnace with more fuel than you need.

Before you know it, the bad habits sneak up and you start backsliding. However, recovery is possible if you just consider exercise and healthy eating as necessary as personal hygiene, like showering or brushing your teeth. Remember, in the final analysis, you are doing this weight-loss thing for yourself.

WHAT SHOULD YOU WEIGH?

The answer to what you should weigh is determined by nature, not by anything that humans come up with. This is often referred to as the "set point," at which your body determines what it is going to weigh regardless of your attempts to bring it lower.

HE SAID: I have a set point of 165 pounds, although all the charts and graphs tell me that I should weigh 158 at the highest range for my height. Even though I have bumped the 160 number with a lower calorie intake and increased exercise, my body regulates its metabolism to keep my weight where it is most comfortable – 165.

SHE SAID: Weight charts are a guide for average weights in North America in terms of height and gender. His efforts to lose those stubborn seven pounds were frustrating because the chart does not take muscle mass into consideration. The 40 minutes of aerobic exercise and daily walks have increased his muscle mass to the point where the higher weight can be justified. We all have to heed our bodies set point.

For those who need some kind of guide to what they should weigh, here's a rule of thumb:

For men, enter 106 pounds for the first five feet of height and add 6 pounds for each additional inch. A 5'7" man should then weigh 106 plus 42 for a total of 148 pounds.

For women, it's 100 pounds for the first five feet of height and 5 pounds for each additional inch. A 5'4" woman should then weigh 100 plus 20 for a total of 120 pounds.

So the question becomes one of overweight or overfat. If you consider Olympic athletes and body builders who weigh considerably more than the weight and BMI tables indicate, the answer lies in lean body mass (muscle, bone, organs and tissue).

Everyone else, though, needs to really consider their body fat as the source of most overweight situations – which translates into overfat rather than overweight.

A certain percentage of body fat is necessary as a normal state of health. Most health professionals agree that women should have about 20 percent body fat, while men need about 15 percent. Women with more than 30 percent fat and men with more than 25 percent fat are considered obese.

How much of your weight is fat can be assessed by a variety of methods, including underwater (hydrostatic) weighing, skinfold thickness measurements and circumference measurements. Each requires a specially trained person to administer the test and perform the calculations. From the numbers obtained, a body fat percentage is determined. Assessing body composition has an advantage over the standard height-weight tables because it can help distinguish between "overweight" and "overfat," a distinction that separates the heavier muscular body from the fat one.

An easy self-test you can do is to pinch the thickness of the fat folds at your waist and abdomen. If you can pinch an inch or more of fat (make sure no muscle is included) chances are you have too much body fat.

Exercise is the key to increasing lean body mass while decreasing the overall fat level. Depending on the amount of fat loss, this can result in a loss of inches without a loss of weight, since muscle weighs more than fat. However, with the proper combination of diet and exercise, both body fat and overall weight can be reduced.

BODY FRAME

The question of body frame type has always been a fuzzy issue. You probably know people who claim to be big-boned. But didn't it always seem like a convenient excuse for being fat?

Some people are tall and obviously have bigger bones than those who are vertically challenged, but how does someone in the medium-height category qualify as big-boned?

Well, after all these years, the information finally comes out of the woodwork. Actually, it comes from Theresa's professional training, which teaches the following:

Form a circle of your thumb and middle finger around the thinnest point of your wrist.

MEDIUM BODY FRAME: Tips of thumb and finger meet.

LARGE BODY FRAME: Tips of thumb and finger don't meet.

SMALL BODY FRAME: Tips of thumb and finger overlap.

For those of you who don't seek professional guidance on your quest to lose weight, and we know you're out there, we dug through the federal government's web sites and came across the body mass index (BMI) table on the opposite page.

BMI measures weight in relation to height. The BMI ranges shown below are for adults. They are not exact ranges of healthy and unhealthy weights. However, health risk increases at higher levels of overweight and obesity. Even within the healthy BMI range, weight gains are associated with health risks for adults.

Healthy Weight:	**BMI from 18.5 up to 24.**
Overweight:	**BMI from 25 up to 29.**
Obese:	**BMI 30 or higher.**

Source: http://www.nhlbi.nih.gov/guidelines/obesity/bmi_tbl.htm

Directions: Find your height at the left edge of the table. Go across until you come to the line that matches your weight. Then look to find your BMI at the top of the table.

BMI	19	20	21	22	23	24	25	26	27	28	29	30	31	32	33	34	35
Height (inches)	**Body Weight (pounds)**																
58	91	96	100	105	110	115	119	124	129	134	138	143	148	153	158	162	167
59	94	99	104	109	114	119	124	128	133	138	143	148	153	158	163	168	173
60	97	102	107	112	118	123	128	133	138	143	148	153	158	163	168	174	179
61	100	106	111	116	122	127	132	137	143	148	153	158	164	169	174	180	185
62	104	109	115	120	126	131	136	142	147	153	158	164	169	175	180	186	191
63	107	113	118	124	130	135	141	146	152	158	163	169	175	180	186	191	197
64	110	116	122	128	134	140	145	151	157	163	169	174	180	186	192	197	204
65	114	120	126	132	138	144	150	156	162	168	174	180	186	192	198	204	210
66	118	124	130	136	142	148	155	161	167	173	179	186	192	198	204	210	216
67	121	127	134	140	146	153	159	166	172	178	185	191	198	204	211	217	223
68	125	131	138	144	151	158	164	171	177	184	190	197	203	210	216	223	230
69	128	135	142	149	155	162	169	176	182	189	196	203	209	216	223	230	236
70	132	139	146	153	160	167	174	181	188	195	202	209	216	222	229	236	243
71	136	143	150	157	165	172	179	186	193	200	208	215	222	229	236	243	250
72	140	147	154	162	169	177	184	191	199	206	213	221	228	235	242	250	258
73	144	151	159	166	174	182	189	197	204	212	219	227	235	242	250	257	265
74	148	155	163	171	179	186	194	202	210	218	225	233	241	249	256	264	272
75	152	160	168	176	184	192	200	208	216	224	232	240	248	256	264	272	279
76	156	164	172	180	189	197	205	213	221	230	238	246	254	263	271	279	287

BMI	36	37	38	39	40	41	42	43	44	45	46	47	48	49	50	51	52	53	54
Height (inches)	**Body Weight (pounds)**																		
58	172	177	181	186	191	196	201	205	210	215	220	224	229	234	239	244	248	253	258
59	178	183	188	193	198	203	208	212	217	222	227	232	237	242	247	252	257	262	267
60	184	189	194	199	204	209	215	220	225	230	235	240	245	250	255	261	266	271	276
61	190	195	201	206	211	217	222	227	232	238	243	248	254	259	264	269	275	280	285
62	196	202	207	213	218	224	229	235	240	246	251	256	262	267	273	278	284	289	295
63	203	208	214	220	225	231	237	242	248	254	259	265	270	278	282	287	293	299	304
64	209	215	221	227	232	238	244	250	256	262	267	273	279	285	291	296	302	308	314
65	216	222	228	234	240	246	252	258	264	270	276	282	288	294	300	306	312	318	324
66	223	229	235	241	247	253	260	266	272	278	284	291	297	303	309	315	322	328	334
67	230	236	242	249	255	261	268	274	280	287	293	299	306	312	319	325	331	338	344
68	236	243	249	256	262	269	276	282	289	295	302	308	315	322	328	335	341	348	354
69	243	250	257	263	270	277	284	291	297	304	311	318	324	331	338	345	351	358	365
70	250	257	264	271	278	285	292	299	306	313	320	327	334	341	348	355	362	369	376
71	257	265	272	279	286	293	301	308	315	322	329	338	343	351	358	365	372	379	386
72	265	272	279	287	294	302	309	316	324	331	338	346	353	361	368	375	383	390	397
73	272	280	288	295	302	310	318	325	333	340	348	355	363	371	378	386	393	401	408
74	280	287	295	303	311	319	326	334	342	350	358	365	373	381	389	396	404	412	420
75	287	295	303	311	319	327	335	343	351	359	367	375	383	391	399	407	415	423	431
76	295	304	312	320	328	336	344	353	361	369	377	385	394	402	410	418	426	435	443

Source: http://www.nhlbi.nih.gov/guidelines/obesity/bmi_tbl.htm

HOW TO EVALUATE YOUR WEIGHT (ADULTS)

Weigh yourself and have your height measured.

Find your BMI category in the table. The higher your BMI category, the greater the risk for health problems.

Measure around your waist, just above your hip bones, while standing. Health risks increase as waist measurement increases, particularly if your waist is greater than 35 inches for women or 40 inches for men. Excess abdominal fat may place you at greater risk of health problems, even if your BMI is about right.

Chapter 10
WEIGHT-LOSS STRATEGIES

Best healthy eating investment – a vegetable steamer (be careful with hot steam)

What follows are a number of strategies Theresa has developed for the transplant center's patients to help them lose excess weight and keep it off long term.

These suggestions reflect the essence of a simple, yet effective, lifestyle of healthy eating that accomplishes both goals. Since Len has implemented all of them, these pages once again take on a first-person narrative flavor to help liven things up a bit and give our readers a bit of the frustrated dieter's point of view – something that we hope brings it closer to home.

KEEP A FOOD DIARY

The best way to determine where your calories are coming from is to keep a food diary. You have to be honest with your entries and committed to doing it for at least three weekdays (include a Friday) and one weekend to establish a baseline. Friday is a must because it often includes an end-of-the-work-week party attitude that includes alcohol and cheesy appetizers.

Weekends also feature more restaurant meals or dinner parties where high-fat/high-calorie foods enter the picture. If these occasions are not recorded, then the whole effort at weight loss becomes a sham. With accurate food records, you can continue to eliminate the villains in your diet and lose weight on a regular basis by chipping away at the problem.

What constitutes a diet villain? Since a gram of fat contains 9 calories compared to the 4 calories per gram of protein or carbohydrate, it's wise to avoid anything fried.

This also includes foods containing butter fat, such as cream, butter, soft cheese, ice cream and whole milk. You'll also want to avoid saturated fats that can clog arteries. These are found in meat, butter and eggs. Health experts recommend that only 30% of your calories should come from fat and less than 10% from saturated fat.

But this doesn't mean that just because a food item has more fat than another, it's necessarily higher in calories. For example, five chicken wings contain 13 grams of fat compared to a slice of cheese pizza or beef burrito, both of which have 9 grams. Consider that, at 209 calories, the wings have a lower calorie content compared to the pizza at 290 and the burrito at a whopping 435.

UNWANTED POSTER BOYS

If I were to put up unwanted posters for the villains in my previous diet, they would include the following:

- Beer
- BBQ ribs
- Bagels & cream cheese
- Bologna sandwiches
- Cheese puffs
- Chips (potato & corn)
- Cookies
- Doughnuts
- Fried foods (chicken, fish, bacon, potatoes, onion rings, etc.)
- Hamburger & onion roll
- Ice cream
- Late night popcorn & wine snacks
- Pancakes & sausage w/syrup
- Pizza
- Pretzels
- Restaurant food
- Salami sandwiches
- Sausages (pork, smoked)

- Take-out food
- Tacos w/sour cream
- Waffles w/butter & whipped cream
- White bread
- White rice
- White pasta

The carb police have put many of these bad boys in front of the firing squad and I, quite frankly, rarely ever visit them anymore. It's basically out of fear that once I let them back into my circle, they're going to spring back to life, set up housekeeping and hang around forever.

The preceding reflects my personal fears and attitudes. However, after reaching your weight goal, you might be strong enough to get back on speaking terms and even set up diplomatic relations with many on the "most unwanted" list. They're not all super criminals, after all.

Popcorn, for example, is recommended by my personal physician – Dr. William P. Bowman – as a healthy snack, but only the air-pop or microwave popped versions without oil or butter toppings. (We prefer kettle-popped popcorn with a tablespoon or so of canola oil in the bottom, but don't tell the good doctor.) If you're not on a salt-restricted diet, buttery flavored salt is a tasty item to sprinkle over the 3-cup serving size.

PUT AWAY THAT DEEP FRYER

Since both authors of this book suffer from the pack-rat syndrome, we have a special place for items we just can't throw away. It's the attic space above the garage. To gain access, the car must be backed out, the stack of plastic milk crates moved aside and the folding stairs pulled down. Then someone has to climb up and deal with the wasps, spiders and other critters that love the rent-free accommodations up there.

This is just the kind of place to stash your deep fryer. Hopefully, you'll forget you even have one after a while. I can't think of one good reason to keep it around, but a few bad reasons come to mind rather quickly.

It doesn't matter how many paper towels you spread out to let your fried chicken, onion rings, doughnuts, etc. drain away the frying oil. It's still there, and those are calories you don't need. That's not to mention the cholesterol, saturated fat and other members of that family that can inflict varying degrees of harm. They're all on the diet villains list.

So do yourself and your loved ones a favor. Deep six that deep fryer or stash it away where the mice love to play. You won't ever catch me on that rickety fold-down ladder trying to retrieve it.

CALORIES AT THE WHEEL

It's amazing how many drivers I see stuffing their faces or sipping on a cup of something while negotiating traffic. Between cell phone use, shaving, farding (applying makeup) and eating behind the wheel, I'm surprised there aren't more pileups on the road.

Need we say that consuming food while driving is a bad idea for a number of reasons? Okay, we'll focus on just the impact it has on your weight. Unless you're drinking water, black coffee, tea or diet soda, there are significant calories going into your body, most of them empty of vital nutrients, and not even registering in your brain as food.

Check out the calorie content of those smoothie drinks at the juice bar or the huge juice portions that many think are so good for them. We're talking 500 to 800 calories in many cases.

So now you grab some fast food along the way, or wait until you get to the office where the box of doughnuts is waiting. This is how more calories with plenty of saturated fats and cholesterol find their way into your system and onto your thighs, waistline and buttocks. Tell us again why drinking and eating behind the wheel makes sense.

NO TIME FOR BREAKFAST?

It's imperative that you have something to break your fast, since the food you ate the previous evening was metabolized and, believe it or not, energy was actually being burned while you were sleeping. So your morning activities are being fueled by a tank that's able to supply little more than fumes.

Here's what happens when you skip breakfast. You deprive your brain of essential nourishment, reduce your performance level and set up a hunger reaction that not only gnaws at your stomach but causes you to overeat at lunch. That, in turn, puts a greater load on your body to metabolize a big noon meal and raises your glucose level, which spikes an insulin response. The result can be a lowered blood sugar level that makes you feel tired and hungry again.

We have a pretty good B.S. detector, and one of the winners in that regard is the excuse from some of Theresa's transplant patients that they "don't have time to eat breakfast in the morning." They're "too busy" to fuel their bodies at this hectic time of day.

Of course, if the tank of their car was near empty, they wouldn't be too busy to stop and buy gas. Some of these same people reply to that analogy by saying they buy gas the night before so they don't have to stop in the morning.

Aha! There's the answer! Prepare your breakfast the night before. In fact, do both your lunch and breakfast at that point, so there's no excuse for "can't find 100% whole wheat" sandwiches at the fast food place or restaurant.

There are probably many of you who read this and shake your head. I can hear it now. "Len, you're being ridiculous. How can you prepare breakfast the night before?" Here's how.

- Slice of 100% whole wheat bread, toasted; 1 tsp. soy butter; slice of soy cheese or low-fat cheese; folded over; wrapped in plastic and eaten at work
- 7-oz. liquid yogurt, 80 calories, sipped at work
- Peeled orange, separated into slices, sealed in plastic bag
- Small banana
- 1-oz. low-fat string cheese.

If you don't have time before you drive to work, wait to eat until you arrive. Otherwise, eat breakfast during your first break on the job. Not so hard, is it?

Do that beautiful machine you were born with a favor. Fuel up every morning, even if it's just whole wheat toast with 1 tsp. of peanut butter and a 4-oz. glass of juice. That's less than five minutes of time invested for a morning's worth of return on that investment. It's certainly better than most of what Wall Street is offering lately.

BARIATRIC NON-SURGERY

Bariatric surgery (often known as stomach stapling) has been getting a lot of media attention in the wake of some celebrities resorting to this procedure as a last resort in confronting obesity. By reducing the size of the stomach, this surgery has been successful in helping the morbidly obese reach satiety (the state of being sated or satisfied) on less food and lose a lot of weight in a relatively short period of time. The smaller stomach requires a much smaller volume of food to feel full and telegraphs the brain that hunger is satisfied.

Conversely, those among us who eat big meals at nearly every sitting with no limits regarding portion sizes are essentially stretching our stomachs to a size that demands a greater level of food volume. If that demand is met with high-density foods, like bacon and potatoes, the calories and carbs that go with them put the weight on and can spike insulin levels. However, if the volume is filled with low-density foods, like vegetables and fruits, you still feel full, but the calories are far fewer and the carbs are absorbed more slowly. Density refers primarily to calories in this regard.

Here's a suggestion: launch your own stomach shrinking process by dividing the amount of food you currently eat at each meal into smaller portions that can be eaten more frequently throughout the day. In other words, you're eating the same amount of food, only more often. Then, start substituting lower calorie alternatives.

HE SAID: These frequent meals also deal with your hunger, keep your blood sugar level at an even keel and cause your stomach to shrink down to a lower "full" level. Your brain will also get an even flow of nourishment, which helps to maximize your performance.

SHE SAID: The idea of "shrinking" one's stomach is a novel one that doesn't hold up to scrutiny. What's actually happening is the stomach is becoming used to less food at each meal and is also sending a "full" signal to the brain on that smaller amount. This is just an extension of that concept to a somewhat exaggerated level.

EAT AT LEAST SIX TIMES DAILY

Bet you never thought a diet book would encourage you to eat more often. Actually, we're not breaking any new ground here. By ingesting the same number of calories and nutrients over six meals instead of the traditional three, you're equalizing the effort it takes your body to metabolize food.

The long-term goal is to gradually reduce the number of calories at each meal until you reach your weight goal. This can be accomplished by substituting foods with lower calorie alternatives found in the USDA Nutrient Database in Appendix C.

What we're proposing is not revolutionary, but it is at the heart of how the DTD can help you take off those unwanted pounds. Instead of your regular breakfast of scrambled eggs, toast, juice and coffee, you eat the eggs with half the toast and take the remainder with you. Trade the juice for an orange that you eat later in the morning as a pre-lunch snack. The toast will go nicely with an early coffee break. Do the same with lunch, which you can divide into two portions whether you brown bag or eat out. Ditto for dinner. Before you know it, your stomach begins demanding less to feel full.

Another bonus: the frequency of food entering your system throughout the day keeps you energized. Instead of big meals that leave you feeling bloated and tired as your body digests a large meal and blood sugar levels gyrate, you now even out the fuel entering your body and moderate the glycemic effect.

While everyone else at work is either zoned out or exhibiting bi-polar symptoms from their traditional eating habits, you just keep on going with energy to spare. And as the weight comes off, your performance levels can really start peaking. Who knows, you could get a promotion, see more money in your pay envelope and be on your way to a new life. When that happens, let us know so we can post your success story on our website: www.ducttapediet.com.

DANGEROUS TO CURVES – VACATIONS!

There are many dangers lurking out there for anyone who's on the pathway to losing weight. Need I spell them out? B-i-r-t-h-d-a-y-s, h-o-l-i-d-a-y-s, a-n-n-i-v-e-r-s-a-r-i-e-s, and – for many of us, the worst of all – v-a-c-a-t-i-o-n-s!

All those special days are bad enough – what with ice cream, cake, candies, pecan pie, alcohol, etc. – but vacations can really knock you off your diet horse. Why? Because we tend to let it all hang out on vacation. After all, this is when we leave our normal work life behind, with its rigid schedules and routines. Consider that if we've made some progress regarding healthy eating habits and then go out on the road with only the most unhealthy options available, we're in trouble.

Take, for example, a trip to Orlando, Florida. If you're shmoozing with Shamu and making goo-goo eyes at Minnie, you're also tempted to overdo the ice cream, caramel corn and fast food that seem to be around every corner. Even the restaurants cater to those who've left their diet scales at home. Just try asking for whole wheat bread, brown rice or steamed veggies. You may luck out, but don't hold your breath.

So here's our **vacation strategy** for getting through one of these highly dangerous outings:

- Call ahead to ensure your resort makes healthy foods available
- Ask for the food service manager to arrange for any special needs
- If you have a car, shop the local markets for healthy foods
- Check out supermarket chains for nutritious prepared meals in the deli section
- Buy easy-to-carry fruits (apples are ideal) as a healthy snack.

If restaurant food is your only option, try these ideas:

- Check out national restaurants on the Internet for calorie content
- Call ahead or ask your hotel if they have sample menus
- Avoid all-you-can-eat buffets
- Order entrees without breading
- Steer clear of cheesy toppings, anything fried
- Avoid entrées with cream sauces; ditto on pasta dishes
- Order non-creamy salad dressings
- Split an entrée with your partner.

Ask the restaurant to:

- Serve soft margarine instead of butter with the meal
- Serve fat-free (skim) milk rather than whole milk or cream
- Trim visible fat from poultry or meat
- Leave all butter, gravy or sauces off a dish
- Serve salad dressing on the side
- Reduce or eliminate oil during cooking.

Look for these descriptions on menu items:

- Steamed
- Lightly sauteed or stir-fried
- Broiled
- Baked
- Roasted
- Poached

Don't be shy about asking for these services. After all, you're paying a hefty premium when patronizing a restaurant and there's no reason to accept someone else's choices for what goes into your body. By following these suggestions, you can survive a vacation without dreading the bathroom scale at home.

If you throw all caution to the wind and take one of those extended sea cruises, you're about to sail off the edge of the Earth (metaphorically). As healthy-eating map makers, we wish you luck.

After a week or two out there where the rules of your new lifestyle go out the window, you can significantly affect your resolve and return to those bad old eating habits, unless you go prepared. What's needed is a reminder of some kind to keep you nutritionally sane when all the signals coming your way are flashing green lights for pedal-to-the-metal food mania.

Let's review. The whole idea of the DTD is that food villains are constantly lurking and need to be avoided while you're trying to lose weight. There is a way, however, for you to protect yourself against the onslaught of these calorie-heavy demons. The answer lies with something that's worked before, but this time the idea is to provide a visual cue. In other words, what you need is a predetermined message delivered at a critical moment.

IT'S ALL IN THE WRIST

A unique method of warding off the villains in your diet is the DTD wrist band. The theory behind it was established many years ago when people used to tie a string around their finger to remind them of something important.

Our version of this classic technique is to tear off a strip of duct tape about 11-inches long, carefully fold the sticky side together and write "The Duct Tape Diet" in indelible ink on the top side. Now use another strip to secure it into a loosely fitting wrist band that slides over your hand.

Wear the DTD wrist band on vacation, around the house or when you're grocery shopping to remind you that the bad boys are out there lurking. When you reach for those chips, cookies or (name your own diet villain), the band is right there, sounding its silent alarm and reminding you that this moment could have grave consequences to your weight-loss resolve.

Let's say you're sniffing around the bakery section at the supermarket where they pipe in the aroma that drives you crazy. There before you is a stack of glazed donuts, 12 to a box, today-only special, $1.99. You know what they taste like, and you've been making progress on the diet, so thoughts of making this compromise start coursing through your brain.

Suddenly, your arm darts out to grab a box and, with that move, your DTD wrist band slides forward with the same effect on you that a crucifix has on Dracula. You recoil in psychic pain, replace the donuts, and skulk away, rich in the knowledge that once again you've been saved by the DTD.

P.S. If you want an official DTD wrist band with "The Duct Tape Diet" printed in bold red letters, please look up our website at: www.ducttapediet.com. You'll not only find this item available, but a host of others that make excellent gifts.

WEIGHT-LOSS EQUIPMENT

I'm a Tim Allen kind of guy who enjoys having the right tools to do the job. If you saw my basement wood shop, you'd see practically everything available in a power and hand tool catalog.

Our kitchen is likewise brimming with useful items, to the point where the drawers and cabinets are sometimes difficult to open or keep closed. So bear with me as we explore the kitchen equipment and gadgets that make our DTD a bit easier to implement.

- Crock pot – slow cooks foods, reduces fat, convenient
- Salad spinner – dries out green leafy vegetables after rinsing
- Food processor – slices, dices veggies, mushrooms, etc.
- Vegetable slicer – thin-slices tomatoes, onions and other veggies
- Vegetable steamer/electric – steams veggies to timed perfection
- Egg slicer – thin-slices hard boiled eggs to add protein to salads
- Food scale – keeps you on track for portion weights
- Knife set & block – corrals knives in one place, protects sharp edges
- Nonstick cookware – reduces need for oils and fats
- Measuring cups – keeps you on track for portion sizes
- Measuring spoons – facilitates accurate amounts of ingredients for recipes
- Cooking grille – cooks fish, meat, poultry w/o fat
- Microwave oven – facilitates quicker and healthier food preparation options
- Meat/fish tongs – facilitates grille cooking

- Slotted spoons – retrieve poached eggs from water, separates fat from food
- Colander – drains veggies, whole wheat pasta, etc.
- Toaster oven – broils small servings of meat/fish/poultry and toasts bread
- Electric can opener – convenient; some have knife sharpener
- Coffee grinder – facilitates freshly ground coffee
- 3-Quart pot with lid – cooks brown rice, pops popcorn, etc.
- Roll of standard gray duct tape – helps win “the battle of the binge” and maintain resolve.

VEGGIES CAN BE YOUR BOSOM BUDDIES

We’ve been trying to figure out why there’s such an aversion to vegetables out there. So in classic “he said/she said” fashion, we thrashed out our own personal histories and came up with a bit of self-discovery that might shed some light on the subject.

We both grew up in ethnic families where vegetables were, more often than not, cooked beyond recognition.

Our mothers really cooked veggies to the point where the consistency was mushy and the flavor was bland. My mother, in particular, was a high-heat specialist. We joke about it now, but this was a household where everything had to be browned or superheated to the point where my lips and tongue had acquired asbestos-level tolerance to hot food. To this day, I can down a cup of coffee right out of the pot while Theresa is still blowing the steam off hers.

Over-cooked vegetables are not only unpalatable, they’ve been stripped of many nutrients. That’s why the best way to eat vegetables is raw (after washing), with perhaps a low-fat salad dressing dip. Next best is steaming. This can be done in a collapsible perforated metal tray that fits into a stove-top pot with an inch of water at the bottom and a loose-fitting cover.

There are plastic versions of this tray for microwaves, or you can just put a half-inch of water in a microwave-safe dish with a plastic lid to seal it semi-tight. About 2-3 minutes on high ought to do it, but you'll have to experiment to get it right for your unit. And be sure to watch out for that hot steam.

The most convenient method is an electric vegetable steamer with a built-in timer. Ours comes with accessories that can accommodate any variety of vegetables, and can steam seafood or other fare without adding any fat to the process.

By the way, we've discovered a zero-calorie, zero-fat, zero-cholesterol, zero trans fat buttery spray flavoring that complements steamed veggies and may bring more converts to the vegetable isle of the supermarket. It's available as *Parkay Buttery Spray* or *I Can't Believe It's Not Butter* spray. I don't know why it's such secret throughout the nutritional community, but it's one that we're more than happy to share.

I'm assuming that everyone reading this is into fresh vegetables. Theresa says no, many of her patients eat only canned vegetables and often cite the lack of taste as to why they don't eat veggies more often. Therein, I believe, lies the problem.

HE SAID: I neglected to mention that our moms prepared a lot of canned vegetables, which is why the only veggies I ate for a long time were canned corn or peas and carrots. We seldom eat canned veggies any more, preferring fresh or frozen. Leftover steamed veggies from the previous night's dinner are now one of my favorite snack foods – and I look forward to having them throughout the day.

SHE SAID: Fresh vegetables are usually the best choice for those who have the time to shop, select and prepare them. Downsides include limited shelf life and availability in quality or selection. Unprocessed frozen vegetables are a good alternative for tight budgets of time or pocketbook – and used in small amounts as-needed – perfect for single people. Canned vegetables are fine if sodium content is within acceptable limits.

ANOTHER BOX OF CANDY?

Think about all the occasions where a box of candy has always been the preferred gift for mother, wife, girlfriend, significant other or whatever the current jargon is for the important females in your life. There's Valentine's Day, Sweetest Day, Mother's Day, Easter, Halloween, Thanksgiving, Christmas, New Year's, her birthday, anniversary, get well gift, etc.

But if we stop and think about the ramifications, the question needs to be asked, is all that candy really necessary? Will it contribute to a weight problem? Will it cause her to backslide from a diet? These questions are yours to ponder and answer.

Alternatives include flowers, jewelry, gift certificate, perfume, bath lotion, professional massage, day at the spa, theater ticket, book, monogrammed stationery, music CD, movie DVD, magazine subscription, etc.

These suggestions tell her that she's in your thoughts, but you've eliminated another calorie temptation from her list of things she doesn't need. By the way, you needn't mention any of this.

SPECIAL DAYS – BEWARE OF ADVERSE REACTIONS

For the truly eccentric (marginally sane) among you, there are a number of ways in which you can spread the word and help those within your sphere of influence to better appreciate the scope of our mission regarding the DTD. Fair warning, there may be some who think you could be just another loose wing-nut on the anchor bolts of society, but true believers won't let these comments bother them in any way.

Here's just a sampling of how you can really make a difference on those special days when the rest of America is letting the diet villains run rampant throughout the land.

• **Valentine's Day/Sweetest Day** – Wrap your lover's box of chocolates in a criss-cross of duct tape. This demonstrates that you remembered this special day, but you have his/her best interests at heart by removing the temptation while at the same time proving you're not a cheapskate. How you deal with the question of "Are you implying I'm fat?" is something beyond the scope of this book, but could lead to chronic celibacy.

• **Easter Sunday** – Wrap those cute chocolate bunnies in duct tape to keep the spirit of the day alive without contributing to the youngster's tooth decay or sugar-buzz. Mom, dad and the kid's teacher will love you for it, but the youngster may use some of that tape for a "kick-me" sign stuck to your back.

• **Halloween** – Respond to those trick-or-treaters with candy wrapped in duct tape and watch the adults write down your address to be sure you receive the proper attention when the authorities make inquiries and the TV crews show up for your perp walk.

• **Columbus Day** – Bring the pizza and pasta for the celebration, just make sure they're made of whole wheat flour. If whole wheat isn't available, then tape off those pizza boxes and stand by for the overwhelming response of the paisanos looking for a fun way of ridding themselves of some over-ripe tomatoes.

• **St. Patrick's Day** – Shop around for some Kelly green duct tape to wrap around the bottle of spirits you bring to the celebration and watch how everyone hoists you up on their shoulders to demonstrate their gratitude. Just beware of low hanging beams and vats of tar and feathers.

• **New Year's Eve** – Wrap the champagne or wine you're bringing to the party in duct tape so everyone there knows your heart is in the right place – next to your back pockets.

Who said that dieting couldn't be fun?

Chapter 11
MIND OVER FATTER

Zap the fats – one tablespoon of oil is 120 calories – more than an average scoop of vanilla ice cream

This chapter provides some perspective on a number of issues relating to weight loss and state of mind. These two factors are so intertwined that it matters little what specific recipes or diet plans are followed. The key is motivation. This could be a candid photo of yourself, an embarrassing incident, a medical event, someone's offensive remark – you name it. Once you've made up your mind to do something about your weight, the strategies outlined within these pages can help you pursue this potentially life-saving objective.

OVERWEIGHT FOREVER? ONLY IN YOUR MIND

There's a certain mindset that haunts all of us who've experienced a weight problem. We tend to believe that we're not really svelte even though the scale and everyone we know tells us differently. We also know that an emotional setback can threaten a return to those bad old days of bingeing on our diet villains – a reality that seems to be lurking around every corner.

So our default setting is often a closet full of clothes in various sizes to accommodate those times when we fall off the wagon and regain our lost weight, often adding another 10% or so.

We're recommending you empty out your closet of those "fat" clothes once you achieve your ideal weight as an incentive to keep yourself trim. During my days as a business executive, I actually had all my suits tailored to fit the downsized body resulting from improved eating habits. The cost and embarrassment of having to reverse that action kept me from straying too far from that smaller size for some time.

Unfortunately, those were the days before Theresa earned her RD, so the temptations of all those business lunches, catered meetings and open bars finally caught up with me and I ended up buying new clothes. I told myself it was to be more in style with suits being worn by the up and coming.

Today, I wear clothing that's chosen more for comfort than style, and my "sense of self" is convinced that the downsized person is here to stay. Why? Because I've discovered the secret to long-term weight management – healthy eating and portion control. Oh – and mummifying the diet villains.

WANT TO BE HAPPY? ACT THE PART!

The man who later became Cary Grant was earlier known as Archibald Leach, a British circus performer from the wrong side of the tracks, who came to Hollywood and played the part of a sophisticated English gentleman in so many films that he actually became the person he never was. That's a lesson in redefining oneself or perhaps a world-class example of self-perception makeover.

Whatever you want to call it, by acting the part of the person you want to be, the habit starts taking hold and you become that person. For me, and many others with weight problems related to emotional and psychological issues, the daily ritual of acting happy is a necessary part of making it through to the next cycle. Conquering one's demons is often the key to weight loss.

Growing up in the post-WWII era, it was almost unheard of to have divorced parents, particularly if they were old enough to be your grandparents and spoke broken English. I found it confusing to be parented by siblings nearly 20 years my senior – and even more dismayed by the hurtful stories of how I came into this world – all of which brought me to understand the meaning of unhappiness. However, I know of people with stories far worse than this, so please don't think I'm whining about something that might seem trivial by those standards. My only purpose is to set the stage for the theme of this chapter.

If you want to uncouple the emotional component of your comfort-food response to anything like what I shared with you just now, you can do it. I was lucky enough to climb my way out of a psychological gravel pit, but it took time and many conversations with myself. I finally discovered some redeeming qualities in my ability to write, and used that to make my way in the world.

You can likewise shed the snakeskin of comfort foods that temporarily solve a hurtful situation or problem. But first you have to tell yourself that – today – you're going to find your solace elsewhere else. Join a neighborhood beautification group. Take a financial basics class. Get on the "friends of the library" staff. Anything that takes you away from all the garbage in your life can help turn things around. Once you find something that clicks, you can concentrate on what's right in your life instead of what's wrong.

IT'S AN INSIDE JOB

Many of us who've lost weight many times over the years realize that taking weight off is a most doable project. Nearly all the fad diets work – for a time – but when you abandon the diet, the old weight comes back, usually with a bonus amount tacked on for good measure.

So the question then becomes – what is the goal we wish to achieve? Do we want to get thin and stay thin? Of course we do, but why? Is it to be more attractive to our mate or maybe to attract someone to eventually become a mate? Is it to be healthier and feel better? Or is it because we've finally hit bottom and want to change our lives for the better?

All are good reasons, but it's becoming more evident that we have to understand ourselves before we can really achieve that elusive "something" that will change our lives. When I say understand, I really mean love ourselves, because that's basically what getting right with yourself is all about.

If you strip it down to the basics, most obesity is the result of some kind of self punishment. Something is driving the need for comfort that food provides. That something could be from one's childhood or current family or work situation. Whatever the cause, it's a subject much deeper than any book on weight loss can address, so we advise those afflicted in this manner to seek counseling as soon as possible.

It stands to reason that most obese people don't really enjoy the lack of mobility, the ostracizing, unkind remarks, chairs collapsing, uncomfortable seating, etc. If these situations don't exactly fit your current weight, they do represent some heartbreaking realities down the road if we don't change our relationship with food.

STRESS IS A WEIGHTY PROBLEM

Since the events of September 11, 2001, Americans have experienced threats to their personal security, as well as that of their loved ones, for perhaps the first time in their lives. Since then, stress levels of modern-day living have escalated, and show no signs of let-up during these times of uncertainty.

It's been a near universal response that during times of stress, humans tend to eat more, particularly carbohydrates, which have been shown to produce a calming effect.

Management consultants advise clients to look at employee weight gain as a sign of emotional distress, which could affect job performance. However, if you see yourself in this situation, don't worry that you might be fired, or you'll only eat more to calm your nerves. If you need something during a stressful episode, have a crunchy apple; only about 80 calories and filling, as well.

KIDS NEED HELP

You can get your kids on the right track to healthy eating by having them prepare their own lunches the night before while you're doing the same for yourself. This will displace the questionable choices that most schools now offer as lunch for their students.

It's shocking to see fast-food franchises operating the lunch counters at many schools. You'll find nearly everything there from fast-food heaven – pizza, burgers, fries, tacos, burritos, shakes, and lots of sugared soda.

The schools answer any objections to this outrage with the constant whine about budget shortfalls, leaving the void to be filled by franchise operators that staff the food service unit and thereby relieve the school of this expense. By the way, they also pay to get the contract, which also puts money in the school's kitty. In light of these kinds of arrangements, is it any wonder why the obesity problem is skyrocketing among children? Look around any school ground and you'll see youngsters puffed up like little balloons.

When kids get to this point, their bodies create additional fat cells that stay with them for the rest of their lives. These cells can shrink, but they're always there just waiting to be restored to their inflated size. Unless you've studied this problem, you have no idea how damaging it is for kids to fight obesity at a young age, not to mention the onset of type 2 diabetes, which is also rampaging throughout America.

The damage to the psyche is as much a problem as what's happening to children's health. The taunts from schoolmates are something that remain with a person until the day he or she dies. Scratch beneath the surface of many obese adults, and you'll find this festering boil.

Since young bodies are growing and developing at a rapid pace, good nuitrition is critically important. That's why fad diets and other approaches that adults might survive without permanent damage is definitely not appropriate for children. Parents need to recognize their youngster's problem and get a pediatrician or family doctor involved to determine the best course of action. Remember, you are responsible for bringing these youngsters into adulthood with good health and a good education. That begins with establishing healthy eating habits early in life. So get rid of the diet villains in the house – now! If they're not in the house, they can't be eaten.

MY DOG WAS EATING HEALTHIER

Tyler – our Irish setter – is the best family dog we've ever had, but has always been a problem eater. We tried just about every combination of dog food out there, and finally settled on a special hypo-allergenic food available only through our veterinarian, who also suggested omega-3 fish oil supplements.

As I was going through all of this, it struck me that Tyler was eating healthier than I was at the time, and that maybe I should reconsider the implications of food on my body.

HE SAID: I thought it was absurd that I was more devoted to my dog's diet than my own. And just like the horse doctor said, anything new going into the diet should be introduced gradually so as not to throw my taste and texture detector for a loop. So that's what I did. It took time, but I acquired a taste for 100% whole wheat bread, brown rice and whole wheat pasta – and now prefer them to the former refined flour versions.

SHE SAID: His epiphany about gradually introducing healthier foods into the diet is something I had been sneaking into our family's diet over many years. We slowly replaced red meat, fried foods and other sources of saturated fat and cholesterol with healthier alternatives, only I never mentioned the changes until much later. If the light bulb over his head went on at the vet's office, so be it, but "surprise, surprise" – we'd been doing so all along.

Okay – so perhaps our food choices were improving long before I became totally aware of what was going on – but now that we're there, let's explore exactly what Theresa was suggesting.

If you often have sausage, eggs and white toast with butter for breakfast, try some of the non-dairy and vegetable-based products that provide the best alternative for taste and preference. Scrambled egg whites, breakfast sausage vegetable substitute and whole wheat toast with zero calorie buttery spray can get you on the road to better choices in food selection. But, again, you don't have to do it all at once. Try making the transitions as uneventful as possible, and you'll be surprised at how many subtle diet changes slip by to become the "normal" food in your diet. Oh – and be sure to include as many fruits and vegetables as you can in your new food regimen.

ACTIVITY – THEN AND NOW

For those of you who eat the way you did years ago, and can't understand why you're gaining weight now but not then, take a stroll down memory lane with us and notice how many things we used to do are now done for us – or done with less work.

<u>Then</u> – we mowed our lawns with manual or gas mowers that at least required you to walk behind, if not push along.
The leaves and grass clippings also had to be raked up and hauled away.
<u>Now</u> – we ride lawn tractors that mow wide swaths and pickup the leaves and clippings. All that's required is steering the machine.

<u>Then</u> – we drove stick-shift cars without power steering, power brakes or power windows. And the radio buttons were a reach away. If you had four-wheel-drive, you had to get out of the vehicle to lock the front hubs.
<u>Now</u> – everything on the vehicle is power operated, with radio buttons on the steering wheel and a transmission that shifts automatically. Four-wheel drive is now a button on the dash.

Then – just about everything was manually operated, including can openers, typewriters, garage doors, TV channel selectors – even refrigerators required defrosting.
Now – well, you get the point.

How about when we were kids?

Then – we walked to school, to the local grocery store, to the library, to after-school events. We rode our bikes when it was too far to walk.
Now – a fleet of minivans with moms at the wheel take the place of those little legs getting the kids to where they need to go. In our neighborhood, youngsters are driven from their homes *within the subdivision* to the school bus pickup area.

Then – sandlot ball games, pickup basketball, street hockey, touch football – all without adult supervision.
Now – many ball fields are empty – and it seems the kids have given up on those spur-of-the-moment games.

Consider the number of calories expended back then compared with now, and you get some idea of what's contributing to the explosion of childhood obesity, not to mention the overall population.

Think about the amount of spare time spent in front of the television or computer in the evening compared with your father working in his woodshop or mother involved with knitting or working in the garden. All those little things add up to a lot at the end of the year.

Years ago, Arthur Murray and his wife had a television show centered around ballroom dancing. The closing line every week was – "Put a little fun in your life – try dancing!" This is a nostalgic way to button this chapter, but let's modify the last part of that line: "– try anything besides sitting on your butt!"

Chapter 12
FOOD FIGHT

Avoid hydrogenated/partially hydrogenated food products, which harbor trans fats – quickly becoming public enemy number one.

We've examined hundreds of processed foods suggested by friends, family, neighbors, newsletters, authors and those visiting our website. By processed foods, we're referring to packaged mixes, canned soups, frozen foods, canned vegetables and salad dressings.

Many of these processed foods are nutritious and can be integrated into your diet without sacrificing the weight-loss goals you've established. However, you need to pay close attention to the food labels and note how much saturated fat, partially hydrogenated vegetable oil and sodium is listed there.

It bears repeating – most Americans over the age of two should limit their intake of saturated fat to less than 10% of total calories, and all fats and oils to less than 30% of total calories.

The evidence is mounting against the use of hydrogenated and partially hydrogenated polyunsaturated oils found in some margarines and commercially prepared baked goods such as crackers, cakes, snack foods, etc. It's been determined that trans fatty acids resulting from this process tend to raise LDL (bad) cholesterol and lower HDL (good) cholesterol. This double whammy facilitates coronary heart disease – the number one cause of death in the U.S.

The FDA has weighed in on this problem with new regulations to require the amount of trans fatty acids in the food item be included in the Nutrition Facts panel – better known as the food label. However, like everything else that goes through the vetting process – the results may not be exactly user friendly.

According to the FDA website – *www.fda.gov/bbs/topics/NEWS/NEW00698.html* – the new regulations:

> "...would require that the amount of *trans* fat per serving be added to the amount of saturated fat per serving so that the amount and percent Daily Value (%DV) per serving on the Nutrition Facts panel will be based on the sum of the two. When *trans* fatty acids are present, an asterisk (or other symbol) would be required after the heading "Saturated fat" to refer to a footnote stating that the product "*Includes __ g trans fat." This footnote would be optional on foods that contain no *trans* fat (i.e. less than 0.5 gram per serving, as analytical methods cannot reliably measure lower levels), except when a fatty acid or cholesterol claim is made.
>
> The FDA notes that it is not proposing a *trans* fat limit for the claim "saturated fat free" because the agency has already defined that claim as less than 0.5 grams of saturated fat and less than 0.5 grams of *trans* fat."

Regardless of the new regulations, it's a good idea to avoid anything made of "partially hydrogenated" oils of any kind.

SODIUM RULES MANY PROCESSED FOODS

We were shocked to find how much sodium was listed for a microwavable can of soup that one might take to work as a convenient lunch. Would you believe 950 milligrams of sodium in a 10-oz serving of soup? That's 40% of a 2,400 milligrams Daily Value of sodium in a 2,000 calorie diet – nearly half of a day's limit in one can!

This blizzard of sodium is common among processed foods, and needs to be accounted for by those with hypertension and other sodium-sensitive ailments. Higher intakes of sodium are associated with the depletion of calcium – something that mature women and teenage girls need to maintain at higher levels. Older adults also need to increase their intake of calcium as bone strength is vitally important with advancing age.

SOME SOURCES OF CALCIUM*

- Yogurt#
- Milk**#
- Natural cheeses – Mozzarella, Cheddar, Swiss, Parmesan#
- Soy-based beverage with added calcium
- Tofu, if made with calcium sulfate (read the ingredient list)
- Breakfast cereal with added calcium
- Canned fish with soft bones such as salmon, sardines†
- Fruit juice with added calcium
- Pudding made with milk#
- Soup made with milk#
- Dark-green leafy vegetables such as spinach, collard greens

* Read food labels for brand-specific information.
** This includes lactose-free and lactose-reduced milk.
# Choose low-fat or fat-free milk products most often.
† High in salt.

Be aware that sodium does not mean just salt, which is sodium chloride. However, just one teaspoon of salt contains 2300 milligrams of sodium – near the limit of 2400 mg for the day. So it's a good idea to put the salt shaker away and limit the amount of sodium in the foods you select.

Sodium is present in many condiments that you might not associate with anything salty, such as ketchup, mustard and soy sauce. It's one of the reasons we recommend more fresh fruits and vegetables over canned varieties, which often have liberal amounts of sodium listed in the food label.

We also recommend that you monitor your restaurant meals, which are notorious for heavy amounts of salt. If you dine out, ask your waiter if the meal can be prepared without added salt. And, by all means, keep the salt shaker away from your food, be it served at a fancy bistro or on a picnic table. That ear of corn with some buttery spray is so good, you'll soon forget the salt.

COMFORT FOOD

We all have childhood memories of good times and maybe some not so good ones, but what really sticks in our brains are the foods we grew up with that evoke good memories. These are often the foods that mother prepared when we were coming off an illness or injury – or maybe just because they represented something important in her life. Whatever the reason, we respond to these foods in such a positive way that when things get stressful, we retreat to them in a big way. It's why they're called comfort foods – and why they are often the most difficult foods to avoid.

For example, in his later years, Elvis ballooned to the point of splitting his pants during performances. Among one of the many villains in his diet was the comfort food from his childhood – fried banana sandwiches – prepared by his housekeeper and cook, who got the recipe from his grandmother. It reminded him of home and better days.

Closer to home, I grew up in a household where my mother would often help cook for Polish weddings. My oldest brother was her favorite and she would prepare many of the foods he grew up with whenever he visited from another state. In fact, he was such a fussy eater as a child that mother would often go behind father's back to feed her son the foods he preferred rather than the standard menu of the day. This created a bond between mother and son that lasted to the day she died. It was a food preference that he carried with him to California, where Polish cooking was such a rarity that he built his life around the few restaurants where it could be found. In some cases, however, his cravings were carried to extreme.

Case in point. Many years ago, my brother visited our home for a holiday weekend. Prior to his arrival, Theresa prepared one of his favorite dishes – homemade tomato soup based on one of my mother's old-world recipes. It was to be a surprise and, since we were all going out to dinner upon his arrival, this huge bowl of soup was tucked away in the fridge overnight to be served for dinner the next day. In the morning, she and I were astonished to find the bowl in the sink – empty. As he told it, one of his "sinus headaches" woke him up and he discovered this "Polish medicine" in the fridge. To help make it through the night, he consumed the entire bowl – about 12 cups. Apparently it was good – we'll never know – but it's an example of comfort food in action.

Chapter 13
MEALS AWAY

Eating while driving – second riskiest behavior according to driver surveys. The riskiest? Speeding.

Current statistics indicate that most Americans eat out or order in more of their meals than ever before. If you're among this group, chances are you've found a key part of your weight problem. Restaurant meals are notorious for humongous portion sizes, along with an abundance of fat, cholesterol, sodium and total calories in the majority of their entrées, appetizers and side dishes.

Don't take our word for it. Enter your favorite restaurant's name in your browser's search engine and click on its website. There you should find postings of their menu items with tabs that provide some, if not all, of the nutritional values, including calories for each item. Fair warning, what you find there could be shocking.

Unfortunately, some of the biggest offenders in the fat/cholesterol/calorie sweepstakes don't list much, if any, of this information. Instead, they're waiting for the government to issue rulings that will force them to do so. If I were you, I'd take this lack of candor and openness as an indicator of just how awful the truth must be. That should give you pause for bringing home anything from those restaurants that don't want you to know what's in their food.

A better alternative would be one of those gorgeous rotisserie chickens that Theresa brings home from the membership warehouse store. A newspaper review voted these the best in the state. We pull the skin off, debone the bird and dine on this luscious poultry for two days – either as a main dish, shredded into a salad or stolen as a quick snack.

As part of my research into the subject of meals away from home, Theresa took me on a tour of a local food emporium located inside a supermarket, where she opened my eyes to the alternatives available to busy people who automatically think of a fast food outlet or takeout window of a restaurant for food on the go.

In the produce section are a large variety of salad "kits" that include croutons, cheese and dressing inside a prepared package of lettuce, tomato, green pepper, carrots, etc. – all ready to take home or to the office for dinner or lunch the next day. They also have "grab and go" packages of sliced turkey, potatoes, green beans and carrots ready for the microwave or toaster oven.

As we toured the facility, it became clear to me that markets are tapping into the busy lifestyles of today's families and single people – all who are so worn out at day's end that they just don't have the energy to cook. But when you can take home stuffed salmon steaks, skewers of tuna/onion/pepper/tomato or shrimp skewers with veggies or mushrooms and other choices – it's easy for you to throw it on the grille and eat healthy instead of suffering the problems we outlined with takeout meals.

Here's another motivation – you SAVE MONEY!

SLIM YOUR BODY AND FATTEN YOUR WALLET

Since we recommend that anyone wanting to lose weight refrain from eating restaurant meals during their initial weight-loss phase, and only dine out occasionally thereafter to maintain their weight loss, our plan <u>saves you money</u> – big time!

Think about this. If you eat lunch out every day, you're lucky to get by with a $10 or $20 meal – exorbinant to anyone who eats fast food – but this is about average. However, if you shop at the market, you can buy a whole bag of prepared salad and a bottle of dressing for under ten dollars. Then you can prepare a bunch of snap-on-lid bowls of salad to lunch on – maybe even throw in some of that rotisserie chicken we talked about earlier.

After a day or so of following our advice, you'll save the price of this book, and – over the months ahead – it adds up to some real money. In lunch alone, you could save $50 a week. That's $2,500 a year – or the start of a college fund for your children. If you eliminate eating restaurant dinners once or twice a week, that's a minimum of $20 per person for another $20 to $40 per week savings – or $1,000 to $2,000 per year.

Now, let's consider takeout dinner 2-3 times per week, which could range from $15 to $20 per person, and $1,500 to $3,000 a year. Add all of this up and it comes to a minimum of $5,000 or maximum of $7,500 – per person! And these are conservative estimates, which I'm sure would be exceeded from time to time, but you get the idea.

For those of us in the "hate to spend money" brigade, it's pure joy to watch the savings mount up and the bathroom scale numbers go down.

EATING OUT/TAKE OUT

Despite the foregoing, we did enjoy eating out at various restaurants and of course had our favorites. Unfortunately, we had to boycott the top restaurant on our list during Phase I – when a dieter needs to reverse direction regarding caloric intake and remove the food villains that make weight loss an uphill battle.

This restaurant was part of a family-run operation that served superb lunches as well as dinners. Patrons were served a multi-course meal starting with focaccia bread dipped in olive oil and garnished with Parmesan cheese, followed with a small plate of pasta topped with tomato meat sauce and more Parmesan.

Then came the entrée, which could be tenderloin beef tips in marsala wine sauce, filet mignon, pan fried walleye – and we're still talking about lunch, mind you.

REGULARS

Not only was the food great at this restaurant, but they had a buy-one-entrée, get-the-second-free coupon, plus – if you purchased four lunches – the fifth was free. So, we became what the trade calls regulars – a status that holds very little promise for anyone trying to lose weight.

We recognized the problem early on, and made some efforts to get around it by stretching the meal. We ate half and took the remainder home for dinner or lunch the next day. That worked some of the time, but – quite frankly – was a less-than-effective strategy. It was tough to duplicate the chef's cooking temperature when reheating in the microwave and the sauce was not as good if overheated. Knowing this, we often just ate it all at one sitting. Not hard to do if you take your time, but a choice we decided was taking us down the wrong road.

So, how does someone get hooked this way? Well, it's not that difficult when you lie to yourself. And what might you say when you do that? Here are some beauties:

- "I'll have a tiny dinner to make up for it."
- "I'll exercise another 30 minutes to work it off."
- "We deserve it because it's the only time we go out."
- "Some people eat like this all the time."

Any of these sound familiar? Chances are, they do. That's why we recommend giving up take-out and restaurant food during the initial phase of the DTD. We did. It's been more than ten months now and, looking back, we didn't start to see much weight coming off until we kissed our favorite place good bye.

We like to travel and have found restaurants in other states that we also enjoyed. Some were chain operations that advertise regularly. They're known as family or casual dining rather than fast food. These operations are famous for serving particular kinds of cuisine – steak, ribs, chicken, seafood, pasta or even old standbys, such as BLTs. What they tend to have in common is the caloric content of the entrées. Quite honestly, it's off-the-charts. For example:

Breakfast – deluxe pancake platter (1,610 calories)
Lunch – roast beef & cheese sandwich (1,641 calories)
Appetizer – deep fried onion fingers w/sauce (2,880 calories)
Dinner – T-bone steak & fried shrimp combo (1,965 calories)
Dessert – apple pie a la Mode (1,205 calories).

You might consider this list as cherry picking the highest calorie items on the menu to make a point, and I don't dispute that contention. Someone else might believe it's okay to try one of these selections for a special occasion, like a birthday or anniversary – and that's okay, too.

But for those who think that no one would ever make a habit of eating at one of these places on a regular basis – better think again. This is based on experiences of a member of our family who managed several of these establishments. He tells us that regulars would come in at least once, sometimes twice a week. A few would show up every day. These folks were easy to recognize due to their size.

Suitable seating for the regulars was problematic. They could not fit into a booth, so table seating was the only option. Many of them confessed that they liked the restaurant's food, but really chose to go there because of its strong chairs that wouldn't collapse and embarrass them.

Bottom line – if you're unhappy with your weight, being a regular in a restaurant that pumps you full of calories is not a good idea. We haven't even touched on the grams of carbohydrates, saturated fat, salt and other problem nutrients that inhabit these foods.

Do yourself a favor. Go to Appendix B in the back of this book for the USDA Nutrient Database for Standard Reference and scope out the profile of any food prior to ordering it at a restaurant or putting it into your shopping basket. This list contains over 6,000 food items and provides the calorie, protein, carbohydrate and fat content for 100 gram portions of each food listed. This portion size can be easily converted with the equivalent measures at the top of each page in Appendix B or with the tables of equivalent measures in Appendix A.

Use the example given there for how you can substitute diet villain foods with diet hero alternatives to reduce your calorie intake and achieve your weight goals.

WATER – NOT JUST WHERE FISH DO THEIR THING

Ever since my days as a broadcast radio newsman and disc jockey, I've been leery of drinking plain water. Those were the psychedelic 60s, and you never knew if someone at the radio station might slip a mind-bending substance in your water to see the effect it would have on your performance – just for laughs, of course.

One day, we had a legend in our business – J.P. McCarthy – stop in at the station in Flint, Michigan to do a commercial voice-over for a friend who owned a local business. When offered a glass of water, J.P. was said to reply, "No way, don't you know that fish make love in that stuff?" Thinking about that off-hand remark for a while, I decided water was fine for everything but drinking.

As I matured, the beverage of choice was usually a regular soda (pop, soft drink, etc.), since beer and wine just didn't appeal to me. However, after a superstar pitcher of the world champion Detroit Tigers baseball team was known to guzzle about a dozen or so colas a day and ended up buying his clothes from the "big-and-bigger" shop, I thought it would be wise to switch to no-cal soft drinks. (see Sugar). That decision saved me from entering the ranks of the obese, but just barely.

Then the great migration toward bottled water emerged. It arrived at our house in California, where the local water was hard and undrinkable by the standards of our former Great Lakes area home. But I still wasn't a convert until we moved back to southeast Michigan and bought a house with well water. That, my friends, is where you separate the men from the boys, because if we were hit with a devastating drought, it would be a flip of the coin to decide between drinking from a muddy hoofprint or well water. I know many of you probably enjoy your well water, but after 20 years, you'd think we'd have acquired a taste for it. Not so.

All this background is offered to establish my credentials as a one-time water-averse person. Today, I'm an avid consumer of bottled water. And nothing fancy here. The supermarket's private label spring water in gallon jugs is plenty fine, and excellent at room temperature.

This whole discussion is necessary because water is essential to keeping your body hydrated, maintaining good kidney function and satisfying any hunger you might experience throughout the day. Sometimes the body disguises its need for water with hunger sensations. So before you reach for food, have a glass of water first to see if food is indeed what your body requires. Eight 8-ounce glasses of water will also help flush your system of the waste products your body excretes when exercising. Basic rule – drink about one quart of water for every 1000 calories you burn during exercise. And be sure you drink before the exercise and before you're thirsty. How do you know how many calories are consumed during various exercises? Am I glad you asked. (See Mandatory Exercise)

Chapter 14
MANDATORY EXERCISE?

If there was an easy way to lose excess weight, why do the rich and famous hire trainers or risk bariatric surgery?

Despite virtually unlimited resources, many overweight celebrities still can't find that magic pill for weight loss. Many of them have personal trainers who drive them mercilessly through arduous exercise programs in order to get them into shape. Some even undergo risky surgery.

Does anyone out there believe these stars purposely avoid those pills, potions, fad diets, etc. just because they prefer to do it the hard way? Does that make any sense?

If that's so, then maybe it's time to bite the bullet and start an exercise program that fits your particular circumstance. But take note, before embarking on any type of exercise, you should consult with your doctor.

Something else needs to be said about exercise. The evidence is just not there to support the idea that exercise by itself will result in significant weight loss. It does help build muscle, which can lead to a more effective calorie burning machine and, therefore, result in some weight loss. But when combined with a healthy diet regimen that includes all the major food groups and eliminates many of the problem foods we've been talking about, exercise works like a catalyst in a chemical reaction.

You might consider starting simple by just walking for exercise. If you check out the Energy Expenditure Chart in this chapter, a leisurely 2-mph walking speed burns 198 cal./hr. Try ballroom dancing, which burns 210 cal./hr. For those who like golfing, a twosome carrying their own bags can burn up to 324 cal./hr. The basic idea is to get away from the couch and enjoy life. Choose whatever activity you like, but just be sure you're up to it physically.

For those who are incapacitated in some way, there are programs run by physical therapy centers that can accommodate you in any number of activities.

Energy Expenditure Chart

A. Sedentary Activities Cal./Hour*	**Energy Costs**
Lying down or sleeping	90
Sitting quietly	84
Sitting and writing, card playing, etc.	114
B. Moderate Activities	**(150-350)**
Bicycling (5 mph)	174
Canoeing (2.5 mph)	174
Dancing (ballroom)	210
Golf (twosome, carrying clubs)	324
Horseback riding (sitting to trot)	246
Light housework, cleaning, etc.	246
Swimming (crawl, 20 yards/min)	288
Tennis (recreational doubles)	312
Volleyball (recreational)	264
Walking (2 mph)	198
C. Vigorous Activities	**More than 350**
Aerobic dancing	546
Basketball (recreational)	450
Bicycling (13 mph)	612
Circuit weight training	756
Cross-country Skiing (5 mph)	690
Football (touch, vigorous)	498
Ice skating (9 mph)	384
Racquetball	588
Roller skating (9 mph)	384
Running (10 minute mile, 6 mph)	654
Scrubbing floors	440
Swimming (crawl, 45 yards/min)	522
Tennis (recreational singles)	450

*Hourly estimates based on values calculated for calories burned per minute for a 150 pound (68 kg) person.

(Sources: William D. McArdle, Frank I. Katch, Victor L. Katch, "Exercise Physiology: Energy, Nutrition and Human Performance" (2nd edition), Lea & Febiger, Philadelphia, 1986; Melvin H. Williams, "Nutrition for Fitness and Sport," William C. Brown Company Publishers, Dubuque, 1983.)

What's interesting about the calories consumed for these activities is that heavier people expend more calories for the same effort than do smaller people. So if you're a 170-pound person engaged in cross-country skiing, you'll burn about the same number of calories in 10 minutes that it takes a 130 pound individual about 13 minutes.

Doesn't seem quite fair, I know, but it does if you consider an analogy with gas mileage and your choice of vehicle. A large car consumes more fuel (calories) than a compact car, which continues on for another 3 minutes after the larger vehicle runs out of gas. Consequently, all SUV-sized folks out there can derive greater benefit from the same exercise

By the way, isn't it good to know that you actually burn calories while sleeping? How about those calories lost during card playing? Now that has some possibilities. For example – instead of making up some kind of excuse about Friday night poker with the guys, all we need to say is: "Going out to exercise, honey. Long session tonight. Be back around 2 a.m." This is a quintessential Tim Allen moment. Of course – if you add the mandatory beer and pretzels – any weight loss will be offset, but the excuse is classic.

EXERCISE II

This may be news to some of us, but research confirms that exercise doesn't necessarily burn fat. It mostly builds muscle. That's why the scale may show minimal weight loss if that's all you're doing to lose weight. In fact, since muscle weighs more than fat, you may see the scale climb higher.

But keep this in mind. If you look at some of our fittest athletes and movie stars on the scene today, many could be considered overweight by standard height/weight tables.

The real measure of your body's fatness is the BMI or Body Mass Index. Tables for determining your BMI are in Chapter 9.

Here's my personal take on exercise. You can seek out the method that makes the most effective use of your time. It could be at home on your own equipment. It might be at a gym where membership fees keep you motivated by appealing to your desire to not waste the money. The simplest and least expensive exercise could be just walking or running outdoors.

The authors have done it all and decided what works best for us is a cross-country skiing machine, stationary bicycle and motorized treadmill – all of which we use in our basement. The reasons why include the privacy and ready access to the equipment when we want to use it. This is not always the case when you join a gym and get crowded out by the same work schedule as most other people.

The computers on our machines are like the gym versions that measure time, distance, pulse rate, resistance level, and calorie consumption. We also can exercise winter or summer without fighting off outdoor menaces that include rain, slippery walkways (victimizing the late Dr. Atkins), mean dogs, black flies, broken concrete and crazy drivers.

Final thoughts on exercise. It fine tunes your body to burn calories more efficiently, improve cardio vascular performance, lower your pulse rate and turbocharge your sex life (after showering, of course). If the last item on the list doesn't happen in your case, we'll refer you to Dr. Ruth.

Chapter 15
PUTTING IT ALL TOGETHER

Eat slowly – the brain needs 20 minutes to get a "full" signal.

So here we are near the close of our adventure in healthy eating. As you've probably realized by now, what we've put together is a non-diet diet plan – about as unorthodox as you can get in this world of highly complex fad diets.

As we said at the outset, our goal is to make weight loss a painless, no-brainer experience, where the whole weight-loss process is broken down into a few simple strategies. Boiled down, here's what we recommend:

- Duct tape your diet villains like mummies or throw them out.

- Tape off "white carbs" in your pantry – replace them with whole grains. Try yams instead of potatoes.

- Never skip breakfast – or any other meal.

- Consume six small meals (or three meals and three snacks) per day instead of three big ones. In other words, divide your three main meals into six, but keep your portions according to serving-size guidelines.

- Eat fish at least three times a week and limit meat to three (or fewer) meals per week.

- Eat out at "healthy food" restaurants where you can get the whole grains, broiled fish/poultry/lean meats and low-fat food preparation – or give up restaurant food until you lose your excess weight.

- Reduce those portions and follow the Food Guide Pyramid for number of servings from all the food groups.

- Factor in soy substitutes that offer lower calories and reduced fats over meats, cheeses and butter. Be aware that some controversy exists over soy products.

- Switch from fructose-sweetened soft drinks known as "liquid candy" to no-cal alternatives.

- After consulting with your doctor, exercise at least 40 minutes per day according to the limits of your physical condition. Exercise includes taking stairs over elevators, walking, cutting the lawn, hand washing the car, etc.

- Limit your alcohol consumption to one or two drinks per day. Better yet, give it up until you lose the excess weight.

- Break those fat-promoting eating habits – such as eating while watching TV or driving.

- Read all food labels and eliminate as much sugar, saturated fat, partially hydrogenated oil and, sodium as possible.

- Always combine a carbohydrate with a protein – particularly a high glycemic carb – to limit the spike in blood sugar and corresponding insulin response.

- Drink plenty of water during the day and at meals.

- Keep your daily intake of saturated fat to less than 10% of total calories, and all fats/oils to less than 30% of total calories.

- Substitute high calorie foods for lower calorie alternatives using the USDA Nutrient Database for Standard Reference.

- Remember – there are no shortcuts to weight loss. If you lose weight quickly, your body will respond by taking every opportunity to regain that weight and then some.

BUT YOU SAID TO K.I.S.S.

Let's clarify this reference, which was established earlier in the book. We promised to Keep It Simple and Successful = K.I.S.S. Of course, we have no objection to the pressing of lips.

So, to live up to our promise, let's see how one day's worth of eating on the DTD can satisfy the palate and the stomach, provide the lower calorie intake of 1,600 calories and supply the whole grains, fruits, vegetables, calcium, protein and fat limits we've recommended. If you adopt this plan, you can't avoid losing weight.

Note that breakfast and lunch are divided to provide an even distribution of calories throughout the work day, and that dinner provides the omega 3 fatty acids necessary for good health. Also be aware that the percent of fat is less than 30% of total calories in this menu and that margarine is non-hydrogenated with no trans fats. These are all important considerations.

Breakfast	**Energy (calories)**	**Fat (grams)**	**% Fat**
Cereal, shredded Wheat, 1 cup	207	2	8
Milk, 1%, 1 cup	102	3	23
Orange juice, 3/4 cup	78	0	0
Coffee, regular, 1 cup	5	0	0
Milk, 1%, 1 oz. (in coffee)	13	0.3	23
2nd-Half Breakfast			
Whole wheat bread, 1 med. slice	70	1.2	15.4
Jelly, regular, 2 tsp.	30	0	.0
Breakfast Total	505	6.5	10

Lunch	**Energy (calories)**	**Fat (grams)**	**% Fat**
½ Roast beef sandwich, whole wheat bread, 1 slice	70.5	1.2	7.5
Lean roast beef, unseasoned, 1.5 oz.	30	0.75	11.5
American cheese, low-fat/low-sodium, ½ slice (3/8 oz.)	23	0.9	18
Lettuce, 1 leaf	1	0	0
Tomato, 3 med. slices	10	0	0
Mayonnaise, low-cal, 2 tsp.	15	1.6	49.5
Apple, ½ med.	40	0	0
Diet soda	0	0	0
2nd-Half Lunch			
½ roast beef sandwich, whole wheat bread, 1 slice	70.5	1.2	7.5
Lean roast beef, unseasoned, 1.5 oz.	30	0.75	11.5
American cheese, low-fat/low-sodium, ½ slice (3/8 oz.)	23	0.9	18
Lettuce, 1 leaf	1	0	0
Tomato, 3 slices	10	0	0
Mayonnaise, low-cal, 2 tsp.	15	1.6	49.5
Apple, ½ med.	40	0	0
Diet soda	0	0	0
Lunch Total	366	9	22

If you have any concerns about going hungry on our weight-loss regimen, just look at how much food we're recommending and how often you're prompted to eat. The key is sticking to the portion sizes. If you start out weighing and measuring, before long you'll be able to eyeball the amounts required and the whole process will be second nature. The weight will begin melting away and your co-workers will wonder how you did it.

Dinner	Energy (calories)	Fat (grams)	% Fat
Salmon, broiled 3 oz.	155	7	40
Vegetable oil, 1.5 tsp.	60	7	100
Baked sweet potato, 3/4 med.	100	0	0
Margarine, 1 tsp.	34	4	100
Green beans, w/margarine 1/2 cup	52	2	4
Carrots w/margarine, 1/2 cup	52	2	4
Whole grain dinner roll, 1 med.	80	3	33
Ice milk, 1/2 cup	92	3	28
Iced tea, unsweetened, 1 cup	0	0	0
Water, 2 cups	0	0	0
Dinner total	625	28	38

Take a 40 minute walk after dinner but don't forget – you still have more food to eat before the day's allotment is complete, so make room for a healthy snack.

Snack	Energy (calories)	Fat (grams)	% Fat
Popcorn, 2 1/2 cups	69	0	0
Margarine, 1 1/2 tsp.	58	6.5	100
Grand Total	1613	50	28

Okay – now you can retire for the evening, knowing that you're body is metabolizing all those whole grains, fruits and vegetables – and taking you along the path of healthy weight management. Sweet dreams – now that those diet villains are wrapped up and silenced with the most effective method we know of keeping them out of your new life – The Duct Tape Diet.

Appendix A
ADDITIONAL READING/ MEASURE EQUIVALENTS

Binge Eating Disorder. NIH Publication No. 94-3589. This fact sheet describes the symptoms, causes, complications, and treatment of binge eating disorder, along with a profile of those at risk for the disorder.

Dieting and Gallstones. NIH Publication No. 94-3677. This fact sheet describes what gallstones are, how weight loss may cause them, and how to lessen the risk of developing them.

Gastric Surgery for Severe Obesity. NIH Publication No. 96-4006. This fact sheet describes the different types of surgery available to treat severe obesity. It explains how gastric surgery promotes weight loss and the benefits and risks of each procedure.

Physical Activity and Weight Control. NIH Publication No. 96-4031. This booklet explains how physical activity helps promote weight control and other ways it benefits one's health. It also describes the different types of physical activity and provides tips on how to become more physically active.

Prescription Medications for the Treatment of Obesity. NIH Publication No. 97-4191. This fact sheet presents information on appetite suppressant medications. These medications may help some obese patients lose more weight than with non-drug treatments. The types of medications and the risks and benefits associated with the use of these medications are described.

Very Low-Calorie Diets. NIH Publication No. 95-3894. Information on who should use a very low-calorie diet (VLCD) and the health benefits and possible adverse effects of VLCDs is provided in this fact sheet.

Weight Cycling. NIH Publication No. 95-3901. Based on research, this fact sheet describes the health effects of weight cycling, also known as "yo-yo" dieting, and how it affects obese individuals' future weight-loss efforts.

http://www.niddk.nih.gov/health/nutrit/nutrit.htm
http://www.nhlbi.nih.gov/health/pubs/index.htm

If you're looking for a good place to start in your hunt for diet villains, take a hard look at the fats. For those who think carbohydrates are the real problem, compare the more than twice as many calories in fat over protein or carbs. Fewer calories burned than eaten = weight gain.

1 teaspoon of protein or carbohydrate	= 16 calories
1 teaspoon of alcohol	= 28 calories
1 teaspoon of fat	= 36 calories

Volume Equivalents

1 tablespoon (tbs.)	= 3 teaspoons (tsp.)
1/16 cup (c)	= 1 tablespoon
1/8 cup	= 2 tablespoons
1/6 cup	= 2 tablespoons + 2 teaspoons
1/4 cup	= 4 tablespoons
1/3 cup	= 5 tablespoons + 1 teaspoon
3/8 cup	= 6 tablespoons
1/2 cup	= 8 tablespoons
2/3 cup	= 10 tablespoons + 2 teaspoons
3/4 cup	= 12 tablespoons
1 cup	= 48 teaspoons
1 cup	= 16 tablespoons
1 cup	= ½ pint
1 fluid ounce	= 2 tablespoons (30 ml)
8 fluid ounces (fl oz)	= 1 cup
1 pint (pt)	= 2 cups
1 quart (qt)	= 2 pints/4 cups (0.946 liter; 946 m)
4 cups	= 1 quart
1 gallon (gal)	= 4 quarts (3.786 liters; 3,786 ml)
1 milliliter (ml)	= 1 cubic centimeter (cc)
1 inch (in)	= 2.54 centimeters (cm)

Weight Equivalents

1 teaspoon	= 5 grams (approx.)
1 cup	= 236.56 grams (240 grams approx.)
1 pound (16 ounces)	= 453.6 grams
3½ ounces	= 100 grams

Metric Conversion Factors		
Multiply	**By**	**To Get**
Fluid Ounces	29.57	grams
Ounces (dry)	28.35	grams
Grams	0.0353	ounces
Grams	0.0022	pounds
Kilograms	2.21	pounds
Pounds	453.6	grams
Pounds	0.4536	kilograms
Quarts	0.946	liters
Quarts (dry)	67.2	cubic inches
Quarts (liquid)	57.7	cubic inches
Liters	1.0567	quarts
Gallons	3,785	cubic centimeters
Gallons	3.785	liters

Appendix B
ABBREVIATIONS IN USDA NUTRIENT DATABASE FOR STANDARD REFERENCE RELEASE 15

All Purpose	ALLPURP	Cholesterol-free	CHOL-FREE
Aluminum	AL	Chopped	CHOPD
And	&	Cinnamon	CINN
Apple	APPL	Coated	COATD
Apples	APPLS	Coconut	COCNT
Applesauce	APPLSAUC	Commercial	COMM
Approximate	APPROX	Commercially	COMMLY
Approximately	APPROX	Commodity	CMDTY
Arm and blade	ARM&BLD	Composite	COMP
Artificial	ART	Concentrate	CONC
Ascorbic acid	VITC	Concentrated	CONCD
Aspartame	ASPRT	Condensed	COND
Aspartame-sweetened	ASPRT-SWTND	Condiment (s)	CONDMNT
Baby food	BABYFD	Cooked	CKD
Baked	BKD	Cottonseed	CTTNSD
Barbequed	BBQ	Cream	CRM
Based	BSD	Creamed	CRMD
Beans	BNS	Dark	DK
Beef	BF	Decorticated	DECORT
Beverage	BEV	Dehydrated	DEHYD
Boiled	BLD	Dessert, desserts	DSSRT
Boneless	BNLESS	Diluted	DIL
Bottled	BTLD	Domestic	DOM
Bottom	BTTM	Drained	DRND
Braised	BRSD	Dressing	DRSNG
Breakfast	BRKFST	Drink	DRK
Broiled	BRLD	Drumstick	DRUMSTK
Buttermilk	BTTRMLK	English	ENG
Calcium	CA	Enriched	ENR
Calorie, calories	CAL	Equal	EQ
Canned	CND	Evaporated	EVAP
Carbonated	CARB	Except	XCPT
Center	CNTR	Extra	EX
Cereal	CRL	Flank steak	FLANKSTK
Cheese	CHS	Flavored	FLAV
Chicken	CHICK	Flour	FLR
Chocolate	CHOC	Food	FD
		Fortified	FORT

French fried	FRENCH FR	Nonfat dry milk	NFDM
French fries	FRENCH FR	Nonfat dry milk solids	NFDMS
Fresh	FRSH	Nonfat milksolids	NFMS
Frosted	FRSTD	Noncarbonated	NONCARB
Frosting	FRSTNG	Not Further Specified	NFS
Frozen	FRZ	Nutrients	NUTR
Grades	GRDS	Nutrition	NUTR
Gram	GM	Ounce	OZ
Green	GRN	Pack	PK
Greens	GRNS	Par fried	PARFR
Heated	HTD	Parboiled	PARBLD
Heavy	HVY	Partial	PART
Hi-meat	HIMT	Partially	PART
High	HI	Partially fried	PARFR
Hour	HR	Pasteurized	PAST
Hydrogenated	HYDR	Peanut	PNUT
Imitation	IMITN	Peanuts	PNUTS
Immature	IMMAT	Phosphate	PO4
Imported	IMP	Phosphorus	P
Includes	INCL	Pineapple	PNAPPL
Including	INCL	Plain	PLN
Infant formula	INFFORMULA	Porterhouse	PRTRHS
Ingredient	ING	Potassium	K
Instant	INST	Powder	PDR
Juice	JUC	Powdered	PDR
Junior	JR	Precooked	PRECKD
Kernels	KRNLS	Preheated	PREHTD
Large	LRG	Prepared	PREP
Lean	LN	Processed	PROC
Lean only	LN	Product code	PROD CD
Leavened	LVND	Propionate	PROP
Light	LT	Protein	PROT
Liquid	LIQ	Pudding	PUDD
Low	LO	Ready-to-bake	RTB
Low fat	LOFAT	Ready-to-cook	RTC
Marshmallow	MARSHMLLW	Ready-to-drink	RTD
Mashed	MSHD	Ready-to-eat	RTE
Mayonnaise	MAYO	Ready-to-feed	RTF
Medium	MED	Ready-to-heat	RTH
Mesquite	MESQ	Ready-to-serve	RTS
Minutes	MIN	Ready-to-use	RTU
Mixed	MXD	Reconstituted	RECON
Moisture	MOIST	Reduced	RED
Natural	NAT	Reduced-calorie	RED-CAL
New Zealand	NZ	Refrigerated	REFR

Regular	REG	Undiluted	UNDIL
Reheated	REHTD	Unenriched	UNENR
Replacement	REPLCMNT	Unheated	UNHTD
Restaurant-prepared	REST-PREP	Unprepared	UNPREP
Retail	RTL	Unspecified	UNSPEC
Roast	RST	Unsweetened	UNSWTND
Roasted	RSTD	Variety, varieties	VAR
Round	RND	Vegetables	VEG
Sandwich	SNDWCH	Vitamin A	VITA
Sauce	SAU	Vitamin C	VITC
Scalloped	SCALLPD	Water	H20
Scrambled	SCRMBLD	Whitener	WHTNR
Seed	SD	Whole	WHL
Select	SEL	Winter	WNTR
Shank & sirloin	SHK&SIRL	With	W/
Short	SHRT	Without	WO/
Shoulder	SHLDR	Yellow	YEL
Simmered	SIMMRD		
Skin	SKN		
Small	SML		
Sodium	NA		
Solids	SOL		
Solution	SOLN		
Soybean	SOYBN		
Special	SPL		
Species	SP		
Spread	SPRD		
Standard	STD		
Steamed	STMD		
Stewed	STWD		
Stick	STK		
Sticks	STKS		
Strained	STR		
Substitute	SUB		
Summer	SMMR		
Supplement	SUPP		
Sweet	SWT		
Sweetened	SWTND		
Sweetener	SWTNR		
Teaspoon	TSP		
Thousand	1000		
Toasted	TSTD		
Toddler	TODD		
Uncooked	UNCKD		
Uncreamed	UNCRMD		

APPENDIX C – USDA NUTRIENT DATABASE FOR STANDARD REFERENCE – RELEASE 15*

Since the Duct Tape Diet focuses on reduced calories as the key to weight loss, we decided to provide the caloric content for 100 gram portions (equivalent to 3½ ounces, 20 tsp. or approximately ½ cup) of more than 6,200 food items listed in the USDA Nutrient Database for Standard Reference – Release 15. To make this reference list even more useful, we also included the protein, carbohydrate, saturated fat, polyunsaturated fat, and monounsaturated fat content of these listed foods.

How to use the list. First, consult your doctor before embarking on any weight-loss diet. Then, look up the foods you entered into your three-day food record, write down the calorie content per portion size, scan the foods you're considering to replace them with, write down their calorie content per portion size, subtract to find the calorie savings and add up the daily savings to get your 3500 calories or one-pound per week weight-loss goal. Be sure to note the carbohydrate and fat content of your alternative foods to ensure the substitution makes sense on all counts.

EXAMPLE: Your dinner entry lists 3½ oz. of beef short ribs. You look up the closest description and find #13148 BEEF, RIB, SHORTRIBS, LN&FAT, CHOIC, CKD, BRSD = 471 calories. Check the abbreviations list to decipher the LN as lean, CHOIC as choice, CKD as cooked, and BRSD as braised. Then you scan down to #15209 SALMON, ATLANTIC, WILD, CKD, DRY HEAT = 182 calories. DRY HEAT means baked or broiled. Enter the numbers in your calculator: 471 calories less 182 calories equals 289 reduced calories by substituting the Atlantic salmon for the beef short ribs. By making these types of substitutions at every meal, you can easily reach your 3500 calorie or one-pound weekly weight loss and eat healthier as well.

* Courtesy of: U.S. Department of Agriculture, Agricultural Research Service. 2002. USDA Nutrient Database for Standard Reference, Release 15. Nutrient Data Laboratory Home Page: http://www.nal.usda.gov/fnic/foodcomp

The complete database — updated with a wider range of foods and nutrients than this abbreviated version — is available on the Internet at: *http://www.nal.usda.gov/fnic/foodcomp/Data/SR16/sr16.html*

NDB #	Food Description (100 gram portions = 3½ ounces = 20 tsp = ½ cup approx.	Calories	Protein	Carbs	Sat Fat
15155	ABALONE, MIXED SPECIES, RAW	105	17.1	6.01	0.149
15156	ABALONE, MXD SP, CKD, FRIED	189	19.63	11.05	1.646
09427	ABIYUCH, RAW	69	1.5	17.6	0.014
09002	ACEROLA JUICE, RAW	23	0.4	4.8	0.068
09001	ACEROLA, (WEST INDIAN CHERRY), RAW	32	0.4	7.69	0.068
12060	ACORN FLOUR, FULL FAT	501	7.49	54.65	3.923
12059	ACORNS, DRIED	509	8.1	53.66	4.084
12058	ACORNS, RAW	387	6.15	40.75	3.102
14006	ALCOHOLIC BEV, BEER, LT	28	0.2	1.3	0
14003	ALCOHOLIC BEV, BEER, REG	41	0.3	3.7	0
14034	ALCOHOLIC BEV, CREME DE MENTHE, 72 PROOF	371	0	41.6	0.014
14009	ALCOHOLIC BEV, DAIQUIRI, CND	125	0	15.7	0
14010	ALCOHOLIC BEV, DAIQUIRI, PREPARED-FROM-RECIPE	186	0.1	6.8	0.007
14037	ALCOHOLIC BEV, DISTILLED, ALL (GIN, RUM, VODKA, WHISKEY) 80 P	231	0	0	0
14550	ALCOHOLIC BEV, DISTILLED, ALL (GIN, RUM, VODKA, WHISKEY) 86 P	250	0	0.1	0
14551	ALCOHOLIC BEV, DISTILLED, ALL (GIN, RUM, VODKA, WHISKEY) 90 P	263	0	0	0
14532	ALCOHOLIC BEV, DISTILLED, ALL (GIN, RUM, VODKA, WHISKEY) 94 P	275	0	0	0
14533	ALCOHOLIC BEV, DISTILLED, ALL 100 PROOF	295	0	0	0
14049	ALCOHOLIC BEV, DISTILLED, GIN, 90 PROOF	263	0	0	0
14050	ALCOHOLIC BEV, DISTILLED, RUM, 80 PROOF	231	0	0	0
14051	ALCOHOLIC BEV, DISTILLED, VODKA, 80 PROOF	231	0	0	0
14052	ALCOHOLIC BEV, DISTILLED, WHISKEY, 86 PROOF	250	0	0.1	0
14415	ALCOHOLIC BEV, LIQUEUR, COFFEE W/CRM, 34 PROOF	327	2.8	20.9	9.664
14414	ALCOHOLIC BEV, LIQUEUR, COFFEE, 53 PROOF	336	0.1	46.8	0.106
14534	ALCOHOLIC BEV, LIQUEUR, COFFEE, 63 PROOF	308	0.1	32.2	0.106
14015	ALCOHOLIC BEV, PINA COLADA, CND	237	0.6	27.6	6.571
14017	ALCOHOLIC BEV, PINA COLADA, PREPARED-FROM-RECIPE	179	0.42	22.64	1.636
14019	ALCOHOLIC BEV, TEQUILA SUNRISE, CND	110	0.3	11.3	0.013
14024	ALCOHOLIC BEV, WHISKEY SOUR MIX, PDR	383	0.6	97.3	0.019
14027	ALCOHOLIC BEV, WHISKEY SOUR, CND	119	0	13.4	0
14029	ALCOHOLIC BEV, WHISKEY SOUR, PREP FROM ITEM 14028	149	0	13.1	0.005
14531	ALCOHOLIC BEV, WHISKEY SOUR, PREP FROM ITEM 14530	149	0	13.1	0.005
14025	ALCOHOLIC BEV, WHISKEY SOUR, PREP W/H2O, WHISKEY&PDR MIX	164	0.1	15.9	0.003
14536	ALCOHOLIC BEV, WINE, DSSRT, DRY	126	0.2	4.1	0
14057	ALCOHOLIC BEV, WINE, DSSRT, SWT	153	0.2	11.8	0

NDB #	Food Description (100 gram portions = 3½ ounces = 20 tsp = ½ cup approx.	Calories	Protein	Carbs	Sat Fat
14084	ALCOHOLIC BEV, WINE, TABLE, ALL	70	0.2	1.4	0
14096	ALCOHOLIC BEV, WINE, TABLE, RED	72	0.2	1.7	0
14104	ALCOHOLIC BEV, WINE, TABLE, ROSE	71	0.2	1.4	0
14106	ALCOHOLIC BEV, WINE, TABLE, WHITE	68	0.1	0.8	0
11001	ALFALFA SEEDS, SPROUTED, RAW	29	3.99	3.78	0.069
02001	ALLSPICE, GROUND	263	6.09	72.12	2.55
12695	ALMOND BUTTER, PLN, W/SALT	633	15.08	21.22	5.602
12195	ALMOND BUTTER, PLN, WO/SALT	633	15.08	21.22	5.602
12071	ALMOND PASTE	458	9	47.81	2.629
12061	ALMONDS	578	21.26	19.74	3.881
12062	ALMONDS, BLANCHED	581	21.94	19.94	3.89
12563	ALMONDS, DRY RSTD, W/SALT	597	22.09	19.29	4.047
12063	ALMONDS, DRY RSTD, WO/SALT	597	22.09	19.29	4.047
12206	ALMONDS, HONEY RSTD, UNBLANCHED	594	18.17	27.9	4.73
12565	ALMONDS, OIL RSTD, W/SALT	607	21.23	17.68	4.208
12065	ALMONDS, OIL RSTD, WO/SALT	607	21.23	17.68	4.208
20001	AMARANTH	374	14.45	66.17	1.662
11700	AMARANTH LEAVES, CKD, BLD, DRND, W/SALT	21	2.11	4.11	0.05
11004	AMARANTH LEAVES, CKD, BLD, DRND, WO/SALT	21	2.11	4.11	0.05
11003	AMARANTH LEAVES, RAW	23	2.46	4.03	0.091
15002	ANCHOVY, EUROPEAN, CND IN OIL, DRND SOL	210	28.89	0	2.203
15001	ANCHOVY, EUROPEAN, RAW	131	20.35	0	1.282
02002	ANISE SEED	337	17.6	50.02	0.586
09400	APPLE JUC, CND OR BTLD, UNSWTND, W/ VIT C	47	0.06	11.68	0.019
09016	APPLE JUC, CND OR BTLD, UNSWTND, WO/ VIT C	47	0.06	11.68	0.019
09018	APPLE JUC, FRZ CONC, UNSWTND, DIL W/3 VOLUME H2O WO/ VIT C	47	0.14	11.54	0.018
09411	APPLE JUC, FRZ CONC, UNSWTND, DIL W/3 VOLUME H2O, W/ VIT C	47	0.14	11.54	0.018
09410	APPLE JUC, FRZ CONC, UNSWTND, UNDIL, W/ VIT C	166	0.51	41	0.06
09017	APPLE JUC, FRZ CONC, UNSWTND, UNDIL, WO/ VIT C	166	0.51	41	0.06
09008	APPLES, CND, SWTND, SLICED, DRND, HTD	67	0.18	16.84	0.07
09007	APPLES, CND, SWTND, SLICED, DRND, UNHTD	67	0.18	16.7	0.08
09010	APPLES, DEHYD (LO MOIST), SULFURED, STWD	74	0.28	19.91	0.02
09009	APPLES, DEHYD (LO MOIST), SULFURED, UNCKD	346	1.32	93.53	0.095
09013	APPLES, DRIED, SULFURED, STWD, W/ SUGAR	83	0.2	20.73	0.011
09012	APPLES, DRIED, SULFURED, STWD, WO/ SUGAR	57	0.22	15.32	0.012

NDB #	Food Description (100 gram portions = 3½ ounces = 20 tsp = ½ cup approx.	Calories	Protein	Carbs	Sat Fat
09011	APPLES, DRIED, SULFURED, UNCKD	243	0.93	65.89	0.052
09015	APPLES, FRZ, UNSWTND, HTD	47	0.29	12	0.053
09014	APPLES, FRZ, UNSWTND, UNHTD	48	0.28	12.31	0.053
09003	APPLES, RAW, WITH SKIN	59	0.19	15.25	0.058
09004	APPLES, RAW, WITHOUT SKIN	57	0.15	14.84	0.051
09005	APPLES, RAW, WO/SKN, CKD, BLD	53	0.26	13.64	0.058
09006	APPLES, RAW, WO/SKN, CKD, MICROWAVE	56	0.28	14.41	0.068
09402	APPLESAUCE, CND, SWTND, W/SALT	76	0.18	19.91	0.03
09020	APPLESAUCE, CND, SWTND, WO/SALT	76	0.18	19.91	0.03
09401	APPLESAUCE, CND, UNSWTND, W/ VIT C	43	0.17	11.29	0.008
09019	APPLESAUCE, CND, UNSWTND, WO/ VIT C	43	0.17	11.29	0.008
09403	APRICOT NECTAR, CND, W/ VIT C	56	0.37	14.39	0.006
09036	APRICOT NECTAR, CND, WO/ VIT C	56	0.37	14.39	0.006
09029	APRICOTS, CND, EX HVY SYRUP PK, WO/SKN, SOL&LIQUIDS	96	0.55	24.85	0.003
09025	APRICOTS, CND, EX LT SYRUP PK, W/SKN, SOL&LIQUIDS	49	0.6	12.5	0.007
09022	APRICOTS, CND, H2O PK, W/SKN, SOL&LIQUIDS	27	0.71	6.39	0.011
09023	APRICOTS, CND, H2O PK, WO/SKN, SOL&LIQUIDS	22	0.69	5.48	0.002
09027	APRICOTS, CND, HVY SYRUP PK, W/SKN, SOL&LIQUIDS	83	0.53	21.47	0.005
09028	APRICOTS, CND, HVY SYRUP PK, WO/SKN, SOL&LIQUIDS	83	0.51	21.45	0.006
09024	APRICOTS, CND, JUC PK, W/SKN, SOL&LIQUIDS	48	0.63	12.34	0.003
09026	APRICOTS, CND, LT SYRUP PK, W/SKN, SOL&LIQUIDS	63	0.53	16.49	0.003
09031	APRICOTS, DEHYD (LOW-MOISTURE), SULFURED, STWD	126	1.93	32.62	0.017
09030	APRICOTS, DEHYD (LOW-MOISTURE), SULFURED, UNCKD	320	4.9	82.89	0.043
09034	APRICOTS, DRIED, SULFURED, STWD, W/ SUGAR	113	1.17	29.26	0.01
09033	APRICOTS, DRIED, SULFURED, STWD, WO/ SUGAR	85	1.3	21.9	0.011
09032	APRICOTS, DRIED, SULFURED, UNCKD	241	3.39	62.64	0.017
09035	APRICOTS, FROZEN, SWEETENED	98	0.7	25.1	0.007
09021	APRICOTS, RAW	48	1.4	11.12	0.027
18516	ARCHWAY HOME STYLE COOKIES, APPL FILLED OATMEAL	394	4.8	65.63	2.97
18517	ARCHWAY HOME STYLE COOKIES, APRICOT FILLED	401	5.06	64.79	5.45
18518	ARCHWAY HOME STYLE COOKIES, AUNT BEA'S POUND CAKE COOKI	402	5.17	60.66	3.85
18519	ARCHWAY HOME STYLE COOKIES, BLACK WALNUT ICE BOX	497	5.25	62	6
18520	ARCHWAY HOME STYLE COOKIES, CHERRY FILLED	401	5.04	64.65	5.44
18521	ARCHWAY HOME STYLE COOKIES, CHOC CHIP DROP	402	5.54	61.87	4.45
18522	ARCHWAY HOME STYLE COOKIES, CHOC CHIP ICE BOX	486	4.79	64.15	7.29

NDB #	Food Description (100 gram portions = 3½ ounces = 20 tsp = ½ cup approx.	Calories	Protein	Carbs	Sat Fat
18523	ARCHWAY HOME STYLE COOKIES, CINN APPL	408	4.99	66.12	3.34
18524	ARCHWAY HOME STYLE COOKIES, COCNT MACAROON	482	3.88	56.15	24.71
18525	ARCHWAY HOME STYLE COOKIES, COOKIES JAR HERMITS	380	5.2	66.5	2.7
18527	ARCHWAY HOME STYLE COOKIES, DATE FILLED OATMEAL	395	5.24	66.53	2.95
18526	ARCHWAY HOME STYLE COOKIES, DK MOLASSES	411	4.23	71.68	2.88
18528	ARCHWAY HOME STYLE COOKIES, DUTCH COCOA	410	4.5	68.8	3.48
18552	ARCHWAY HOME STYLE COOKIES, FAT FREE CINN HONEY HEARTS	352	4.61	82.27	0.21
18553	ARCHWAY HOME STYLE COOKIES, FAT FREE DEVIL'S FD COOKIE	338	4.82	79.27	0.32
18554	ARCHWAY HOME STYLE COOKIES, FAT FREE LEMON NUGGETS	358	4.22	84.14	0.19
18555	ARCHWAY HOME STYLE COOKIES, FAT FREE OATMEAL RAISIN	343	4.63	78.59	0.34
18556	ARCHWAY HOME STYLE COOKIES, FAT FREE OATMEAL RASPBERRY	351	4.63	80.42	0.34
18557	ARCHWAY HOME STYLE COOKIES, FAT FREE SUGAR COOKIES	354	4.4	82.9	0.26
18529	ARCHWAY HOME STYLE COOKIES, FROSTY LEMON	430	4.41	64.78	5.83
18530	ARCHWAY HOME STYLE COOKIES, FROSTY ORANGE	434	4.53	64.86	5.24
18531	ARCHWAY HOME STYLE COOKIES, FRUIT&HONEY BAR	398	4.69	67.33	3.01
18549	ARCHWAY HOME STYLE COOKIES, GOURMET APPLE'N RAISIN	425	5.43	65.68	3.54
18550	ARCHWAY HOME STYLE COOKIES, GOURMET CARROT CAKE	430	3.97	64.24	5.26
18551	ARCHWAY HOME STYLE COOKIES, GOURMET CHOC CHIP N' TOFFEE	468	4.4	64	6.36
18560	ARCHWAY HOME STYLE COOKIES, GOURMET OATMEAL PECAN	477	6.09	57.56	8.62
18561	ARCHWAY HOME STYLE COOKIES, GOURMET OL'FASHION PNUT BU	469	9.09	57.25	5.19
18563	ARCHWAY HOME STYLE COOKIES, GOURMET ROCKY ROAD	455	5.88	62.62	5.28
18564	ARCHWAY HOME STYLE COOKIES, GOURMET RUTH'S GOLDEN OAT	434	5.84	63.19	3.49
18558	ARCHWAY HOME STYLE COOKIES, ICED GINGER SNAPS	466	3.66	70.85	5.73
18532	ARCHWAY HOME STYLE COOKIES, ICED MOLASSES	407	3.72	69.9	4.1
18533	ARCHWAY HOME STYLE COOKIES, ICED OATMEAL	439	5.22	65.99	5.32
18534	ARCHWAY HOME STYLE COOKIES, LEMON DROP	389	5.15	61.66	3.35
18559	ARCHWAY HOME STYLE COOKIES, LEMON SNAPS	489	5.02	64.77	5.64
18535	ARCHWAY HOME STYLE COOKIES, MOLASSES	398	4.53	69.94	2.82
18536	ARCHWAY HOME STYLE COOKIES, MUD PIE	429	5.3	59.69	8.6
18537	ARCHWAY HOME STYLE COOKIES, OATMEAL	424	6.05	66.84	3.51
18538	ARCHWAY HOME STYLE COOKIES, OATMEAL RAISIN	410	5.7	67.24	3.15
18539	ARCHWAY HOME STYLE COOKIES, OLD FASHIONED MOLASSES	402	4.61	70.93	2.79
18540	ARCHWAY HOME STYLE COOKIES, OLD FASHIONED WINDMILL COO	455	5.52	70.97	3.7
18543	ARCHWAY HOME STYLE COOKIES, PECAN ICE BOX	500	4.49	62.05	5.71
18541	ARCHWAY HOME STYLE COOKIES, PNUT BUTTER	480	9	58.48	5.39

NDB #	Food Description (100 gram portions = 3½ ounces = 20 tsp = ½ cup approx.	Calories	Protein	Carbs	Sat Fat
18542	ARCHWAY HOME STYLE COOKIES, PNUT JUMBLE	484	9.09	55.6	6.83
18544	ARCHWAY HOME STYLE COOKIES, RASPBERRY FILLED	404	5.01	65.21	5.45
18562	ARCHWAY HOME STYLE COOKIES, RED FAT GINGER SNAPS	425	4.23	76.92	2.87
18545	ARCHWAY HOME STYLE COOKIES, RUTH'S OATMEAL	428	5.94	66.15	3.53
18546	ARCHWAY HOME STYLE COOKIES, SOFT SUGAR DROP	390	5.2	62.98	3.34
18547	ARCHWAY HOME STYLE COOKIES, STRAWBERRY FILLED	401	5.01	64.67	5.44
18548	ARCHWAY HOME STYLE COOKIES, SUGAR	410	5.13	68.98	3.17
18565	ARCHWAY HOME STYLE COOKIES, SUGAR FREE CHOC CHIP	448	4.51	66.87	6.23
18513	ARCHWAY HOME STYLE COOKIES, SUGAR FREE OATMEAL	442	5.54	67.2	4.9
18514	ARCHWAY HOME STYLE COOKIES, SUGAR FREE ROCKY ROAD	421	5.64	64.4	4.88
18515	ARCHWAY HOME STYLE COOKIES, SUGAR FREE SHORTBREAD	445	4.66	65.94	5.26
22692	ARMOUR CORNED BF HASH, CND ENTREE	211	10.1	5.1	6.63
11701	ARROWHEAD, CKD, BLD, DRND, W/SALT	78	4.49	16.14	
11006	ARROWHEAD, CKD, BLD, DRND, WO/SALT	78	4.49	16.14	
11005	ARROWHEAD, RAW	99	5.33	20.23	
20003	ARROWROOT FLOUR	357	0.3	88.15	0.019
11697	ARROWROOT, RAW	65	4.24	13.38	0.039
11702	ARTICHOKES, (GLOBE OR FRENCH), CKD, BLD, DRND, W/SALT	50	3.48	11.18	0.037
11008	ARTICHOKES, (GLOBE OR FRENCH), CKD, BLD, DRND, WO/SALT	50	3.48	11.18	0.037
11703	ARTICHOKES, (GLOBE OR FRENCH), FRZ, CKD, BLD, DRND, W/SALT	45	3.11	9.18	0.117
11010	ARTICHOKES, (GLOBE OR FRENCH), FRZ, CKD, BLD, DRND, WO/SAL	45	3.11	9.18	0.117
11009	ARTICHOKES, (GLOBE OR FRENCH), FRZ, UNPREP	38	2.63	7.76	0.099
11007	ARTICHOKES, (GLOBE OR FRENCH), RAW	47	3.27	10.51	0.035
18566	ARTIFICIAL BLUEBERRY MUFFIN MIX, DRY	407	4.7	77.45	1.865
11959	ARUGULA, RAW	25	2.58	3.65	0.086
11012	ASPARAGUS, CKD, BLD, DRND	24	2.59	4.23	0.071
11705	ASPARAGUS, CKD, BLD, DRND, W/SALT	24	2.59	4.23	0.071
11015	ASPARAGUS, CND, DRND SOL	19	2.14	2.48	0.147
11707	ASPARAGUS, CND, NO SALT, SOL&LIQUIDS	15	1.8	2.47	0.044
11013	ASPARAGUS, CND, REG PK, SOL&LIQUIDS	15	1.8	2.47	0.044
11709	ASPARAGUS, FRZ, CKD, BLD, DRND, W/SALT	28	2.95	4.87	0.095
11019	ASPARAGUS, FRZ, CKD, BLD, DRND, WO/SALT	28	2.95	4.87	0.095
11018	ASPARAGUS, FRZ, UNPREP	24	3.23	4.1	0.052
11011	ASPARAGUS, RAW	23	2.28	4.54	0.046
09037	AVOCADOS, RAW, ALL COMM VAR	161	1.98	7.39	2.437

NDB #	Food Description (100 gram portions = 3½ ounces = 20 tsp = ½ cup approx.	Calories	Protein	Carbs	Sat Fat
09038	AVOCADOS, RAW, CALIFORNIA	177	2.11	6.91	2.59
09039	AVOCADOS, RAW, FLORIDA	112	1.59	8.91	1.755
03167	BABYFOOD, APPLE-BANANA JUC	51	0.2	12.3	0.018
03169	BABYFOOD, APPLE-CRANBERRY JUC	47	0	11.4	0.007
03289	BABYFOOD, APPLS W/HAM, STR	62	2.6	10.9	0.25
03294	BABYFOOD, APPLS&TURKEY, STR	65	2.9	10.5	0.34
03115	BABYFOOD, APPLS, DICES, TODD	51	0.2	12.1	0.02
03290	BABYFOOD, CARROTS&BF, STR	59	3.4	5.7	0.96
03185	BABYFOOD, CEREAL, MIXED, DRY	379	12.2	73.3	0.769
03194	BABYFOOD, CEREAL, RICE, DRY	391	7.1	77.6	0.919
03222	BABYFOOD, CHERRY COBBLER, JR	78	0.3	19.2	0.02
03213	BABYFOOD, COOKIES	433	11.8	67.1	3.7
03214	BABYFOOD, COOKIES, ARROWROOT	442	7.6	71.2	3.33
03181	BABYFOOD, CRL, BARLEY, DRY	365	11.1	75.3	0.418
03681	BABYFOOD, CRL, BARLEY, PREP W/WHL MILK	111	4.6	16.3	
03201	BABYFOOD, CRL, EGG YOLKS&BACON, JR	79	2.5	6.2	1.64
03182	BABYFOOD, CRL, HI PROT, DRY	362	36	46.7	0.876
03682	BABYFOOD, CRL, HI PROT, PREP W/WHL MILK	111	8.7	11.6	
03211	BABYFOOD, CRL, HI PROT, W/APPL&ORANGE, DRY	374	25.4	57.6	0.96
03711	BABYFOOD, CRL, HI PROT, W/APPL&ORANGE, PREP W/WHL MILK	112	6.9	13.4	
03685	BABYFOOD, CRL, MXD, PREP W/WHL MILK	113	4.8	15.9	1.927
03188	BABYFOOD, CRL, MXD, W/APPLSAUC&BANANAS, JR	83	1.2	18.4	0.072
03187	BABYFOOD, CRL, MXD, W/APPLSAUC&BANANAS, STR	82	1.2	17.9	0.09
03186	BABYFOOD, CRL, MXD, W/BANANAS, DRY	391	10.7	77.1	0.846
03686	BABYFOOD, CRL, MXD, W/BANANAS, PREP W/WHL MILK	115	4.5	16.6	1.982
03704	BABYFOOD, CRL, MXD, W/HONEY, PREP W/WHL MILK	115	5	15.9	
03189	BABYFOOD, CRL, OATMEAL, DRY	398	13.6	69.2	1.353
03689	BABYFOOD, CRL, OATMEAL, PREP W/WHL MILK	116	5	15.3	2.258
03192	BABYFOOD, CRL, OATMEAL, W/APPLSAUC&BANANAS, JR	75	1.3	15.7	0.126
03191	BABYFOOD, CRL, OATMEAL, W/APPLSAUC&BANANAS, STR	73	1.3	15.4	0.125
03190	BABYFOOD, CRL, OATMEAL, W/BANANAS, DRY	393	12	73.4	1.267
03690	BABYFOOD, CRL, OATMEAL, W/BANANAS, PREP W/WHL MILK	116	4.7	16	
03193	BABYFOOD, CRL, OATMEAL, W/HONEY, DRY	391	13.5	69.3	
03693	BABYFOOD, CRL, OATMEAL, W/HONEY, PREP W/WHL MILK	115	5	15.3	
03694	BABYFOOD, CRL, RICE, PREP W/WHL MILK	115	3.9	16.7	2.325

NDB #	Food Description (100 gram portions = 3½ ounces = 20 tsp = ½ cup approx.	Calories	Protein	Carbs	Sat Fat
03195	BABYFOOD, CRL, RICE, W/APPLSAUC&BANANAS, STR	79	1.2	17.1	0.114
03212	BABYFOOD, CRL, RICE, W/BANANAS, DRY	404	8.7	79.9	0.978
03712	BABYFOOD, CRL, RICE, W/BANANAS, PREP W/WHL MILK	117	4.2	17	2.261
03696	BABYFOOD, CRL, RICE, W/HONEY, PREP W/WHL MILK	115	3.9	17.1	
03210	BABYFOOD, CRL, RICE, W/MXD FRUIT, JR	79	0.9	18.3	0.06
03198	BABYFOOD, CRL, W/EGG YOLKS, JR	52	1.9	7.1	0.61
03197	BABYFOOD, CRL, W/EGG YOLKS, STR	51	1.9	7	0.61
03199	BABYFOOD, CRL, W/EGGS, STR	58	2.2	8	0.49
03297	BABYFOOD, DINNER, APPLS&CHICK, STR	65	2.16	10.87	0.347
03043	BABYFOOD, DINNER, BF LASAGNA, TODD	77	4.2	10	
03287	BABYFOOD, DINNER, BF NOODLE, JR	57	2.5	7.4	0.766
03047	BABYFOOD, DINNER, BF NOODLE, STR	63	2.44	8.18	0.937
03052	BABYFOOD, DINNER, BF STEW, TODD	51	5.1	5.5	0.58
03049	BABYFOOD, DINNER, BF&RICE, TODD	82	5	8.8	
03298	BABYFOOD, DINNER, BROCCOLI&CHICK, STR	42	3.93	3.22	0.414
03069	BABYFOOD, DINNER, CHICK NOODLE, JR	55	2.37	8.79	0.338
03068	BABYFOOD, DINNER, CHICK NOODLE, STR	66	2.69	9.08	0.595
03070	BABYFOOD, DINNER, CHICK SOUP, STR	50	1.6	7.2	0.278
03072	BABYFOOD, DINNER, CHICK STEW, TODD	78	5.2	6.4	1.1
03284	BABYFOOD, DINNER, GRN BNS&TURKEY, STR	53	3.8	5.41	0.481
03090	BABYFOOD, DINNER, MACARONI&CHS, JR	61	2.6	8.2	1.175
03089	BABYFOOD, DINNER, MACARONI&CHS, STR	67	3.14	8.95	1.291
03045	BABYFOOD, DINNER, MACARONI&TOMATO&BF, JR	59	2.5	9.4	0.411
03044	BABYFOOD, DINNER, MACARONI&TOMATO&BF, STR	61	2.36	9.45	0.486
03279	BABYFOOD, DINNER, MXD VEG, JR	33	1	7.9	
03278	BABYFOOD, DINNER, MXD VEG, STR	41	1.2	9.5	
03077	BABYFOOD, DINNER, PASTA W/VEG	60	1.7	8.4	1.23
03050	BABYFOOD, DINNER, SPAGHETTI&TOMATO&MEAT, JR	68	2.57	11.42	0.543
03051	BABYFOOD, DINNER, SPAGHETTI&TOMATO&MEAT, TODD	75	5.3	10.8	
03303	BABYFOOD, DINNER, SWT POTATOES&CHICK, STR	74	2.51	11.04	0.572
03083	BABYFOOD, DINNER, TURKEY&RICE, JR	56	2.37	9.57	0.239
03082	BABYFOOD, DINNER, TURKEY&RICE, STR	52	2.27	7.94	0.338
03073	BABYFOOD, DINNER, VEG CHICK, STR	59	2.47	8.42	0.496
03060	BABYFOOD, DINNER, VEG&BACON, JR	71	1.8	7.6	1.4
03059	BABYFOOD, DINNER, VEG&BACON, STR	71	1.92	8.81	1.063

NDB #	Food Description (100 gram portions = 3½ ounces = 20 tsp = ½ cup approx.	Calories	Protein	Carbs	Sat Fat
03054	BABYFOOD, DINNER, VEG&BF, JR	62	2.3	9	0.683
03053	BABYFOOD, DINNER, VEG&BF, STR	63	2.59	7.7	1.029
03274	BABYFOOD, DINNER, VEG&CHICK, JR	53	2.04	8.66	0.302
03042	BABYFOOD, DINNER, VEG&DUMPLINGS&BF, JR	48	2.1	8	
03041	BABYFOOD, DINNER, VEG&DUMPLINGS&BF, STR	48	2	7.7	
03062	BABYFOOD, DINNER, VEG&HAM, JR	60	2.02	8.65	0.483
03061	BABYFOOD, DINNER, VEG&HAM, STR	59	2.19	7.8	0.764
03067	BABYFOOD, DINNER, VEG&LAMB, JR	51	2.1	7.1	0.696
03066	BABYFOOD, DINNER, VEG&LAMB, STR	52	2	6.9	0.828
03081	BABYFOOD, DINNER, VEG&NOODLES&TURKEY, JR	52	1.8	7.6	
03079	BABYFOOD, DINNER, VEG&NOODLES&TURKEY, STR	44	1.2	6.8	
03085	BABYFOOD, DINNER, VEG&TURKEY, JR	53	1.72	7.55	0.485
03084	BABYFOOD, DINNER, VEG&TURKEY, STR	48	2.32	7.62	0.236
03086	BABYFOOD, DINNER, VEG&TURKEY, TODD	80	4.8	8	
03076	BABYFOOD, DINNER, VEG, NOODLES&CHICK, JR	64	1.7	9.1	
03075	BABYFOOD, DINNER, VEG, NOODLES&CHICK, STR	63	2	7.9	
03285	BABYFOOD, DINNER, VEG, TURKEY, &BARLEY	53	2.5	8.3	0.313
03225	BABYFOOD, DSSRT, CHERRY VANILLA PUDD, JR	69	0.2	18.4	0.058
03224	BABYFOOD, DSSRT, CHERRY VANILLA PUDD, STR	68	0.2	17.8	0.087
03246	BABYFOOD, DSSRT, CUSTARD PUDD, VANILLA, JR	86	1.76	17.59	0.325
03245	BABYFOOD, DSSRT, CUSTARD PUDD, VANILLA, STR	85	1.6	16.1	1.01
03221	BABYFOOD, DSSRT, DUTCH APPL, JR	79	0.2	19.18	0.025
03220	BABYFOOD, DSSRT, DUTCH APPL, STR	68	0	16.7	0.58
03236	BABYFOOD, DSSRT, FRUIT DSSRT, WO/VIT C, JR	63	0.3	17.2	0
03235	BABYFOOD, DSSRT, FRUIT DSSRT, WO/VIT C, STR	59	0.3	16	0
03226	BABYFOOD, DSSRT, FRUIT PUDD, ORANGE, STR	80	1.1	17.7	0.545
03234	BABYFOOD, DSSRT, FRUIT PUDD, PNAPPL, JR	87	1.4	21.6	0.13
03233	BABYFOOD, DSSRT, FRUIT PUDD, PNAPPL, STR	81	1.3	20.3	0.099
03228	BABYFOOD, DSSRT, PEACH COBBLER, JR	67	0.3	18.3	0
03227	BABYFOOD, DSSRT, PEACH COBBLER, STR	65	0.3	17.8	0
03238	BABYFOOD, DSSRT, TROPICAL FRUIT, JR	60	0.2	16.4	
03154	BABYFOOD, FRUIT&VEG, APPL&SWT POTATO	63	0.3	15.3	0.041
03165	BABYFOOD, FRUIT, APPL&BLUEBERRY, JR	62	0.2	16.6	0.024
03164	BABYFOOD, FRUIT, APPL&BLUEBERRY, STR	61	0.2	16.3	0.024
03153	BABYFOOD, FRUIT, APPL&RASPBERRY, W/SUGAR, JR	58	0.2	15.5	0.032

NDB #	Food Description (100 gram portions = 3½ ounces = 20 tsp = ½ cup approx.	Calories	Protein	Carbs	Sat Fat
03152	BABYFOOD, FRUIT, APPL&RASPBERRY, W/SUGAR, STR	58	0.2	15.7	0.033
03147	BABYFOOD, FRUIT, APPLSAUC W/BANANA, JR	66	0.37	16.16	0.04
03143	BABYFOOD, FRUIT, APPLSAUC&APRICOTS, JR	47	0.2	12.4	0.028
03142	BABYFOOD, FRUIT, APPLSAUC&APRICOTS, STR	45	0.2	11.6	0.024
03145	BABYFOOD, FRUIT, APPLSAUC&CHERRIES, JR	56	0	14.1	0
03144	BABYFOOD, FRUIT, APPLSAUC&CHERRIES, STR	51	0	14.1	0
03151	BABYFOOD, FRUIT, APPLSAUC&PNAPPL, JR	39	0.1	10.5	0.011
03150	BABYFOOD, FRUIT, APPLSAUC&PNAPPL, STR	37	0.1	10.1	0.01
03117	BABYFOOD, FRUIT, APPLSAUC, JR	37	0	10.3	0
03116	BABYFOOD, FRUIT, APPLSAUC, STR	41	0.2	10.9	0.032
03128	BABYFOOD, FRUIT, APRICOT W/TAPIOCA, JR	63	0.3	17.3	0
03118	BABYFOOD, FRUIT, APRICOT W/TAPIOCA, STR	60	0.3	16.3	0
03280	BABYFOOD, FRUIT, BANANAS W/TAPIOCA, JR	67	0.4	17.8	0.076
03129	BABYFOOD, FRUIT, BANANAS W/TAPIOCA, STR	57	0.4	15.3	0.035
03156	BABYFOOD, FRUIT, BANANAS&PNAPPL W/TAPIOCA, JR	68	0.2	18.4	0.036
03157	BABYFOOD, FRUIT, BANANAS&PNAPPL W/TAPIOCA, STR	65	0.2	17.8	0
03138	BABYFOOD, FRUIT, GUAVA W/TAPIOCA, STR	67	0.3	18.3	
03160	BABYFOOD, FRUIT, GUAVA&PAPAYA W/TAPIOCA, STR	63	0.2	17	
03140	BABYFOOD, FRUIT, MANGO W/TAPIOCA, STR	80	0.3	21.6	0.049
03162	BABYFOOD, FRUIT, PAPAYA&APPLSAUC W/TAPIOCA, STR	70	0.2	18.9	
03131	BABYFOOD, FRUIT, PEACHES W/SUGAR, JR	71	0.5	18.9	0.02
03130	BABYFOOD, FRUIT, PEACHES W/SUGAR, STR	71	0.5	18.9	0.02
03159	BABYFOOD, FRUIT, PEARS&PNAPPL, JR	44	0.3	11.4	0.013
03158	BABYFOOD, FRUIT, PEARS&PNAPPL, STR	41	0.3	10.9	0.007
03133	BABYFOOD, FRUIT, PEARS, JR	43	0.3	11.6	0.006
03132	BABYFOOD, FRUIT, PEARS, STR	41	0.3	10.8	0.012
03135	BABYFOOD, FRUIT, PLUMS W/TAPIOCA, WO/VIT C, JR	74	0.1	20.4	0
03134	BABYFOOD, FRUIT, PLUMS W/TAPIOCA, WO/VIT C, STR	71	0.1	19.7	0
03137	BABYFOOD, FRUIT, PRUNES W/TAPIOCA, WO/VIT C, JR	70	0.6	18.7	0.008
03136	BABYFOOD, FRUIT, PRUNES W/TAPIOCA, WO/VIT C, STR	70	0.6	18.5	0.008
03093	BABYFOOD, GRN BNS, DICES, TODD	29	1.2	5.7	0.044
03266	BABYFOOD, JUC, APPL GRAPE, W/CA	52	0.2	12.7	0.019
03268	BABYFOOD, JUC, APPL&CHERRY	41	0.1	9.9	0.035
03265	BABYFOOD, JUC, APPL&GRAPE	46	0.1	11.4	0.04
03168	BABYFOOD, JUC, APPL&PEACH	42	0.2	10.5	0.018

NDB #	Food Description (100 gram portions = 3½ ounces = 20 tsp = ½ cup approx.	Calories	Protein	Carbs	Sat Fat
03170	BABYFOOD, JUC, APPL&PLUM	49	0.1	12.3	0
03171	BABYFOOD, JUC, APPL&PRUNE	73	0.2	18	0.018
03267	BABYFOOD, JUC, FRUIT PUNCH, W/CA	52	0.2	12.7	0.02
03179	BABYFOOD, JUC, MXD FRUIT	47	0.1	11.6	0.015
03173	BABYFOOD, JUC, ORANGE&APPL	43	0.4	10.1	
03174	BABYFOOD, JUC, ORANGE&APPL&BANANA	47	0.4	11.5	0.016
03175	BABYFOOD, JUC, ORANGE&APRICOT	46	0.8	10.9	0.011
03176	BABYFOOD, JUC, ORANGE&BANANA	50	0.7	11.9	
03177	BABYFOOD, JUC, ORANGE&PNAPPL	48	0.5	11.7	0.01
03178	BABYFOOD, JUC, PRUNE&ORANGE	70	0.6	16.8	
03166	BABYFOOD, JUICE, APPLE	47	0	11.7	0.018
03172	BABYFOOD, JUICE, ORANGE	44	0.6	10.2	0.035
03003	BABYFOOD, MEAT, BEEF, JUNIOR	106	14.5	0	2.59
03002	BABYFOOD, MEAT, BF, STR	107	13.6	0	2.58
03014	BABYFOOD, MEAT, CHICK STKS, JR	188	14.6	1.4	4.094
03013	BABYFOOD, MEAT, CHICK, JR	149	14.7	0	2.47
03012	BABYFOOD, MEAT, CHICK, STR	130	13.7	0.1	2.03
03009	BABYFOOD, MEAT, HAM, JUNIOR	125	15.1	0	2.24
03008	BABYFOOD, MEAT, HAM, STR	111	13.9	0	1.94
03011	BABYFOOD, MEAT, LAMB, JUNIOR	112	15.2	0	2.56
03010	BABYFOOD, MEAT, LAMB, STR	103	14.1	0.1	2.31
03021	BABYFOOD, MEAT, MEAT STKS, JR	184	13.4	1.1	5.82
03007	BABYFOOD, MEAT, PORK, STR	124	14	0	2.4
03017	BABYFOOD, MEAT, TURKEY STKS, JR	182	13.7	1.4	4.143
03016	BABYFOOD, MEAT, TURKEY, JR	129	15.4	0	2.31
03015	BABYFOOD, MEAT, TURKEY, STR	114	14.3	0.1	1.91
03006	BABYFOOD, MEAT, VEAL, JUNIOR	110	15.3	0	2.39
03005	BABYFOOD, MEAT, VEAL, STR	101	13.5	0	2.29
03205	BABYFOOD, OATMEAL CRL W/FRUIT, DRY, INST, TODD	402	10.5	74.15	1.572
03161	BABYFOOD, PEACHES, DICES, TODD	51	0.5	11.8	0.016
03141	BABYFOOD, PEARS, DICES, TODD	57	0.3	13.6	0.01
03122	BABYFOOD, PEAS, DICES, TODD	64	3.9	10.3	0.14
03112	BABYFOOD, POTATOES, TODDLER	51	1	11.8	0.015
03215	BABYFOOD, PRETZELS	397	10.8	82.2	0.316
03216	BABYFOOD, TEETHING BISCUITS	392	10.7	76.4	1.534

NDB #	Food Description (100 gram portions = 3½ ounces = 20 tsp = ½ cup approx.	Calories	Protein	Carbs	Sat Fat
03296	BABYFOOD, TURKEY, RICE&VEG, TODD	59	3.8	7.5	0.5
03098	BABYFOOD, VEG, BEETS, STR	34	1.3	7.7	0.016
03114	BABYFOOD, VEG, BUTTERNUT SQUASH&CORN	50	2	9.3	0.095
03100	BABYFOOD, VEG, CARROTS, JR	32	0.8	7.2	0.036
03099	BABYFOOD, VEG, CARROTS, STR	27	0.8	6	0.018
03120	BABYFOOD, VEG, CORN, CRMD, JR	65	1.4	16.3	0.074
03119	BABYFOOD, VEG, CORN, CRMD, STR	57	1.4	14.1	0.076
03283	BABYFOOD, VEG, GARDEN VEG, STR	37	2.3	6.8	0.035
03096	BABYFOOD, VEG, GRN BNS&POTATOES	63	2.2	9.3	1.117
03097	BABYFOOD, VEG, GRN BNS, CRMD, JR	32	1	7.2	0.072
03092	BABYFOOD, VEG, GRN BNS, JR	25	1.2	5.7	0.023
03091	BABYFOOD, VEG, GRN BNS, STR	25	1.3	5.9	0.023
03282	BABYFOOD, VEG, MIX VEG JR	41	1.4	8.2	0.079
03286	BABYFOOD, VEG, MIX VEG STR	41	1.2	8	0.089
03125	BABYFOOD, VEG, PEAS, CRMD, STR	53	2.2	8.9	0.42
03121	BABYFOOD, VEG, PEAS, STR	40	3.5	8.1	0.054
03127	BABYFOOD, VEG, SPINACH, CRMD, STR	37	2.5	5.7	0.702
03105	BABYFOOD, VEG, SQUASH, JR	24	0.8	5.6	0.041
03104	BABYFOOD, VEG, SQUASH, STR	24	0.8	5.6	0.041
03109	BABYFOOD, VEG, SWT POTATOES, JR	60	1.1	13.9	0.021
03108	BABYFOOD, VEG, SWT POTATOES, STR	57	1.1	13.2	0.021
07921	BACON & BF STKS	520	29.1	0.8	16
16104	BACON, MEATLESS	310	10.68	6.33	4.622
18005	BAGELS, CINNAMON-RAISIN	274	9.8	55.2	0.274
18006	BAGELS, CINNAMON-RAISIN, TSTD	294	10.6	59.3	0.295
18003	BAGELS, EGG	278	10.6	53	0.421
18007	BAGELS, OAT BRAN	255	10.7	53.3	0.191
18001	BAGELS, PLN, ENR, W/CA PROP (INCL ONION, POPPY, SESAME)	275	10.5	53.4	0.22
18406	BAGELS, PLN, ENR, WO/CA PROP (INCL ONION, POPPY, SESAME)	275	10.5	53.4	0.22
18002	BAGELS, PLN, TSTD, ENR, W/CA PROP (INCL ONION, POPPY, SESAME	295	11.3	57.5	0.236
18407	BAGELS, PLN, UNENR, W/CA PROP (INCL ONION, POPPY, SESAME)	275	10.5	53.4	0.22
18408	BAGELS, PLN, UNENR, WO/CA PROP (INCL ONION, POPPY, SESAME)	275	10.5	53.4	0.22
19146	BAKING CHOC, M&M MARS, "M&M'S"MILK CHOC MINI BAKING BITS	498	4.78	67.3	14.452
19139	BAKING CHOC, M&M MARS, "M&M'S"SEMISWEET CHOC MINI BAKING	518	4.42	65.96	15.655
19124	BAKING CHOC, MEXICAN, SQUARES	426	3.64	77.41	8.606

NDB #	Food Description (100 gram portions = 3½ ounces = 20 tsp = ½ cup approx.	Calories	Protein	Carbs	Sat Fat
19077	BAKING CHOC, UNSWTND, LIQ	472	12.1	33.9	25.29
19078	BAKING CHOC, UNSWTND, SQUARES	522	10.3	28.3	32.6
11710	BALSAM-PEAR (BITTER GOURD), LEAFY TIPS, CKD, BLD, DRND, W/S	35	3.6	6.78	
11023	BALSAM-PEAR (BITTER GOURD), LEAFY TIPS, CKD, BLD, DRND, WO/	35	3.6	6.78	0.032
11022	BALSAM-PEAR (BITTER GOURD), LEAFY TIPS, RAW	30	5.3	3.29	
11711	BALSAM-PEAR (BITTER GOURD), PODS, CKD, BLD, DRND, W/SALT	19	0.84	4.32	
11025	BALSAM-PEAR (BITTER GOURD), PODS, CKD, BLD, DRND, WO/SALT	19	0.84	4.32	0.014
11024	BALSAM-PEAR (BITTER GOURD), PODS, RAW	17	1	3.7	
11712	BAMBOO SHOOTS, CKD, BLD, DRND, W/SALT	12	1.53	1.92	0.051
11027	BAMBOO SHOOTS, CKD, BLD, DRND, WO/SALT	12	1.53	1.92	0.051
11028	BAMBOO SHOOTS, CND, DRND SOL	19	1.72	3.22	0.092
11026	BAMBOO SHOOTS, RAW	27	2.6	5.2	0.069
19400	BANANA CHIPS	519	2.3	58.4	28.97
09041	BANANAS, DEHYD, OR BANANA PDR	346	3.89	88.28	0.698
09040	BANANAS, RAW	92	1.03	23.43	0.185
22525	BANQUET CHICK POT PIE, FRZ ENTREE	193	5	18.16	4.5
22675	BANQUET EX HELP MT LOAF DIN, TOM SAU, MSH POT&CAR W/SAU, F	135	6.42	7.41	3.42
22689	BANQUET EX HELP SALSBRY STK DIN, GRVY, MSH POT&CORN, SAU,	167	5.78	10.06	4.56
22711	BANQUET SALISBURY STK ML, GRVY, SALSBRY STK, MSH POT, COR	148	5.7	10.3	3.17
22691	BANQUET SLICED BF MEAL, W/GRAVY, MSHD POT&PEAS W/SAU, FR	106	10.35	7.37	1.7
22607	BANQUET TURKEY&GRAVY W/DRSNG MEAL, MSHD POT&CORN W/S	107	5.34	12.97	0.97
22605	BANQUET VEAL PARMIGIANA ML, TOM SAU, MSHD POT&PEAS&SAU,	142	4.95	13.66	2.43
22571	BANQUET, OUR ORIGINAL FRIED CHICK MEAL, MSHD POT, CORN, FR	206	9.41	15.39	4.06
07001	BARBECUE LOAF, PORK, BEEF	173	15.84	6.4	3.17
22575	BARBER FOODS CHICK CORDON BLEU, FILLED W/CHS&HAM, FRZ E	205	15.2	8.7	3.39
20004	BARLEY	354	12.48	73.48	0.482
20130	BARLEY FLOUR OR MEAL	345	10.5	74.52	0.335
20131	BARLEY MALT FLOUR	361	10.28	78.3	0.386
20006	BARLEY, PEARLED, COOKED	123	2.26	28.22	0.093
20005	BARLEY, PEARLED, RAW	352	9.91	77.72	0.244
02044	BASIL, FRESH	27	2.54	4.34	0.041
15187	BASS, FRESHWATER, MXD SP, CKD, DRY HEAT	146	24.18	0	1.001
15003	BASS, FRSH H2O, MXD SP, RAW	114	18.86	0	0.78
15188	BASS, STRIPED, CKD, DRY HEAT	124	22.73	0	0.65
15004	BASS, STRIPED, RAW	97	17.73	0	0.507

NDB #	Food Description (100 gram portions = 3½ ounces = 20 tsp = ½ cup approx.	Calories	Protein	Carbs	Sat Fat
16302	BEANS, ADZUKI, MATURE SD, CKD, BLD, W/SALT	128	7.52	24.77	0.036
16002	BEANS, ADZUKI, MATURE SEEDS, CKD, BLD, WO/SALT	128	7.52	24.77	0.036
16003	BEANS, ADZUKI, MATURE SEEDS, CND, SWTND	237	3.8	55.01	0.011
16001	BEANS, ADZUKI, MATURE SEEDS, RAW	329	19.87	62.9	0.191
16004	BEANS, ADZUKI, YOKAN, MATURE SEEDS	260	3.29	60.72	0.043
16005	BEANS, BAKED, HOME PREPARED	151	5.54	21.39	1.948
16006	BEANS, BKD, CND, PLN OR VEGETARIAN	93	4.79	20.51	0.116
16007	BEANS, BKD, CND, W/BF	121	6.38	16.91	1.677
16008	BEANS, BKD, CND, W/FRANKS	142	6.75	15.39	2.352
16009	BEANS, BKD, CND, W/PORK	106	5.19	19.98	0.599
16010	BEANS, BKD, CND, W/PORK&SWT SAU	111	5.31	20.99	0.563
16011	BEANS, BKD, CND, W/PORK&TOMATO SAU	98	5.16	19.39	0.395
16317	BEANS, BLACK TURTLE SOUP, MATURE SEEDS, CKD, BLD, W/SALT	130	8.18	24.35	0.089
16017	BEANS, BLACK TURTLE SOUP, MATURE SEEDS, CKD, BLD, WO/SALT	130	8.18	24.35	0.089
16018	BEANS, BLACK TURTLE SOUP, MATURE SEEDS, CND	91	6.03	16.56	0.075
16016	BEANS, BLACK TURTLE SOUP, MATURE SEEDS, RAW	339	21.25	63.25	0.232
16315	BEANS, BLACK, MATURE SEEDS, CKD, BLD, W/SALT	132	8.86	23.71	0.139
16015	BEANS, BLACK, MATURE SEEDS, CKD, BLD, WO/SALT	132	8.86	23.71	0.139
16014	BEANS, BLACK, MATURE SEEDS, RAW	341	21.6	62.37	0.366
16320	BEANS, CRANBERRY (ROMAN), MATURE SEEDS, CKD, BLD, W/SALT	136	9.34	24.46	0.119
16020	BEANS, CRANBERRY (ROMAN), MATURE SEEDS, CKD, BLD, WO/SALT	136	9.34	24.46	0.119
16021	BEANS, CRANBERRY (ROMAN), MATURE SEEDS, CND	83	5.54	15.12	0.072
16019	BEANS, CRANBERRY (ROMAN), MATURE SEEDS, RAW	335	23.03	60.05	0.316
11973	BEANS, FAVA, IN POD, RAW	88	7.92	17.62	0.118
16323	BEANS, FRENCH, MATURE SEEDS, CKD, BLD, W/SALT	129	7.05	24.02	0.083
16023	BEANS, FRENCH, MATURE SEEDS, CKD, BLD, WO/SALT	129	7.05	24.02	0.083
16022	BEANS, FRENCH, MATURE SEEDS, RAW	343	18.81	64.11	0.221
16325	BEANS, GREAT NORTHERN, MATURE SEEDS, CKD, BLD, W/SALT	118	8.33	21.09	0.14
16025	BEANS, GREAT NORTHERN, MATURE SEEDS, CKD, BLD, WO/SALT	118	8.33	21.09	0.14
16026	BEANS, GREAT NORTHERN, MATURE SEEDS, CND	114	7.37	21.03	0.12
16024	BEANS, GREAT NORTHERN, MATURE SEEDS, RAW	339	21.86	62.37	0.356
16328	BEANS, KIDNEY, ALL TYPES, MATURE SEEDS, CKD, BLD, W/SALT	127	8.67	22.81	0.072
16028	BEANS, KIDNEY, ALL TYPES, MATURE SEEDS, CKD, BLD, WO/SALT	127	8.67	22.81	0.072
16029	BEANS, KIDNEY, ALL TYPES, MATURE SEEDS, CND	81	5.2	14.88	0.045
16027	BEANS, KIDNEY, ALL TYPES, MATURE SEEDS, RAW	333	23.58	60.01	0.12

NDB #	Food Description (100 gram portions = 3½ ounces = 20 tsp = ½ cup approx.	Calories	Protein	Carbs	Sat Fat
16331	BEANS, KIDNEY, CALIFORNIA RED, MATURE SEEDS, CKD, BLD, W/SA	124	9.13	22.41	0.014
16031	BEANS, KIDNEY, CALIFORNIA RED, MATURE SEEDS, CKD, BLD, WO/S	124	9.13	22.41	0.014
16030	BEANS, KIDNEY, CALIFORNIA RED, MATURE SEEDS, RAW	330	24.37	59.8	0.036
11713	BEANS, KIDNEY, MATURE SEEDS, SPROUTED, CKD, BLD, DRND, W/S	33	4.83	4.72	0.083
11030	BEANS, KIDNEY, MATURE SEEDS, SPROUTED, CKD, BLD, DRND, WO/	33	4.83	4.72	0.083
11029	BEANS, KIDNEY, MATURE SEEDS, SPROUTED, RAW	29	4.2	4.1	0.072
16333	BEANS, KIDNEY, RED, MATURE SEEDS, CKD, BLD, W/SALT	127	8.67	22.81	0.072
16033	BEANS, KIDNEY, RED, MATURE SEEDS, CKD, BLD, WO/SALT	127	8.67	22.81	0.072
16034	BEANS, KIDNEY, RED, MATURE SEEDS, CND	85	5.25	15.6	0.05
16032	BEANS, KIDNEY, RED, MATURE SEEDS, RAW	337	22.53	61.3	0.154
16336	BEANS, KIDNEY, ROYAL RED, MATURE SEEDS, CKD, BLD W/SALT	123	9.49	21.85	0.024
16036	BEANS, KIDNEY, ROYAL RED, MATURE SEEDS, CKD, BLD, WO/SALT	123	9.49	21.85	0.024
16035	BEANS, KIDNEY, ROYAL RED, MATURE SEEDS, RAW	329	25.33	58.33	0.065
11033	BEANS, LIMA, IMMAT SEEDS, CND, REG PK, SOL&LIQUIDS	71	4.07	13.33	0.066
11626	BEANS, MUNG, MATURE SEEDS, SPROUTED, CND, DRND SOL	12	1.4	2.15	0.016
16338	BEANS, NAVY, MATURE SEEDS, CKD, BLD, W/SALT	142	8.7	26.31	0.148
16038	BEANS, NAVY, MATURE SEEDS, CKD, BLD, WO/SALT	142	8.7	26.31	0.148
16039	BEANS, NAVY, MATURE SEEDS, CND	113	7.53	20.45	0.112
16037	BEANS, NAVY, MATURE SEEDS, RAW	335	22.33	60.65	0.331
11719	BEANS, NAVY, MATURE SEEDS, SPROUTED, CKD, BLD, DRND, W/SAL	78	7.07	15.01	0.098
11047	BEANS, NAVY, MATURE SEEDS, SPROUTED, CKD, BLD, DRND, WO/S	78	7.07	15.01	0.098
11046	BEANS, NAVY, MATURE SEEDS, SPROUTED, RAW	67	6.15	13.05	0.085
16341	BEANS, PINK, MATURE SEEDS, CKD, BLD, W/SALT	149	9.06	27.91	0.126
16041	BEANS, PINK, MATURE SEEDS, CKD, BLD, WO/SALT	149	9.06	27.91	0.126
16040	BEANS, PINK, MATURE SEEDS, RAW	343	20.96	64.19	0.292
11720	BEANS, PINTO, IMMAT SEEDS, FRZ, CKD, BLD, DRND, W/SALT	162	9.31	30.88	0.058
11049	BEANS, PINTO, IMMAT SEEDS, FRZ, CKD, BLD, DRND, WO/SALT	162	9.31	30.88	0.058
11048	BEANS, PINTO, IMMAT SEEDS, FRZ, UNPREP	170	9.8	32.5	0.061
16343	BEANS, PINTO, MATURE SEEDS, CKD, BLD, W/SALT	137	8.21	25.65	0.109
16043	BEANS, PINTO, MATURE SEEDS, CKD, BLD, WO/SALT	137	8.21	25.65	0.109
16044	BEANS, PINTO, MATURE SEEDS, CND	86	4.86	15.25	0.167
16042	BEANS, PINTO, MATURE SEEDS, RAW	340	20.88	63.41	0.235
11721	BEANS, PINTO, MATURE SEEDS, SPROUTED, CKD, BLD, DRND, W/SA	22	1.86	4.1	0.039
11654	BEANS, PINTO, MATURE SEEDS, SPROUTED, CKD, BLD, DRND, WO/S	22	1.86	4.1	0.039
11653	BEANS, PINTO, MATURE SEEDS, SPROUTED, RAW	62	5.25	11.6	0.109

NDB #	Food Description (100 gram portions = 3½ ounces = 20 tsp = ½ cup approx.	Calories	Protein	Carbs	Sat Fat
11050	BEANS, SHELL, CND, SOL&LIQUIDS	30	1.76	6.19	0.023
16346	BEANS, SML WHITE, MATURE SEEDS, CKD, BLD, W/SALT	142	8.97	25.81	0.166
16046	BEANS, SML WHITE, MATURE SEEDS, CKD, BLD, WO/SALT	142	8.97	25.81	0.166
16045	BEANS, SML WHITE, MATURE SEEDS, RAW	336	21.11	62.25	0.304
11058	BEANS, SNAP, CND, ALL STYLES, SEASONED, SOL&LIQUIDS	16	0.83	3.49	0.045
11052	BEANS, SNAP, GREEN, RAW	31	1.82	7.14	0.026
11054	BEANS, SNAP, GRN VAR, CND, REG PK, SOL&LIQUIDS	15	0.8	3.5	0.023
11723	BEANS, SNAP, GRN, CKD, BLD, DRND, W/SALT	35	1.89	7.89	0.064
11053	BEANS, SNAP, GRN, CKD, BLD, DRND, WO/SALT	35	1.89	7.89	0.064
11729	BEANS, SNAP, GRN, CND, NO SALT, DRND SOL	20	1.15	4.5	0.022
11726	BEANS, SNAP, GRN, CND, NO SALT, SOL&LIQUIDS	15	0.8	3.5	0.023
11056	BEANS, SNAP, GRN, CND, REG PK, DRND SOL	20	1.15	4.5	0.022
11060	BEANS, SNAP, GRN, FRZ, ALL STYLES, UNPREP	33	1.8	7.57	0.047
11061	BEANS, SNAP, GRN, FRZ, CKD, BLD, DRND WO/SALT	28	1.49	6.45	0.044
11731	BEANS, SNAP, GRN, FRZ, CKD, BLD, DRND, W/SALT	28	1.49	6.45	0.044
11725	BEANS, SNAP, YEL, CKD, BLD, DRND, W/SALT	35	1.89	7.89	0.064
11724	BEANS, SNAP, YEL, CKD, BLD, DRND, WO/SALT	35	1.89	7.89	0.064
11933	BEANS, SNAP, YEL, CND, NO SALT, DRND SOL	20	1.15	4.5	0.022
11728	BEANS, SNAP, YEL, CND, NO SALT, SOL&LIQUIDS	15	0.8	3.5	0.023
11932	BEANS, SNAP, YEL, CND, REG PK, DRND SOL	20	1.15	4.5	0.022
11727	BEANS, SNAP, YEL, CND, REG PK, SOL&LIQUIDS	15	0.8	3.5	0.023
11730	BEANS, SNAP, YEL, FRZ, ALL STYLES, UNPREP	33	1.8	7.57	0.047
11733	BEANS, SNAP, YEL, FRZ, CKD, BLD, DRND, W/SALT	28	1.49	6.45	0.044
11732	BEANS, SNAP, YEL, FRZ, CKD, BLD, DRND, WO/SALT	28	1.49	6.45	0.044
11722	BEANS, SNAP, YELLOW, RAW	31	1.82	7.14	0.026
16350	BEANS, WHITE, MATURE SEEDS, CKD, BLD, W/SALT	139	9.73	25.1	0.091
16050	BEANS, WHITE, MATURE SEEDS, CKD, BLD, WO/SALT	139	9.73	25.1	0.091
16051	BEANS, WHITE, MATURE SEEDS, CND	117	7.26	21.94	0.074
16049	BEANS, WHITE, MATURE SEEDS, RAW	333	23.36	60.27	0.219
16136	BEANS, WINGED, MATURE SEEDS, CKD, BLD, WO/SALT	147	10.62	14.94	0.825
16348	BEANS, YEL, MATURE SEEDS, CKD, BLD, W/SALT	144	9.16	25.27	0.279
16048	BEANS, YEL, MATURE SEEDS, CKD, BLD, WO/SALT	144	9.16	25.27	0.279
16047	BEANS, YEL, MATURE SEEDS, RAW	345	22	60.7	0.671
12077	BEECHNUTS, DRIED	576	6.2	33.5	5.719
13204	BEEF RND TIP RND LN ONLY TO 1/4" FAT SEL CKD RSTD	180	28.71	0	2.24

NDB #	Food Description (100 gram portions = 3½ ounces = 20 tsp = ½ cup approx.	Calories	Protein	Carbs	Sat Fat
14114	BEEF BROTH&TOMATO JUC, CND	37	0.6	8.5	0.032
19002	BEEF JERKY, CHOPD&FORMED	410	33.2	11	10.85
22529	BEEF POT PIE, FRZ ENTREE	227	6.7	22.3	4.3
22905	BEEF STEW, CANNED ENTREE	94	4.94	6.77	2.22
13462	BEEF, LOIN, PRTRHS STEAK, LN & FAT, 1/4" FAT, USDA SEL, CKD, BR	311	23.47	0	9.463
13369	BEEF, BRISKET, FLAT HALF, LN&FAT, 0"FAT, ALL GRDS, CKD, BRSD	215	30.48	0	3.35
13026	BEEF, BRISKET, FLAT HALF, LN&FAT, 1/4"FAT, ALL GRDS, CKD, BRSD	364	25.05	0	11.02
13025	BEEF, BRISKET, FLAT HALF, LN&FAT, 1/4"FAT, ALL GRDS, RAW	290	17.88	0	9.4
13806	BEEF, BRISKET, FLAT HALF, LN&FAT, 1/8"FAT, ALL GRDS, CKD, BRSD	309	27.55	0	7.98
13805	BEEF, BRISKET, FLAT HALF, LN&FAT, 1/8"FAT, ALL GRDS, RAW	235	19.25	0	6.55
13370	BEEF, BRISKET, FLAT HALF, LN, 0"FAT, ALL GRDS, CKD, BRSD	191	31.52	0	2.03
13028	BEEF, BRISKET, FLAT HALF, LN, 1/4"FAT, ALL GRDS, CKD, BRSD	222	31.52	0	3.17
13027	BEEF, BRISKET, FLAT HALF, LN, 1/4"FAT, ALL GRDS, RAW	148	21.45	0	1.99
13371	BEEF, BRISKET, POINT HALF, LN&FAT, 0"FAT, ALL GRDS, CKD, BRSD	358	23.53	0	11.24
13030	BEEF, BRISKET, POINT HALF, LN&FAT, 1/4"FAT, ALL GRDS, CKD, BRS	404	22.13	0	13.58
13029	BEEF, BRISKET, POINT HALF, LN&FAT, 1/4"FAT, ALL GRDS, RAW	331	16.12	0	11.84
13808	BEEF, BRISKET, POINT HALF, LN&FAT, 1/8"FAT, ALL GRDS, CKD, BRS	349	24.4	0	10.64
13807	BEEF, BRISKET, POINT HALF, LN&FAT, 1/8"FAT, ALL GRDS, RAW	265	17.65	0	8.42
13372	BEEF, BRISKET, POINT HALF, LN, 0"FAT, ALL GRDS, CKD, BRSD	244	28.05	0	5.18
13032	BEEF, BRISKET, POINT HALF, LN, 1/4"FAT, ALL GRDS, CKD, BRSD	261	28.05	0	5.89
13031	BEEF, BRISKET, POINT HALF, LN, 1/4"FAT, ALL GRDS, RAW	162	20.01	0	3.17
13367	BEEF, BRISKET, WHL, LN&FAT, 0"FAT, ALL GRDS, CKD, BRSD	291	26.79	0	7.53
13022	BEEF, BRISKET, WHL, LN&FAT, 1/4"FAT, ALL GRDS, CKD, BRSD	385	23.5	0	12.38
13021	BEEF, BRISKET, WHL, LN&FAT, 1/4"FAT, ALL GRDS, RAW	312	16.94	0	10.69
13804	BEEF, BRISKET, WHL, LN&FAT, 1/8"FAT, ALL GRDS, CKD, BRSD	331	25.85	0	9.44
13803	BEEF, BRISKET, WHL, LN&FAT, 1/8"FAT, ALL GRDS, RAW	251	18.42	0	7.53
13368	BEEF, BRISKET, WHL, LN, 0"FAT, ALL GRDS, CKD, BRSD	218	29.75	0	3.63
13024	BEEF, BRISKET, WHL, LN, 1/4"FAT, ALL GRDS, CKD, BRSD	242	29.75	0	4.56
13023	BEEF, BRISKET, WHL, LN, ALL GRDS, RAW	155	20.72	0	2.59
23543	BEEF, BTTM SIRLOIN, TRI-TIP RST, LN & FAT, 1/4" FAT, ALL GRDS, RA	165	20.43	0	3.185
13985	BEEF, BTTM SIRLOIN, TRI-TIP RST, LN, 0" FAT, ALL GRDS, CKD, RSTD	208	28.24	0	3.52
13987	BEEF, BTTM SIRLOIN, TRI-TIP STEAK, LN, 0" FAT, ALL GRDS, CKD, BRL	250	30.68	0	4.87
23546	BEEF, BTTM SIRLOIN, TRI-TIP STK, LN & FAT, 1/4" FAT, ALL GRDS, RA	199	20.78	0	4.668
13001	BEEF, CARCASS, LN&FAT, CHOIC, RAW	291	17.32	0	9.75
13002	BEEF, CARCASS, LN&FAT, SEL, RAW	278	17.48	0	9.16

NDB #	Food Description (100 gram portions = 3½ ounces = 20 tsp = ½ cup approx.	Calories	Protein	Carbs	Sat Fat
13033	BEEF, CHUCK, ARM POT RST, LN & FAT, 1/4" FAT, ALL GRDS, RAW	245	18.52	0	7.44
13373	BEEF, CHUCK, ARM POT RST, LN&FAT, 0"FAT, ALL GRDS, CKD, BRSD	280	29.66	0	6.62
13374	BEEF, CHUCK, ARM POT RST, LN&FAT, 0"FAT, CHOIC, CKD, BRSD	293	29.44	0	7.21
13375	BEEF, CHUCK, ARM POT RST, LN&FAT, 0"FAT, SEL, CKD, BRSD	260	30.11	0	5.69
13540	BEEF, CHUCK, ARM POT RST, LN&FAT, 1/2"FAT, PRIME, CKD, BRSD	391	26.11	0	12.69
13539	BEEF, CHUCK, ARM POT RST, LN&FAT, 1/2"FAT, PRIME, RAW	294	17.75	0	10.31
13034	BEEF, CHUCK, ARM POT RST, LN&FAT, 1/4"FAT, ALL GRDS, CKD, BRS	332	27.43	0	9.38
13036	BEEF, CHUCK, ARM POT RST, LN&FAT, 1/4"FAT, CHOIC, CKD, BRSD	348	26.98	0	10.16
13035	BEEF, CHUCK, ARM POT RST, LN&FAT, 1/4"FAT, CHOIC, RAW	255	18.39	0	7.92
13038	BEEF, CHUCK, ARM POT RST, LN&FAT, 1/4"FAT, SEL, CKD, BRSD	315	27.87	0	8.57
13037	BEEF, CHUCK, ARM POT RST, LN&FAT, 1/4"FAT, SEL, RAW	234	18.65	0	6.93
13810	BEEF, CHUCK, ARM POT RST, LN&FAT, 1/8"FAT, ALL GRDS, CKD, BRS	309	28.54	0	8.11
13809	BEEF, CHUCK, ARM POT RST, LN&FAT, 1/8"FAT, ALL GRDS, RAW	234	18.78	0	6.88
13812	BEEF, CHUCK, ARM POT RST, LN&FAT, 1/8"FAT, CHOIC, CKD, BRSD	323	28.19	0	8.8
13811	BEEF, CHUCK, ARM POT RST, LN&FAT, 1/8"FAT, CHOIC, RAW	244	18.65	0	7.36
13814	BEEF, CHUCK, ARM POT RST, LN&FAT, 1/8"FAT, SEL, CKD, BRSD	291	28.99	0	7.27
13813	BEEF, CHUCK, ARM POT RST, LN&FAT, 1/8"FAT, SEL, RAW	220	18.97	0	6.25
13376	BEEF, CHUCK, ARM POT RST, LN, 0"FAT, ALL GRDS, CKD, BRSD	210	33.02	0	2.76
13377	BEEF, CHUCK, ARM POT RST, LN, 0"FAT, CHOIC, CKD, BRSD	219	33.02	0	3.16
13378	BEEF, CHUCK, ARM POT RST, LN, 0"FAT, SEL, CKD, BRSD	198	33.02	0	2.29
13548	BEEF, CHUCK, ARM POT RST, LN, 1/2"FAT, PRIME, CKD, BRSD	261	33.02	0	5.07
13547	BEEF, CHUCK, ARM POT RST, LN, 1/2"FAT, PRIME, RAW	154	21.26	0	2.7
13042	BEEF, CHUCK, ARM POT RST, LN, 1/4" FAT, ALL GRDS, CKD, BRSD	216	33.02	0	3.01
13044	BEEF, CHUCK, ARM POT RST, LN, 1/4" FAT, CHOIC, CKD, BRSD	225	33.02	0	3.37
13046	BEEF, CHUCK, ARM POT RST, LN, 1/4" FAT, SEL, CKD, BRSD	206	33.02	0	2.61
13041	BEEF, CHUCK, ARM POT RST, LN, 1/4"FAT, ALL GRDS, RAW	130	21.26	0	1.59
13043	BEEF, CHUCK, ARM POT RST, LN, 1/4"FAT, CHOIC, RAW	137	21.26	0	1.84
13045	BEEF, CHUCK, ARM POT RST, LN, 1/4"FAT, SEL, RAW	123	21.26	0	1.3
13379	BEEF, CHUCK, BLADE RST, LN&FAT, 0"FAT, ALL GRDS, CKD, BRSD	334	27.18	0	9.59
13380	BEEF, CHUCK, BLADE RST, LN&FAT, 0"FAT, CHOIC, CKD, BRSD	348	26.98	0	10.26
13381	BEEF, CHUCK, BLADE RST, LN&FAT, 0"FAT, SEL, CKD, BRSD	313	27.59	0	8.61
13556	BEEF, CHUCK, BLADE RST, LN&FAT, 1/2"FAT, PRIME, CKD, BRSD	417	25.49	0	14.2
13555	BEEF, CHUCK, BLADE RST, LN&FAT, 1/2"FAT, PRIME, RAW	328	16.33	0	12.15
13050	BEEF, CHUCK, BLADE RST, LN&FAT, 1/4"FAT, ALL GRDS, CKD, BRSD	345	26.57	0	10.23
13049	BEEF, CHUCK, BLADE RST, LN&FAT, 1/4"FAT, ALL GRDS, RAW	254	17.04	0	8.11

NDB #	Food Description (100 gram portions = 3½ ounces = 20 tsp = ½ cup approx.	Calories	Protein	Carbs	Sat Fat
13052	BEEF, CHUCK, BLADE RST, LN&FAT, 1/4"FAT, CHOIC, CKD, BRSD	363	26.16	0	11.08
13051	BEEF, CHUCK, BLADE RST, LN&FAT, 1/4"FAT, CHOIC, RAW	272	16.82	0	8.97
13054	BEEF, CHUCK, BLADE RST, LN&FAT, 1/4"FAT, SEL, CKD, BRSD	326	26.98	0	9.3
13053	BEEF, CHUCK, BLADE RST, LN&FAT, 1/4"FAT, SEL, RAW	235	17.26	0	7.24
13816	BEEF, CHUCK, BLADE RST, LN&FAT, 1/8"FAT, ALL GRDS, CKD, BRSD	341	26.78	0	10
13815	BEEF, CHUCK, BLADE RST, LN&FAT, 1/8"FAT, ALL GRDS, RAW	248	17.16	0	7.82
13818	BEEF, CHUCK, BLADE RST, LN&FAT, 1/8"FAT, CHOIC, CKD, BRSD	359	26.37	0	10.86
13817	BEEF, CHUCK, BLADE RST, LN&FAT, 1/8"FAT, CHOIC, RAW	265	16.98	0	8.59
13820	BEEF, CHUCK, BLADE RST, LN&FAT, 1/8"FAT, SEL, CKD, BRSD	318	27.33	0	8.89
13819	BEEF, CHUCK, BLADE RST, LN&FAT, 1/8"FAT, SEL, RAW	230	17.37	0	6.99
13382	BEEF, CHUCK, BLADE RST, LN, 0"FAT, ALL GRDS, CKD, BRSD	253	31.06	0	5.16
13383	BEEF, CHUCK, BLADE RST, LN, 0"FAT, CHOIC, CKD, BRSD	265	31.06	0	5.7
13384	BEEF, CHUCK, BLADE RST, LN, 0"FAT, SEL, CKD, BRSD	238	31.06	0	4.54
13564	BEEF, CHUCK, BLADE RST, LN, 1/2"FAT, PRIME, CKD, BRSD	318	31.06	0	8.37
13563	BEEF, CHUCK, BLADE RST, LN, 1/2"FAT, PRIME, RAW	203	19.25	0	5.3
13058	BEEF, CHUCK, BLADE RST, LN, 1/4" FAT, ALL GRDS, CKD, BRSD	251	31.06	0	5.08
13060	BEEF, CHUCK, BLADE RST, LN, 1/4" FAT, CHOIC, CKD, BRSD	263	31.06	0	5.58
13062	BEEF, CHUCK, BLADE RST, LN, 1/4" FAT, SEL, CKD, BRSD	237	31.06	0	4.5
13057	BEEF, CHUCK, BLADE RST, LN, 1/4"FAT, ALL GRDS, RAW	149	19.25	0	2.78
13059	BEEF, CHUCK, BLADE RST, LN, 1/4"FAT, CHOIC, RAW	159	19.25	0	3.19
13061	BEEF, CHUCK, BLADE RST, LN, 1/4"FAT, SEL, RAW	139	19.25	0	2.37
23552	BEEF, CHUCK, CLOD RST, LN & FAT, 0" FAT, ALL GRDS, CKD, RSTD	207	25.7	0	3.904
23528	BEEF, CHUCK, CLOD RST, LN & FAT, 0" FAT, USDA CHOIC, CKD, RSTD	216	24.61	0	4.285
23531	BEEF, CHUCK, CLOD RST, LN & FAT, 0" FAT, USDA SEL, CKD, RSTD	196	27.3	0	3.349
23553	BEEF, CHUCK, CLOD RST, LN & FAT, 1/4" FAT, ALL GRDS, CKD, RSTD	242	24.22	0	5.738
23551	BEEF, CHUCK, CLOD RST, LN & FAT, 1/4" FAT, ALL GRDS, RAW	162	18.94	0	3.101
23529	BEEF, CHUCK, CLOD RST, LN & FAT, 1/4" FAT, USDA CHOIC, CKD, RST	242	24.13	0	5.705
23527	BEEF, CHUCK, CLOD RST, LN & FAT, 1/4" FAT, USDA CHOIC, RAW	161	18.81	0	2.975
23532	BEEF, CHUCK, CLOD RST, LN & FAT, 1/4" FAT, USDA SEL, CKD, RSTD	243	24.35	0	5.786
23530	BEEF, CHUCK, CLOD RST, LN & FAT, 1/4" FAT, USDA SEL, RAW	163	19.14	0	3.286
13937	BEEF, CHUCK, CLOD RST, LN ONLY, TO 0" FAT, USDA CHOIC, CKD, RS	171	25.95	0	1.96
13940	BEEF, CHUCK, CLOD RST, LN ONLY, TO 0" FAT, USDA SEL, CKD, RST	172	28.09	0	2.15
23515	BEEF, CHUCK, CLOD RST, LN ONLY, TO 1/4" FAT, ALL GRDS, CKD, RS	173	26.36	0	2.144
13938	BEEF, CHUCK, CLOD RST, LN ONLY, TO 1/4" FAT, USDA CHOIC, CKD,	178	26.1	0	2.38
13936	BEEF, CHUCK, CLOD RST, LN ONLY, TO 1/4" FAT, USDA CHOIC, RAW	129	19.48	0	1.3

NDB #	Food Description (100 gram portions = 3½ ounces = 20 tsp = ½ cup approx.	Calories	Protein	Carbs	Sat Fat
13941	BEEF, CHUCK, CLOD RST, LN ONLY, TO 1/4" FAT, USDA SEL, CKD, RS	166	26.75	0	1.8
13939	BEEF, CHUCK, CLOD RST, LN ONLY, TO 1/4" FAT, USDA SEL, RAW	130	19.85	0	1.58
23514	BEEF, CHUCK, CLOD RST, LN, 0" FAT, ALL GRDS, CKD, RSTD	172	26.82	0	2.037
23513	BEEF, CHUCK, CLOD RST, LN, 1/4" FAT, ALL GRDS, RAW	129	19.63	0	1.414
23554	BEEF, CHUCK, CLOD STEAK, LN & FAT, 0" FAT, ALL GRDS, CKD, BRSD	220	28.79	0	3.76
23533	BEEF, CHUCK, CLOD STEAK, LN & FAT, 0" FAT, USDA CHOIC, CKD, BR	231	28.06	0	4.157
23536	BEEF, CHUCK, CLOD STEAK, LN & FAT, 0" FAT, USDA SEL, CKD, BRSD	205	29.84	0	3.183
23555	BEEF, CHUCK, CLOD STEAK, LN & FAT, 1/4" FAT, ALL GRDS, CKD, BRS	272	26.19	0	6.699
23556	BEEF, CHUCK, CLOD STEAK, LN & FAT, 1/4" FAT, ALL GRDS, RAW	154	20.52	0	2.649
23534	BEEF, CHUCK, CLOD STEAK, LN & FAT, 1/4" FAT, USDA CHOIC, CKD, B	272	26.44	0	6.42
23535	BEEF, CHUCK, CLOD STEAK, LN & FAT, 1/4" FAT, USDA CHOIC, RAW	151	20.43	0	2.368
23537	BEEF, CHUCK, CLOD STEAK, LN & FAT, 1/4" FAT, USDA SEL, CKD, BRS	271	25.81	0	7.107
23538	BEEF, CHUCK, CLOD STEAK, LN & FAT, 1/4" FAT, USDA SEL, RAW	159	20.64	0	3.06
13944	BEEF, CHUCK, CLOD STEAK, LN ONLY, 1/4" FAT, USDA CHOIC, CKD, B	193	29.52	0	2.12
23516	BEEF, CHUCK, CLOD STEAK, LN ONLY, TO 0" FAT, ALL GRDS, CKD, B	192	29.87	0	2.267
13943	BEEF, CHUCK, CLOD STEAK, LN ONLY, TO 0" FAT, USDA CHOIC, CKD,	193	29.52	0	2.12
13946	BEEF, CHUCK, CLOD STEAK, LN ONLY, TO 0" FAT, USDA SEL, CKD, BR	191	30.37	0	2.48
23517	BEEF, CHUCK, CLOD STEAK, LN ONLY, TO 1/4" FAT, ALL GRDS, CKD,	189	29.34	0	2.271
23518	BEEF, CHUCK, CLOD STEAK, LN ONLY, TO 1/4" FAT, ALL GRDS, RAW	129	21.13	0	1.323
13942	BEEF, CHUCK, CLOD STEAK, LN ONLY, TO 1/4" FAT, USDA CHOIC, RA	132	20.88	0	1.38
13947	BEEF, CHUCK, CLOD STEAK, LN ONLY, TO 1/4" FAT, USDA SEL, CKD,	183	29.08	0	2.49
13945	BEEF, CHUCK, CLOD STEAK, LN ONLY, TO 1/4" FAT, USDA SEL, RAW	124	21.5	0	1.24
23547	BEEF, CHUCK, TENDER STEAK, LN & FAT, 0" FAT, ALL GRDS, CKD, BR	160	25.87	0	1.871
23519	BEEF, CHUCK, TENDER STEAK, LN & FAT, 0" FAT, USDA CHOIC, CKD,	161	25.73	0	1.721
23521	BEEF, CHUCK, TENDER STEAK, LN & FAT, 0" FAT, USDA SEL, CKD, BR	159	26.08	0	2.09
23548	BEEF, CHUCK, TENDER STEAK, LN & FAT, 1/4" FAT, ALL GRDS, RAW	113	19	0	1.196
23520	BEEF, CHUCK, TENDER STEAK, LN & FAT, 1/4" FAT, USDA CHOIC, RA	114	18.89	0	1.334
23522	BEEF, CHUCK, TENDER STEAK, LN & FAT, 1/4" FAT, USDA SEL, RAW	110	19.16	0	0.994
13961	BEEF, CHUCK, TENDER STEAK, LN ONLY, 0" FAT, USDA CHOIC, CKD,	161	25.74	0	1.71
13963	BEEF, CHUCK, TENDER STEAK, LN ONLY, TO 0" FAT, USDA SEL, CKD,	157	26.13	0	2
13960	BEEF, CHUCK, TENDER STEAK, LN ONLY, TO 1/4" FAT, USDA CHOIC,	114	18.9	0	1.3
13962	BEEF, CHUCK, TENDER STEAK, LN ONLY, TO 1/4" FAT, USDA SEL, RA	109	19.18	0	0.94
23509	BEEF, CHUCK, TENDER STEAK, LN, 0" FAT, ALL GRDS, CKD, BRLD	160	25.9	0	1.828
23510	BEEF, CHUCK, TENDER STEAK, LN, 1/4" FAT, ALL GRDS, RAW	107	19.01	0	1.153
23549	BEEF, CHUCK, TOP BLADE, LN & FAT, 0" FAT, ALL GRDS, CKD, BRLD	216	25.73	0	3.906

NDB #	Food Description (100 gram portions = 3½ ounces = 20 tsp = ½ cup approx.	Calories	Protein	Carbs	Sat Fat
23523	BEEF, CHUCK, TOP BLADE, LN & FAT, 0" FAT, USDA CHOIC, CKD, BRL	227	25.77	0	4.162
23525	BEEF, CHUCK, TOP BLADE, LN & FAT, 0" FAT, USDA SEL, CKD, BRLD	200	25.67	0	3.533
23550	BEEF, CHUCK, TOP BLADE, LN & FAT, 1/4" FAT, ALL GRDS, RAW	149	19.07	0	2.382
23524	BEEF, CHUCK, TOP BLADE, LN & FAT, 1/4" FAT, USDA CHOIC, RAW	162	19.25	0	2.842
23526	BEEF, CHUCK, TOP BLADE, LN & FAT, 1/4" FAT, USDA SEL, RAW	131	18.82	0	1.711
23511	BEEF, CHUCK, TOP BLADE, LN ONLY, TO 0" FAT, ALL GRDS, CKD, BRL	203	26.13	0	3.25
13965	BEEF, CHUCK, TOP BLADE, LN ONLY, TO 0" FAT, USDA CHOIC, CKD, B	217	26.11	0	3.62
13967	BEEF, CHUCK, TOP BLADE, LN ONLY, TO 0" FAT, USDA SEL, CKD, BRL	184	26.16	0	2.71
13964	BEEF, CHUCK, TOP BLADE, LN ONLY, TO 1/4" FAT, USDA CHOIC, RAW	150	19.5	0	2.23
13966	BEEF, CHUCK, TOP BLADE, LN ONLY, TO 1/4" FAT, USDA SEL, RAW	129	18.84	0	1.65
23512	BEEF, CHUCK, TOP BLADE, LN, 1/4" FAT, ALL GRDS, RAW	136	19.23	0	1.994
13361	BEEF, COMP OF RTL CUTS, LN&FAT, 0"FAT, ALL GRDS, CKD	273	27.33	0	6.85
13362	BEEF, COMP OF RTL CUTS, LN&FAT, 0"FAT, CHOIC, CKD	283	27.21	0	7.31
13363	BEEF, COMP OF RTL CUTS, LN&FAT, 0"FAT, SEL, CKD	261	27.47	0	6.27
13510	BEEF, COMP OF RTL CUTS, LN&FAT, 1/2"FAT, PRIME, CKD	405	23.4	0	14.01
13509	BEEF, COMP OF RTL CUTS, LN&FAT, 1/2"FAT, PRIME, RAW	344	16.55	0	12.98
13004	BEEF, COMP OF RTL CUTS, LN&FAT, 1/4"FAT, ALL GRDS, CKD	305	25.94	0	8.54
13003	BEEF, COMP OF RTL CUTS, LN&FAT, 1/4"FAT, ALL GRDS, RAW	251	18.24	0	7.8
13006	BEEF, COMP OF RTL CUTS, LN&FAT, 1/4"FAT, CHOIC, CKD	322	25.48	0	9.38
13005	BEEF, COMP OF RTL CUTS, LN&FAT, 1/4"FAT, CHOIC, RAW	259	18.17	0	8.16
13010	BEEF, COMP OF RTL CUTS, LN&FAT, 1/4"FAT, PRIME, CKD	322	25.62	0	9.49
13009	BEEF, COMP OF RTL CUTS, LN&FAT, 1/4"FAT, PRIME, RAW	288	18.28	0	9.56
13008	BEEF, COMP OF RTL CUTS, LN&FAT, 1/4"FAT, SEL, CKD	291	26.17	0	7.88
13007	BEEF, COMP OF RTL CUTS, LN&FAT, 1/4"FAT, SEL, RAW	236	18.47	0	7.07
13796	BEEF, COMP OF RTL CUTS, LN&FAT, 1/8"FAT, ALL GRDS, CKD	291	26.42	0	7.77
13795	BEEF, COMP OF RTL CUTS, LN&FAT, 1/8"FAT, ALL GRDS, RAW	234	18.68	0	6.91
13798	BEEF, COMP OF RTL CUTS, LN&FAT, 1/8"FAT, CHOIC, CKD	301	26.21	0	8.24
13797	BEEF, COMP OF RTL CUTS, LN&FAT, 1/8"FAT, CHOIC, RAW	243	18.57	0	7.32
13802	BEEF, COMP OF RTL CUTS, LN&FAT, 1/8"FAT, PRIME, CKD	299	26.22	0	8.32
13801	BEEF, COMP OF RTL CUTS, LN&FAT, 1/8"FAT, PRIME, RAW	265	18.72	0	8.37
13800	BEEF, COMP OF RTL CUTS, LN&FAT, 1/8"FAT, SEL, CKD	278	26.63	0	7.2
13799	BEEF, COMP OF RTL CUTS, LN&FAT, 1/8"FAT, SEL, RAW	223	18.87	0	6.37
13364	BEEF, COMP OF RTL CUTS, LN, 0" FAT, ALL GRDS, CKD	211	29.88	0	3.54
13365	BEEF, COMP OF RTL CUTS, LN, 0"FAT, CHOIC, CKD	219	29.88	0	3.87
13366	BEEF, COMP OF RTL CUTS, LN, 0"FAT, SEL, CKD	201	29.89	0	3.09

NDB #	Food Description (100 gram portions = 3½ ounces = 20 tsp = ½ cup approx.	Calories	Protein	Carbs	Sat Fat
13518	BEEF, COMP OF RTL CUTS, LN, 1/2"FAT, PRIME, CKD	252	30.49	0	5.26
13517	BEEF, COMP OF RTL CUTS, LN, 1/2"FAT, PRIME, RAW	169	20.97	0	3.41
13012	BEEF, COMP OF RTL CUTS, LN, 1/4" FAT, ALL GRDS, CKD	216	29.58	0	3.79
13011	BEEF, COMP OF RTL CUTS, LN, 1/4" FAT, ALL GRDS, RAW	144	20.78	0	2.32
13014	BEEF, COMP OF RTL CUTS, LN, 1/4"FAT, CHOIC, CKD	222	29.58	0	4.07
13013	BEEF, COMP OF RTL CUTS, LN, 1/4"FAT, CHOIC, RAW	150	20.78	0	2.56
13018	BEEF, COMP OF RTL CUTS, LN, 1/4"FAT, PRIME, CKD	241	29.04	0	5.2
13017	BEEF, COMP OF RTL CUTS, LN, 1/4"FAT, PRIME, RAW	178	21.16	0	3.87
13016	BEEF, COMP OF RTL CUTS, LN, 1/4"FAT, SEL, CKD	205	29.59	0	3.35
13015	BEEF, COMP OF RTL CUTS, LN, 1/4"FAT, SEL, RAW	141	20.67	0	2.23
13345	BEEF, CURED, BRKFST STRIPS, CKD	449	31.3	1.4	14.35
13344	BEEF, CURED, BRKFST STRIPS, RAW OR UNHTD	406	12.5	0.7	15.95
13347	BEEF, CURED, CORNED BF, BRISKET, CKD	251	18.17	0.47	6.34
13346	BEEF, CURED, CORNED BF, BRISKET, RAW	198	14.68	0.14	4.73
13348	BEEF, CURED, CORNED BF, CND	250	27.1	0	6.18
13350	BEEF, CURED, DRIED BEEF	165	29.1	1.56	1.59
13353	BEEF, CURED, LUNCHEON MEAT, JELLIED	111	19	0	1.41
13355	BEEF, CURED, PASTRAMI	349	17.24	3.05	10.42
13357	BEEF, CURED, SAUSAGE, CKD, SMOKED	312	14.11	2.42	11.44
13358	BEEF, CURED, SMOKED, CHOPD BF	133	20.19	1.86	1.81
13360	BEEF, CURED, THIN-SLICED BF	177	28.11	5.71	1.65
13067	BEEF, FLANK, LN&FAT, 0"FAT, CHOIC, CKD, BRLD	226	26.42	0	5.32
13066	BEEF, FLANK, LN&FAT, 0"FAT, CHOIC, CKD, BRSD	263	26.98	0	6.92
13065	BEEF, FLANK, LN&FAT, 0"FAT, CHOIC, RAW	180	19.7	0	4.52
13069	BEEF, FLANK, LN, 0" FAT, CHOIC, CKD, BRSD	237	28.02	0	5.54
13068	BEEF, FLANK, LN, 0" FAT, CHOIC, RAW	154	20.31	0	3.21
13070	BEEF, FLANK, LN, 0"FAT, CHOIC, CKD, BRLD	207	27.07	0	4.36
23580	BEEF, GROUND, 75% LN MEAT / 25% FAT, CRUMBLES, CKD, PAN-BRO	277	26.28	0	7.007
23581	BEEF, GROUND, 75% LN MEAT / 25% FAT, LOAF, CKD, BKD	254	24.56	0	6.348
23578	BEEF, GROUND, 75% LN MEAT / 25% FAT, PATTY, CKD, BRLD	278	25.56	0	7.208
23579	BEEF, GROUND, 75% LN MEAT / 25% FAT, PATTY, CKD, PAN-BROILED	248	23.45	0	6.326
23577	BEEF, GROUND, 75% LN MEAT / 25% FAT, RAW	293	15.76	0	9.617
23575	BEEF, GROUND, 80% LN MEAT / 20% FAT, CRUMBLES, CKD, PAN-BRO	272	27	0	6.734
23576	BEEF, GROUND, 80% LN MEAT / 20% FAT, LOAF, CKD, BKD	254	25.25	0	6.27
23573	BEEF, GROUND, 80% LN MEAT / 20% FAT, PATTY, CKD, BRLD	271	25.75	0	6.911

NDB #	Food Description (100 gram portions = 3½ ounces = 20 tsp = ½ cup approx.	Calories	Protein	Carbs	Sat Fat
23574	BEEF, GROUND, 80% LN MEAT / 20% FAT, PATTY, CKD, PAN-BROILED	246	24.04	0	6.181
23572	BEEF, GROUND, 80% LN MEAT / 20% FAT, RAW	254	17.17	0	7.757
23570	BEEF, GROUND, 85% LN MEAT / 15% FAT, CRUMBLES, CKD, PAN-BRO	256	27.73	0	6.017
23571	BEEF, GROUND, 85% LN MEAT / 15% FAT, LOAF, CKD, BKD	240	25.93	0	5.647
23568	BEEF, GROUND, 85% LN MEAT / 15% FAT, PATTY, CKD, BRLD	250	25.93	0	6.087
23569	BEEF, GROUND, 85% LN MEAT / 15% FAT, PATTY, CKD, PAN-BROILED	232	24.62	0	5.51
23567	BEEF, GROUND, 85% LN MEAT / 15% FAT, RAW	215	18.59	0	5.897
23565	BEEF, GROUND, 90% LN MEAT / 10% FAT, CRUMBLES, CKD, PAN-BRO	230	28.45	0	4.862
23566	BEEF, GROUND, 90% LN MEAT / 10% FAT, LOAF, CKD, BKD	214	26.62	0	4.48
23563	BEEF, GROUND, 90% LN MEAT / 10% FAT, PATTY, CKD, BRLD	217	26.11	0	4.734
23564	BEEF, GROUND, 90% LN MEAT / 10% FAT, PATTY, CKD, PAN-BROILED	204	25.21	0	4.313
23562	BEEF, GROUND, 90% LN MEAT / 10% FAT, RAW	176	20	0	4.037
23560	BEEF, GROUND, 95% LN MEAT / 5% FAT, CRUMBLES, CKD, PAN-BRO	193	29.17	0	3.3
23561	BEEF, GROUND, 95% LN MEAT / 5% FAT, LOAF, CKD, BKD	174	27.31	0	2.772
23558	BEEF, GROUND, 95% LN MEAT / 5% FAT, PATTY, CKD, BRLD	171	26.29	0	2.854
23559	BEEF, GROUND, 95% LN MEAT / 5% FAT, PATTY, CKD, PAN-BROILED	164	25.8	0	2.587
23557	BEEF, GROUND, 95% LN MEAT / 5% FAT, RAW	137	21.41	0	2.177
13316	BEEF, GROUND, PATTIES, FRZ, (APPROX 23% FAT), RAW	282	17.11	0	9.36
13317	BEEF, GROUND, PATTIES, FRZ, CKD, BRLD, MED	282	24.5	0	7.72
13984	BEEF, LOIN, BTTM SIRLOIN, TRI-TIP RST, LN, 1/4" FAT, ALL GRDS, RA	154	20.7	0	2.6
13458	BEEF, LOIN, PRTRHS STEAK, LN & FAT, 1/4" FAT, ALL GRDS, CKD, BRL	329	22.51	0	10.167
13230	BEEF, LOIN, PRTRHS STEAK, LN & FAT, 1/4" FAT, USDA CHOIC, CKD, B	342	21.84	0	10.65
13460	BEEF, LOIN, PRTRHS STK, LN & FAT, 0" FAT, USDA CHOIC, CKD, BRLD	283	23.61	0	7.43
13986	BEEF, LOIN, SIRLOIN, TRI-TIP STEAK, LN, 1/4" FAT, ALL GRDS, RAW	167	21.62	0	3.01
13474	BEEF, LOIN, T-BONE STEAK, LN & FAT, 0" FAT, USDA CHOIC, CKD, BR	258	24.05	0	6.449
13472	BEEF, LOIN, T-BONE STEAK, LN & FAT, 1/4" FAT, ALL GRDS, CKD, BRL	306	23.47	0	8.92
13234	BEEF, LOIN, T-BONE STEAK, LN & FAT, 1/4" FAT, USDA CHOIC, CKD, B	322	22.79	0	9.748
13476	BEEF, LOIN, T-BONE STEAK, LN & FAT, 1/4" FAT, USDA SEL, CKD, BRL	281	24.45	0	7.713
23544	BEEF, LOIN, TRI-TIP RST, LN & FAT, 0" FAT, ALL GRDS, CKD, RSTD	217	27.9	0	4.007
23539	BEEF, PLATE, INSIDE SKIRT STEAK, LN & FAT, 1/4" FAT, ALL GRDS, RA	204	20.07	0	5.197
13976	BEEF, PLATE, INSIDE SKIRT STEAK, LN ONLY, 1/4" FAT, ALL GRDS, RA	164	21.08	0	3.14
13977	BEEF, PLATE, INSIDE SKIRT STEAK, LN, 0" FAT, ALL GRDS, CKD, BRLD	205	26.66	0	3.85
13978	BEEF, PLATE, OUTSIDE SKIRT STEAK, LN ONLY, 1/4" FAT, ALL GRDS,	165	19.62	0	3.47
13979	BEEF, PLATE, OUTSIDE SKIRT STEAK, LN, 0" FAT, ALL GRDS, CKD, BR	233	24.18	0	5.97
23541	BEEF, PLATE, OUTSIDE SKIRT, LN & FAT, 0" FAT, ALL GRDS, CKD, BRL	255	23.51	0	7.083

NDB #	Food Description (100 gram portions = 3½ ounces = 20 tsp = ½ cup approx.	Calories	Protein	Carbs	Sat Fat
23542	BEEF, PLATE, OUTSIDE SKIRT, LN & FAT, 1/4" FAT, ALL GRDS, RAW	204	18.74	0	5.473
23540	BEEF, PLATE, SKIRT STEAK, LN & FAT, 0" FAT, ALL GRDS, CKD, BRLD	220	26.13	0	4.666
13096	BEEF, RIB, EYE, SML END (10-12), LN&FAT, 0"FAT, CHOIC, CKD, BRLD	307	24.91	0	9.01
13095	BEEF, RIB, EYE, SML END (RIBS 10-12), LN&FAT, 0"FAT, CHOIC, RAW	274	17.51	0	9
13098	BEEF, RIB, EYE, SML END (RIBS 10-12), LN, 0"FAT, CHOIC, CKD, BRLD	225	28.04	0	4.73
13097	BEEF, RIB, EYE, SML END (RIBS 10-12), LN, 0"FAT, CHOIC, RAW	161	20.13	0	3.23
13385	BEEF, RIB, LRG END (RIBS 6-9), LN&FAT, 0"FAT, ALL GRDS, CKD, RST	353	23.14	0	11.37
13386	BEEF, RIB, LRG END (RIBS 6-9), LN&FAT, 0"FAT, CHOIC, CKD, RSTD	372	22.8	0	12.29
13387	BEEF, RIB, LRG END (RIBS 6-9), LN&FAT, 0"FAT, SEL, CKD, RSTD	331	23.48	0	10.3
13609	BEEF, RIB, LRG END (RIBS 6-9), LN&FAT, 1/2"FAT, PRIME, CKD, BRLD	425	19.87	0	16.03
13610	BEEF, RIB, LRG END (RIBS 6-9), LN&FAT, 1/2"FAT, PRIME, CKD, RSTD	407	22.24	0	14.7
13608	BEEF, RIB, LRG END (RIBS 6-9), LN&FAT, 1/2"FAT, PRIME, RAW	383	15.38	0	15.32
13100	BEEF, RIB, LRG END (RIBS 6-9), LN&FAT, 1/4"FAT, ALL GRDS, CKD, BR	347	21.25	0	11.55
13101	BEEF, RIB, LRG END (RIBS 6-9), LN&FAT, 1/4"FAT, ALL GRDS, CKD, RS	365	22.64	0	12.01
13099	BEEF, RIB, LRG END (RIBS 6-9), LN&FAT, 1/4"FAT, ALL GRDS, RAW	323	16.09	0	11.66
13103	BEEF, RIB, LRG END (RIBS 6-9), LN&FAT, 1/4"FAT, CHOIC, CKD, BRLD	367	20.96	0	12.51
13104	BEEF, RIB, LRG END (RIBS 6-9), LN&FAT, 1/4"FAT, CHOIC, CKD, RSTD	383	22.3	0	12.89
13102	BEEF, RIB, LRG END (RIBS 6-9), LN&FAT, 1/4"FAT, CHOIC, RAW	345	15.75	0	12.76
13109	BEEF, RIB, LRG END (RIBS 6-9), LN&FAT, 1/4"FAT, PRIME, CKD, BRLD	413	20.3	0	15
13110	BEEF, RIB, LRG END (RIBS 6-9), LN&FAT, 1/4"FAT, PRIME, CKD, RSTD	402	22.47	0	14.06
13108	BEEF, RIB, LRG END (RIBS 6-9), LN&FAT, 1/4"FAT, PRIME, RAW	377	15.52	0	14.47
13106	BEEF, RIB, LRG END (RIBS 6-9), LN&FAT, 1/4"FAT, SEL, CKD, BRLD	324	21.54	0	10.46
13107	BEEF, RIB, LRG END (RIBS 6-9), LN&FAT, 1/4"FAT, SEL, CKD, RSTD	340	23.14	0	10.78
13105	BEEF, RIB, LRG END (RIBS 6-9), LN&FAT, 1/4"FAT, SEL, RAW	304	16.32	0	10.74
13839	BEEF, RIB, LRG END (RIBS 6-9), LN&FAT, 1/8"FAT, ALL GRDS, CKD, BR	338	21.55	0	11.06
13840	BEEF, RIB, LRG END (RIBS 6-9), LN&FAT, 1/8"FAT, ALL GRDS, CKD, RS	355	23.01	0	11.5
13838	BEEF, RIB, LRG END (RIBS 6-9), LN&FAT, 1/8"FAT, ALL GRDS, RAW	316	16.26	0	11.29
13842	BEEF, RIB, LRG END (RIBS 6-9), LN&FAT, 1/8"FAT, CHOIC, CKD, BRLD	370	20.86	0	12.67
13843	BEEF, RIB, LRG END (RIBS 6-9), LN&FAT, 1/8"FAT, CHOIC, CKD, RSTD	378	22.5	0	12.62
13841	BEEF, RIB, LRG END (RIBS 6-9), LN&FAT, 1/8"FAT, CHOIC, RAW	333	16.03	0	12.13
13848	BEEF, RIB, LRG END (RIBS 6-9), LN&FAT, 1/8"FAT, PRIME, CKD, BRLD	404	20.65	0	14.51
13849	BEEF, RIB, LRG END (RIBS 6-9), LN&FAT, 1/8"FAT, PRIME, CKD, RSTD	393	22.86	0	13.59
13847	BEEF, RIB, LRG END (RIBS 6-9), LN&FAT, 1/8"FAT, PRIME, RAW	367	15.77	0	13.96
13845	BEEF, RIB, LRG END (RIBS 6-9), LN&FAT, 1/8"FAT, SEL, CKD, BRLD	324	21.55	0	10.43
13846	BEEF, RIB, LRG END (RIBS 6-9), LN&FAT, 1/8"FAT, SEL, CKD, RSTD	333	23.4	0	10.42

NDB #	Food Description (100 gram portions = 3½ ounces = 20 tsp = ½ cup approx.	Calories	Protein	Carbs	Sat Fat
13844	BEEF, RIB, LRG END (RIBS 6-9), LN&FAT, 1/8"FAT, SEL, RAW	295	16.52	0	10.28
13388	BEEF, RIB, LRG END (RIBS 6-9), LN, 0"FAT, ALL GRDS, CKD, RSTD	238	27.53	0	5.35
13389	BEEF, RIB, LRG END (RIBS 6-9), LN, 0"FAT, CHOIC, CKD, RSTD	253	27.53	0	5.99
13390	BEEF, RIB, LRG END (RIBS 6-9), LN, 0"FAT, SEL, CKD, RSTD	220	27.53	0	4.55
13621	BEEF, RIB, LRG END (RIBS 6-9), LN, 1/2"FAT, PRIME, CKD, BRLD	294	24.64	0	8.94
13622	BEEF, RIB, LRG END (RIBS 6-9), LN, 1/2"FAT, PRIME, CKD, RSTD	283	27.53	0	7.85
13113	BEEF, RIB, LRG END (RIBS 6-9), LN, 1/4" FAT, ALL GRDS, CKD, RSTD	237	27.53	0	5.27
13112	BEEF, RIB, LRG END (RIBS 6-9), LN, 1/4"FAT, ALL GRDS, CKD, BRLD	224	25.17	0	5.28
13111	BEEF, RIB, LRG END (RIBS 6-9), LN, 1/4"FAT, ALL GRDS, RAW	165	19.63	0	3.67
13115	BEEF, RIB, LRG END (RIBS 6-9), LN, 1/4"FAT, CHOIC, CKD, BRLD	240	25.17	0	5.98
13116	BEEF, RIB, LRG END (RIBS 6-9), LN, 1/4"FAT, CHOIC, CKD, RSTD	250	27.53	0	5.87
13114	BEEF, RIB, LRG END (RIBS 6-9), LN, 1/4"FAT, CHOIC, RAW	176	19.63	0	4.16
13121	BEEF, RIB, LRG END (RIBS 6-9), LN, 1/4"FAT, PRIME, CKD, BRLD	294	24.64	0	8.94
13122	BEEF, RIB, LRG END (RIBS 6-9), LN, 1/4"FAT, PRIME, CKD, RSTD	283	27.53	0	7.88
13120	BEEF, RIB, LRG END (RIBS 6-9), LN, 1/4"FAT, PRIME, RAW	210	19.63	0	6.05
13118	BEEF, RIB, LRG END (RIBS 6-9), LN, 1/4"FAT, SEL, CKD, BRLD	206	25.17	0	4.44
13119	BEEF, RIB, LRG END (RIBS 6-9), LN, 1/4"FAT, SEL, CKD, RSTD	220	27.53	0	4.55
13117	BEEF, RIB, LRG END (RIBS 6-9), LN, 1/4"FAT, SEL, RAW	152	19.63	0	3.1
13149	BEEF, RIB, SHORTRIBS, LN ONLY, CHOIC, RAW	173	19.05	0	4.33
13148	BEEF, RIB, SHORTRIBS, LN&FAT, CHOIC, CKD, BRSD	471	21.57	0	17.8
13147	BEEF, RIB, SHORTRIBS, LN&FAT, CHOIC, RAW	388	14.4	0	15.76
13150	BEEF, RIB, SHORTRIBS, LN, CHOIC, CKD, BRSD	295	30.76	0	7.74
13124	BEEF, RIB, SML END (10-12), LN&FAT, 1/4"FAT, ALL GRDS, CKD, BRLD	336	23.69	0	10.52
13125	BEEF, RIB, SML END (10-12), LN&FAT, 1/4"FAT, ALL GRDS, CKD, RSTD	347	22.31	0	11.26
13391	BEEF, RIB, SML END (RIBS 10-12), LN&FAT, 0"FAT, ALL GRDS, CKD, B	297	24.91	0	8.54
13392	BEEF, RIB, SML END (RIBS 10-12), LN&FAT, 0"FAT, CHOIC, CKD, BRLD	312	24.73	0	9.24
13393	BEEF, RIB, SML END (RIBS 10-12), LN&FAT, 0"FAT, SEL, CKD, BRLD	285	24.91	0	8.01
13633	BEEF, RIB, SML END (RIBS 10-12), LN&FAT, 1/2"FAT, PRIME, CKD, BRL	364	23.72	0	12.33
13634	BEEF, RIB, SML END (RIBS 10-12), LN&FAT, 1/2"FAT, PRIME, CKD, RST	420	21.78	0	15.34
13632	BEEF, RIB, SML END (RIBS 10-12), LN&FAT, 1/2"FAT, PRIME, RAW	349	16.39	0	13.33
13123	BEEF, RIB, SML END (RIBS 10-12), LN&FAT, 1/4"FAT, ALL GRDS, RAW	298	16.79	0	10.29
13127	BEEF, RIB, SML END (RIBS 10-12), LN&FAT, 1/4"FAT, CHOIC, CKD, BRL	349	23.52	0	11.18
13128	BEEF, RIB, SML END (RIBS 10-12), LN&FAT, 1/4"FAT, CHOIC, CKD, RST	367	21.98	0	12.19
13126	BEEF, RIB, SML END (RIBS 10-12), LN&FAT, 1/4"FAT, CHOIC, RAW	315	16.56	0	11.09
13133	BEEF, RIB, SML END (RIBS 10-12), LN&FAT, 1/4"FAT, PRIME, CKD, BRL	361	23.86	0	11.84

NDB #	Food Description (100 gram portions = 3½ ounces = 20 tsp = ½ cup approx.	Calories	Protein	Carbs	Sat Fat
13134	BEEF, RIB, SML END (RIBS 10-12), LN&FAT, 1/4"FAT, PRIME, CKD, RST	417	21.91	0	14.81
13132	BEEF, RIB, SML END (RIBS 10-12), LN&FAT, 1/4"FAT, PRIME, RAW	342	16.56	0	12.45
13130	BEEF, RIB, SML END (RIBS 10-12), LN&FAT, 1/4"FAT, SEL, CKD, BRLD	321	23.86	0	9.82
13131	BEEF, RIB, SML END (RIBS 10-12), LN&FAT, 1/4"FAT, SEL, CKD, RSTD	331	22.47	0	10.49
13129	BEEF, RIB, SML END (RIBS 10-12), LN&FAT, 1/4"FAT, SEL, RAW	286	16.91	0	9.71
13851	BEEF, RIB, SML END (RIBS 10-12), LN&FAT, 1/8"FAT, ALL GRDS, CKD,	330	23.92	0	10.21
13852	BEEF, RIB, SML END (RIBS 10-12), LN&FAT, 1/8"FAT, ALL GRDS, CKD,	341	22.54	0	10.92
13850	BEEF, RIB, SML END (RIBS 10-12), LN&FAT, 1/8"FAT, ALL GRDS, RAW	291	16.96	0	9.91
13854	BEEF, RIB, SML END (RIBS 10-12), LN&FAT, 1/8"FAT, CHOIC, CKD, BRL	343	23.76	0	10.85
13855	BEEF, RIB, SML END (RIBS 10-12), LN&FAT, 1/8"FAT, CHOIC, CKD, RST	359	22.28	0	11.78
13853	BEEF, RIB, SML END (RIBS 10-12), LN&FAT, 1/8"FAT, CHOIC, RAW	304	16.81	0	10.53
13860	BEEF, RIB, SML END (RIBS 10-12), LN&FAT, 1/8"FAT, PRIME, CKD, BRL	354	24.13	0	11.51
13861	BEEF, RIB, SML END (RIBS 10-12), LN&FAT, 1/8"FAT, PRIME, CKD, RST	411	22.15	0	14.51
13859	BEEF, RIB, SML END (RIBS 10-12), LN&FAT, 1/8"FAT, PRIME, RAW	335	16.74	0	12.07
13857	BEEF, RIB, SML END (RIBS 10-12), LN&FAT, 1/8"FAT, SEL, CKD, BRLD	315	24.07	0	9.52
13858	BEEF, RIB, SML END (RIBS 10-12), LN&FAT, 1/8"FAT, SEL, CKD, RSTD	323	22.76	0	10.05
13856	BEEF, RIB, SML END (RIBS 10-12), LN&FAT, 1/8"FAT, SEL, RAW	276	17.12	0	9.24
13394	BEEF, RIB, SML END (RIBS 10-12), LN, 0"FAT, ALL GRDS, CKD, BRLD	213	28.04	0	4.16
13395	BEEF, RIB, SML END (RIBS 10-12), LN, 0"FAT, CHOIC, CKD, BRLD	225	28.04	0	4.73
13396	BEEF, RIB, SML END (RIBS 10-12), LN, 0"FAT, SEL, CKD, BRLD	198	28.04	0	3.51
13645	BEEF, RIB, SML END (RIBS 10-12), LN, 1/2"FAT, PRIME, CKD, BRLD	260	28.04	0	6.58
13646	BEEF, RIB, SML END (RIBS 10-12), LN, 1/2"FAT, PRIME, CKD, RSTD	304	26.74	0	8.94
13136	BEEF, RIB, SML END (RIBS 10-12), LN, 1/4" FAT, ALL GRDS, CKD, BRLD	221	28.04	0	4.52
13143	BEEF, RIB, SML END (RIBS 10-12), LN, 1/4" FAT, SEL, CKD, RSTD	203	26.84	0	3.83
13137	BEEF, RIB, SML END (RIBS 10-12), LN, 1/4"FAT, ALL GRDS, CKD, RSTD	218	26.84	0	4.55
13135	BEEF, RIB, SML END (RIBS 10-12), LN, 1/4"FAT, ALL GRDS, RAW	152	20.13	0	2.84
13139	BEEF, RIB, SML END (RIBS 10-12), LN, 1/4"FAT, CHOIC, CKD, BRLD	233	28.04	0	5.09
13140	BEEF, RIB, SML END (RIBS 10-12), LN, 1/4"FAT, CHOIC, CKD, RSTD	232	26.84	0	5.21
13138	BEEF, RIB, SML END (RIBS 10-12), LN, 1/4"FAT, CHOIC, RAW	161	20.13	0	3.23
13145	BEEF, RIB, SML END (RIBS 10-12), LN, 1/4"FAT, PRIME, CKD, BRLD	260	28.04	0	6.58
13146	BEEF, RIB, SML END (RIBS 10-12), LN, 1/4"FAT, PRIME, CKD, RSTD	304	26.74	0	8.94
13144	BEEF, RIB, SML END (RIBS 10-12), LN, 1/4"FAT, PRIME, RAW	200	20.13	0	5.16
13142	BEEF, RIB, SML END (RIBS 10-12), LN, 1/4"FAT, SEL, CKD, BRLD	207	28.04	0	3.92
13141	BEEF, RIB, SML END (RIBS 10-12), LN, 1/4"FAT, SEL, RAW	142	20.13	0	2.41
13581	BEEF, RIB, WHL (RIBS 6-12), LN&FAT, 1/2"FAT, PRIME, CKD, BRLD	408	21.11	0	14.94

NDB #	Food Description (100 gram portions = 3½ ounces = 20 tsp = ½ cup approx.	Calories	Protein	Carbs	Sat Fat
13582	BEEF, RIB, WHL (RIBS 6-12), LN&FAT, 1/2"FAT, PRIME, CKD, RSTD	425	21.53	0	15.65
13580	BEEF, RIB, WHL (RIBS 6-12), LN&FAT, 1/2"FAT, PRIME, RAW	370	15.75	0	14.58
13072	BEEF, RIB, WHL (RIBS 6-12), LN&FAT, 1/4"FAT, ALL GRDS, CKD, BRLD	342	22.24	0	11.13
13073	BEEF, RIB, WHL (RIBS 6-12), LN&FAT, 1/4"FAT, ALL GRDS, CKD, RSTD	358	22.5	0	11.7
13071	BEEF, RIB, WHL (RIBS 6-12), LN&FAT, 1/4"FAT, ALL GRDS, RAW	313	16.37	0	11.13
13075	BEEF, RIB, WHL (RIBS 6-12), LN&FAT, 1/4"FAT, CHOIC, CKD, BRLD	360	21.98	0	11.98
13076	BEEF, RIB, WHL (RIBS 6-12), LN&FAT, 1/4"FAT, CHOIC, CKD, RSTD	376	22.17	0	12.6
13074	BEEF, RIB, WHL (RIBS 6-12), LN&FAT, 1/4"FAT, CHOIC, RAW	333	16.06	0	12.11
13081	BEEF, RIB, WHL (RIBS 6-12), LN&FAT, 1/4"FAT, PRIME, CKD, BRLD	392	21.72	0	13.72
13082	BEEF, RIB, WHL (RIBS 6-12), LN&FAT, 1/4"FAT, PRIME, CKD, RSTD	409	22.21	0	14.41
13080	BEEF, RIB, WHL (RIBS 6-12), LN&FAT, 1/4"FAT, PRIME, RAW	364	15.91	0	13.72
13078	BEEF, RIB, WHL (RIBS 6-12), LN&FAT, 1/4"FAT, SEL, CKD, BRLD	323	22.49	0	10.2
13079	BEEF, RIB, WHL (RIBS 6-12), LN&FAT, 1/4"FAT, SEL, CKD, RSTD	336	22.86	0	10.66
13077	BEEF, RIB, WHL (RIBS 6-12), LN&FAT, 1/4"FAT, SEL, RAW	297	16.55	0	10.34
13825	BEEF, RIB, WHL (RIBS 6-12), LN&FAT, 1/8"FAT, ALL GRDS, CKD, BRLD	337	22.42	0	10.85
13826	BEEF, RIB, WHL (RIBS 6-12), LN&FAT, 1/8"FAT, ALL GRDS, CKD, RSTD	351	22.77	0	11.33
13824	BEEF, RIB, WHL (RIBS 6-12), LN&FAT, 1/8"FAT, ALL GRDS, RAW	306	16.53	0	10.76
13828	BEEF, RIB, WHL (RIBS 6-12), LN&FAT, 1/8"FAT, CHOIC, CKD, BRLD	352	22.26	0	11.57
13829	BEEF, RIB, WHL (RIBS 6-12), LN&FAT, 1/8"FAT, CHOIC, CKD, RSTD	365	22.6	0	12.01
13827	BEEF, RIB, WHL (RIBS 6-12), LN&FAT, 1/8"FAT, CHOIC, RAW	322	16.34	0	11.51
13834	BEEF, RIB, WHL (RIBS 6-12), LN&FAT, 1/8"FAT, PRIME, CKD, BRLD	386	21.95	0	13.42
13835	BEEF, RIB, WHL (RIBS 6-12), LN&FAT, 1/8"FAT, PRIME, CKD, RSTD	400	22.57	0	13.96
13833	BEEF, RIB, WHL (RIBS 6-12), LN&FAT, 1/8"FAT, PRIME, RAW	355	16.15	0	13.22
13831	BEEF, RIB, WHL (RIBS 6-12), LN&FAT, 1/8"FAT, SEL, CKD, BRLD	315	22.73	0	9.81
13832	BEEF, RIB, WHL (RIBS 6-12), LN&FAT, 1/8"FAT, SEL, CKD, RSTD	330	23.1	0	10.32
13830	BEEF, RIB, WHL (RIBS 6-12), LN&FAT, 1/8"FAT, SEL, RAW	288	16.75	0	9.88
13593	BEEF, RIB, WHL (RIBS 6-12), LN, 1/2"FAT, PRIME, CKD, BRLD	280	26.03	0	7.97
13594	BEEF, RIB, WHL (RIBS 6-12), LN, 1/2"FAT, PRIME, CKD, RSTD	292	27.21	0	8.29
13088	BEEF, RIB, WHL (RIBS 6-12), LN, 1/4" FAT, CHOIC, CKD, RSTD	243	27.25	0	5.6
13084	BEEF, RIB, WHL (RIBS 6-12), LN, 1/4"FAT, ALL GRDS, CKD, BRLD	223	26.34	0	4.97
13085	BEEF, RIB, WHL (RIBS 6-12), LN, 1/4"FAT, ALL GRDS, CKD, RSTD	229	27.25	0	4.98
13083	BEEF, RIB, WHL (RIBS 6-12), LN, 1/4"FAT, ALL GRDS, RAW	160	19.83	0	3.35
13087	BEEF, RIB, WHL (RIBS 6-12), LN, 1/4"FAT, CHOIC, CKD, BRLD	237	26.34	0	5.62
13086	BEEF, RIB, WHL (RIBS 6-12), LN, 1/4"FAT, CHOIC, RAW	170	19.83	0	3.78
13093	BEEF, RIB, WHL (RIBS 6-12), LN, 1/4"FAT, PRIME, CKD, BRLD	280	26.03	0	7.98

NDB #	Food Description (100 gram portions = 3½ ounces = 20 tsp = ½ cup approx.	Calories	Protein	Carbs	Sat Fat
13094	BEEF, RIB, WHL (RIBS 6-12), LN, 1/4"FAT, PRIME, CKD, RSTD	292	27.21	0	8.31
13092	BEEF, RIB, WHL (RIBS 6-12), LN, 1/4"FAT, PRIME, RAW	206	19.83	0	5.69
13090	BEEF, RIB, WHL (RIBS 6-12), LN, 1/4"FAT, SEL, CKD, BRLD	206	26.33	0	4.23
13091	BEEF, RIB, WHL (RIBS 6-12), LN, 1/4"FAT, SEL, CKD, RSTD	213	27.25	0	4.26
13089	BEEF, RIB, WHL (RIBS 6-12), LN, 1/4"FAT, SEL, RAW	148	19.83	0	2.82
13398	BEEF, RND, BTTM RND, LN&FAT, 0"FAT, ALL GRDS, CKD, BRSD	213	31.17	0	3.08
13399	BEEF, RND, BTTM RND, LN&FAT, 0"FAT, ALL GRDS, CKD, RSTD	188	28.59	0	2.5
13401	BEEF, RND, BTTM RND, LN&FAT, 0"FAT, CHOIC, CKD, BRSD	227	30.96	0	3.7
13402	BEEF, RND, BTTM RND, LN&FAT, 0"FAT, CHOIC, CKD, RSTD	203	28.41	0	3.12
13404	BEEF, RND, BTTM RND, LN&FAT, 0"FAT, SEL, CKD, BRSD	201	31.17	0	2.65
13405	BEEF, RND, BTTM RND, LN&FAT, 0"FAT, SEL, CKD, RSTD	177	28.59	0	2.05
13666	BEEF, RND, BTTM RND, LN&FAT, 1/2"FAT, PRIME, CKD, BRSD	297	29.24	0	7.32
13665	BEEF, RND, BTTM RND, LN&FAT, 1/2"FAT, PRIME, RAW	225	20.13	0	6.29
13160	BEEF, RND, BTTM RND, LN&FAT, 1/4"FAT, ALL GRDS, CKD, BRSD	275	28.66	0	6.37
13397	BEEF, RND, BTTM RND, LN&FAT, 1/4"FAT, ALL GRDS, CKD, RSTD	248	26.6	0	5.63
13159	BEEF, RND, BTTM RND, LN&FAT, 1/4"FAT, ALL GRDS, RAW	208	20.23	0	5.21
13162	BEEF, RND, BTTM RND, LN&FAT, 1/4"FAT, CHOIC, CKD, BRSD	284	28.66	0	6.72
13400	BEEF, RND, BTTM RND, LN&FAT, 1/4"FAT, CHOIC, CKD, RSTD	260	26.42	0	6.16
13161	BEEF, RND, BTTM RND, LN&FAT, 1/4"FAT, CHOIC, RAW	218	20.09	0	5.7
13164	BEEF, RND, BTTM RND, LN&FAT, 1/4"FAT, SEL, CKD, BRSD	259	28.87	0	5.7
13403	BEEF, RND, BTTM RND, LN&FAT, 1/4"FAT, SEL, CKD, RSTD	234	26.78	0	5.01
13163	BEEF, RND, BTTM RND, LN&FAT, 1/4"FAT, SEL, RAW	195	20.37	0	4.67
13869	BEEF, RND, BTTM RND, LN&FAT, 1/8"FAT, ALL GRDS, CKD, BRSD	256	29.49	0	5.34
13870	BEEF, RND, BTTM RND, LN&FAT, 1/8"FAT, ALL GRDS, CKD, RSTD	229	27.3	0	4.63
13868	BEEF, RND, BTTM RND, LN&FAT, 1/8"FAT, ALL GRDS, RAW	191	20.65	0	4.37
13872	BEEF, RND, BTTM RND, LN&FAT, 1/8"FAT, CHOIC, CKD, BRSD	268	29.37	0	5.86
13873	BEEF, RND, BTTM RND, LN&FAT, 1/8"FAT, CHOIC, CKD, RSTD	241	27.14	0	5.14
13871	BEEF, RND, BTTM RND, LN&FAT, 1/8"FAT, CHOIC, RAW	200	20.58	0	4.72
13875	BEEF, RND, BTTM RND, LN&FAT, 1/8"FAT, SEL, CKD, BRSD	245	29.49	0	4.92
13876	BEEF, RND, BTTM RND, LN&FAT, 1/8"FAT, SEL, CKD, RSTD	219	27.32	0	4.22
13874	BEEF, RND, BTTM RND, LN&FAT, 1/8"FAT, SEL, RAW	181	20.72	0	3.95
13407	BEEF, RND, BTTM RND, LN, 0"FAT, ALL GRDS, CKD, BRSD	203	31.59	0	2.57
13408	BEEF, RND, BTTM RND, LN, 0"FAT, ALL GRDS, CKD, RSTD	183	28.77	0	2.24
13410	BEEF, RND, BTTM RND, LN, 0"FAT, CHOIC, CKD, BRSD	213	31.59	0	2.94
13411	BEEF, RND, BTTM RND, LN, 0"FAT, CHOIC, CKD, RSTD	193	28.77	0	2.61

NDB #	Food Description (100 gram portions = 3½ ounces = 20 tsp = ½ cup approx.	Calories	Protein	Carbs	Sat Fat
13413	BEEF, RND, BTTM RND, LN, 0"FAT, SEL, CKD, BRSD	192	31.59	0	2.13
13414	BEEF, RND, BTTM RND, LN, 0"FAT, SEL, CKD, RSTD	171	28.77	0	1.78
13674	BEEF, RND, BTTM RND, LN, 1/2"FAT, PRIME, CKD, BRSD	249	31.59	0	4.49
13673	BEEF, RND, BTTM RND, LN, 1/2"FAT, PRIME, RAW	159	21.87	0	2.61
13168	BEEF, RND, BTTM RND, LN, 1/4" FAT, ALL GRDS, CKD, BRSD	209	31.59	0	2.77
13406	BEEF, RND, BTTM RND, LN, 1/4"FAT, ALL GRDS, CKD, RSTD	189	28.77	0	2.51
13167	BEEF, RND, BTTM RND, LN, 1/4"FAT, ALL GRDS, RAW	144	21.87	0	1.91
13170	BEEF, RND, BTTM RND, LN, 1/4"FAT, CHOIC, CKD, BRSD	220	31.59	0	3.17
13409	BEEF, RND, BTTM RND, LN, 1/4"FAT, CHOIC, CKD, RSTD	198	28.77	0	2.83
13169	BEEF, RND, BTTM RND, LN, 1/4"FAT, CHOIC, RAW	150	21.87	0	2.15
13172	BEEF, RND, BTTM RND, LN, 1/4"FAT, SEL, CKD, BRSD	196	31.59	0	2.3
13412	BEEF, RND, BTTM RND, LN, 1/4"FAT, SEL, CKD, RSTD	179	28.77	0	2.11
13171	BEEF, RND, BTTM RND, LN, 1/4"FAT, SEL, RAW	136	21.87	0	1.6
13415	BEEF, RND, EYE OF RND, LN&FAT, 0"FAT, ALL GRDS, CKD, RSTD	171	28.8	0	1.97
13416	BEEF, RND, EYE OF RND, LN&FAT, 0"FAT, CHOIC, CKD, RSTD	180	28.8	0	2.33
13417	BEEF, RND, EYE OF RND, LN&FAT, 0"FAT, SEL, CKD, RSTD	161	28.8	0	1.54
13682	BEEF, RND, EYE OF RND, LN&FAT, 1/2"FAT, PRIME, CKD, RSTD	250	27.01	0	6.02
13681	BEEF, RND, EYE OF RND, LN&FAT, 1/2"FAT, PRIME, RAW	221	19.91	0	6.27
13176	BEEF, RND, EYE OF RND, LN&FAT, 1/4"FAT, ALL GRDS, CKD, RSTD	229	26.79	0	4.98
13175	BEEF, RND, EYE OF RND, LN&FAT, 1/4"FAT, ALL GRDS, RAW	213	19.72	0	5.68
13178	BEEF, RND, EYE OF RND, LN&FAT, 1/4"FAT, CHOIC, CKD, RSTD	241	26.6	0	5.5
13177	BEEF, RND, EYE OF RND, LN&FAT, 1/4"FAT, CHOIC, RAW	218	19.72	0	5.85
13180	BEEF, RND, EYE OF RND, LN&FAT, 1/4"FAT, SEL, CKD, RSTD	217	26.97	0	4.43
13179	BEEF, RND, EYE OF RND, LN&FAT, 1/4"FAT, SEL, RAW	202	19.85	0	5.19
13878	BEEF, RND, EYE OF RND, LN&FAT, 1/8"FAT, ALL GRDS, CKD, RSTD	194	28.07	0	3.11
13877	BEEF, RND, EYE OF RND, LN&FAT, 1/8"FAT, ALL GRDS, RAW	166	20.89	0	3.26
13880	BEEF, RND, EYE OF RND, LN&FAT, 1/8"FAT, CHOIC, CKD, RSTD	200	28.07	0	3.39
13879	BEEF, RND, EYE OF RND, LN&FAT, 1/8"FAT, CHOIC, RAW	173	20.85	0	3.53
13882	BEEF, RND, EYE OF RND, LN&FAT, 1/8"FAT, SEL, CKD, RSTD	186	28.07	0	2.8
13881	BEEF, RND, EYE OF RND, LN&FAT, 1/8"FAT, SEL, RAW	159	20.93	0	2.94
13418	BEEF, RND, EYE OF RND, LN, 0"FAT, ALL GRDS, CKD, RSTD	166	28.99	0	1.7
13419	BEEF, RND, EYE OF RND, LN, 0"FAT, CHOIC, CKD, RSTD	175	28.99	0	2.07
13420	BEEF, RND, EYE OF RND, LN, 0"FAT, SEL, CKD, RSTD	155	28.99	0	1.27
13690	BEEF, RND, EYE OF RND, LN, 1/2"FAT, PRIME, CKD, RSTD	198	28.99	0	3.16
13689	BEEF, RND, EYE OF RND, LN, 1/2"FAT, PRIME, RAW	149	21.75	0	2.28

NDB #	Food Description (100 gram portions = 3½ ounces = 20 tsp = ½ cup approx.	Calories	Protein	Carbs	Sat Fat
13184	BEEF, RND, EYE OF RND, LN, 1/4" FAT, ALL GRDS, CKD, RSTD	168	28.99	0	1.78
13183	BEEF, RND, EYE OF RND, LN, 1/4"FAT, ALL GRDS, RAW	132	21.75	0	1.48
13186	BEEF, RND, EYE OF RND, LN, 1/4"FAT, CHOIC, CKD, RSTD	175	28.99	0	2.07
13185	BEEF, RND, EYE OF RND, LN, 1/4"FAT, CHOIC, RAW	137	21.75	0	1.69
13188	BEEF, RND, EYE OF RND, LN, 1/4"FAT, SEL, CKD, RSTD	160	28.99	0	1.45
13187	BEEF, RND, EYE OF RND, LN, 1/4"FAT, SEL, RAW	125	21.75	0	1.24
13152	BEEF, RND, FULL CUT, LN&FAT, 1/4"FAT, CHOIC, CKD, BRLD	240	27.35	0	5.16
13151	BEEF, RND, FULL CUT, LN&FAT, 1/4"FAT, CHOIC, RAW	203	20.37	0	5
13154	BEEF, RND, FULL CUT, LN&FAT, 1/4"FAT, SEL, CKD, BRLD	223	27.39	0	4.13
13153	BEEF, RND, FULL CUT, LN&FAT, 1/4"FAT, SEL, RAW	191	20.37	0	4.59
13865	BEEF, RND, FULL CUT, LN&FAT, 1/8"FAT, CHOIC, CKD, BRLD	235	27.54	0	4.9
13864	BEEF, RND, FULL CUT, LN&FAT, 1/8"FAT, CHOIC, RAW	195	20.56	0	4.63
13867	BEEF, RND, FULL CUT, LN&FAT, 1/8"FAT, SEL, CKD, BRLD	218	27.58	0	4.23
13866	BEEF, RND, FULL CUT, LN&FAT, 1/8"FAT, SEL, RAW	184	20.56	0	4.2
13155	BEEF, RND, FULL CUT, LN, 1/4" FAT, CHOIC, RAW	138	22.03	0	1.67
13156	BEEF, RND, FULL CUT, LN, 1/4"FAT, CHOIC, CKD, BRLD	191	29.21	0	2.56
13158	BEEF, RND, FULL CUT, LN, 1/4"FAT, SEL, CKD, BRLD	172	29.25	0	1.83
13157	BEEF, RND, FULL CUT, LN, 1/4"FAT, SEL, RAW	126	22.03	0	1.2
13196	BEEF, RND, TIP RND, LN & FAT, 1/4" FAT, SEL, CKD, RSTD	225	27.09	0	4.6
13421	BEEF, RND, TIP RND, LN&FAT, 0"FAT, ALL GRDS, CKD, RSTD	191	28.17	0	2.86
13422	BEEF, RND, TIP RND, LN&FAT, 0"FAT, CHOIC, CKD, RSTD	200	27.99	0	3.29
13423	BEEF, RND, TIP RND, LN&FAT, 0"FAT, SEL, CKD, RSTD	186	28.17	0	2.65
13698	BEEF, RND, TIP RND, LN&FAT, 1/2"FAT, PRIME, CKD, RSTD	284	25.96	0	7.64
13697	BEEF, RND, TIP RND, LN&FAT, 1/2"FAT, PRIME, RAW	223	19.14	0	6.71
13192	BEEF, RND, TIP RND, LN&FAT, 1/4"FAT, ALL GRDS, CKD, RSTD	234	26.91	0	5.02
13191	BEEF, RND, TIP RND, LN&FAT, 1/4"FAT, ALL GRDS, RAW	201	19.31	0	5.24
13194	BEEF, RND, TIP RND, LN&FAT, 1/4"FAT, CHOIC, CKD, RSTD	247	26.54	0	5.67
13193	BEEF, RND, TIP RND, LN&FAT, 1/4"FAT, CHOIC, RAW	212	19.18	0	5.69
13198	BEEF, RND, TIP RND, LN&FAT, 1/4"FAT, PRIME, CKD, RSTD	274	26.36	0	6.92
13197	BEEF, RND, TIP RND, LN&FAT, 1/4"FAT, PRIME, RAW	214	19.44	0	5.75
13195	BEEF, RND, TIP RND, LN&FAT, 1/4"FAT, SEL, RAW	186	19.56	0	4.49
13884	BEEF, RND, TIP RND, LN&FAT, 1/8"FAT, ALL GRDS, CKD, RSTD	219	27.45	0	4.24
13883	BEEF, RND, TIP RND, LN&FAT, 1/8"FAT, ALL GRDS, RAW	189	19.6	0	4.6
13886	BEEF, RND, TIP RND, LN&FAT, 1/8"FAT, CHOIC, CKD, RSTD	228	27.27	0	4.63
13885	BEEF, RND, TIP RND, LN&FAT, 1/8"FAT, CHOIC, RAW	199	19.48	0	5.04

NDB #	Food Description (100 gram portions = 3½ ounces = 20 tsp = ½ cup approx.	Calories	Protein	Carbs	Sat Fat
13888	BEEF, RND, TIP RND, LN&FAT, 1/8"FAT, SEL, CKD, RSTD	210	27.63	0	3.81
13887	BEEF, RND, TIP RND, LN&FAT, 1/8"FAT, SEL, RAW	178	19.74	0	4.1
13424	BEEF, RND, TIP RND, LN, 0"FAT, ALL GRDS, CKD, RSTD	176	28.71	0	2.06
13425	BEEF, RND, TIP RND, LN, 0"FAT, CHOIC, CKD, RSTD	180	28.71	0	2.24
13426	BEEF, RND, TIP RND, LN, 0"FAT, SEL, CKD, RSTD	170	28.71	0	1.85
13706	BEEF, RND, TIP RND, LN, 1/2"FAT, PRIME, CKD, RSTD	213	28.71	0	3.69
13200	BEEF, RND, TIP RND, LN, 1/4" FAT, ALL GRDS, CKD, RSTD	185	28.71	0	2.41
13202	BEEF, RND, TIP RND, LN, 1/4" FAT, CHOIC, CKD, RSTD	188	28.71	0	2.55
13199	BEEF, RND, TIP RND, LN, 1/4"FAT, ALL GRDS, RAW	124	21.11	0	1.29
13201	BEEF, RND, TIP RND, LN, 1/4"FAT, CHOIC, RAW	130	21.11	0	1.5
13206	BEEF, RND, TIP RND, LN, 1/4"FAT, PRIME, CKD, RSTD	213	28.71	0	3.69
13205	BEEF, RND, TIP RND, LN, 1/4"FAT, PRIME, RAW	146	21.11	0	2.21
13203	BEEF, RND, TIP RND, LN, 1/4"FAT, SEL, RAW	119	21.11	0	1.09
13428	BEEF, RND, TOP RND, LN&FAT, 0"FAT, ALL GRDS, CKD, BRSD	209	35.62	0	2.25
13430	BEEF, RND, TOP RND, LN&FAT, 0"FAT, CHOIC, CKD, BRSD	216	35.62	0	2.52
13432	BEEF, RND, TOP RND, LN&FAT, 0"FAT, SEL, CKD, BRSD	200	35.62	0	1.92
13715	BEEF, RND, TOP RND, LN&FAT, 1/2"FAT, PRIME, CKD, BRLD	237	30.73	0	4.32
13714	BEEF, RND, TOP RND, LN&FAT, 1/2"FAT, PRIME, RAW	188	21.81	0	4.28
13208	BEEF, RND, TOP RND, LN&FAT, 1/4"FAT, ALL GRDS, CKD, BRLD	216	30.17	0	3.62
13427	BEEF, RND, TOP RND, LN&FAT, 1/4"FAT, ALL GRDS, CKD, BRSD	248	33.83	0	4.32
13207	BEEF, RND, TOP RND, LN&FAT, 1/4"FAT, ALL GRDS, RAW	176	21.48	0	3.68
13210	BEEF, RND, TOP RND, LN&FAT, 1/4"FAT, CHOIC, CKD, BRLD	224	30.17	0	3.94
13429	BEEF, RND, TOP RND, LN&FAT, 1/4"FAT, CHOIC, CKD, BRSD	260	33.58	0	4.86
13211	BEEF, RND, TOP RND, LN&FAT, 1/4"FAT, CHOIC, CKD, PAN-FRIED	277	32.38	0	5.29
13209	BEEF, RND, TOP RND, LN&FAT, 1/4"FAT, CHOIC, RAW	181	21.48	0	3.87
13215	BEEF, RND, TOP RND, LN&FAT, 1/4"FAT, PRIME, CKD, BRLD	229	31.06	0	3.86
13214	BEEF, RND, TOP RND, LN&FAT, 1/4"FAT, PRIME, RAW	180	22.06	0	3.63
13213	BEEF, RND, TOP RND, LN&FAT, 1/4"FAT, SEL, CKD, BRLD	206	30.17	0	3.24
13431	BEEF, RND, TOP RND, LN&FAT, 1/4"FAT, SEL, CKD, BRSD	234	34.09	0	3.73
13212	BEEF, RND, TOP RND, LN&FAT, 1/4"FAT, SEL, RAW	164	21.62	0	3.14
13893	BEEF, RND, TOP RND, LN&FAT, 1/8"FAT, ALL GRDS, CKD, BRLD	207	30.53	0	3.16
13892	BEEF, RND, TOP RND, LN&FAT, 1/8"FAT, ALL GRDS, CKD, BRSD	238	34.34	0	3.78
13891	BEEF, RND, TOP RND, LN&FAT, 1/8"FAT, ALL GRDS, RAW	163	21.83	0	3
13896	BEEF, RND, TOP RND, LN&FAT, 1/8"FAT, CHOIC, CKD, BRLD	216	30.53	0	3.48
13895	BEEF, RND, TOP RND, LN&FAT, 1/8"FAT, CHOIC, CKD, BRSD	250	34.09	0	4.33

NDB #	Food Description (100 gram portions = 3½ ounces = 20 tsp = ½ cup approx.	Calories	Protein	Carbs	Sat Fat
13897	BEEF, RND, TOP RND, LN&FAT, 1/8"FAT, CHOIC, CKD, PAN-FRIED	266	32.99	0	4.64
13894	BEEF, RND, TOP RND, LN&FAT, 1/8"FAT, CHOIC, RAW	169	21.81	0	3.22
13902	BEEF, RND, TOP RND, LN&FAT, 1/8"FAT, PRIME, CKD, BRLD	225	31.27	0	3.61
13901	BEEF, RND, TOP RND, LN&FAT, 1/8"FAT, PRIME, RAW	173	22.24	0	3.3
13900	BEEF, RND, TOP RND, LN&FAT, 1/8"FAT, SEL, CKD, BRLD	196	30.55	0	2.74
13899	BEEF, RND, TOP RND, LN&FAT, 1/8"FAT, SEL, CKD, BRSD	225	34.6	0	3.2
13898	BEEF, RND, TOP RND, LN&FAT, 1/8"FAT, SEL, RAW	156	21.85	0	2.7
13434	BEEF, RND, TOP RND, LN, 0"FAT, ALL GRDS, CKD, BRSD	199	36.12	0	1.72
13436	BEEF, RND, TOP RND, LN, 0"FAT, CHOIC, CKD, BRSD	207	36.12	0	1.99
13438	BEEF, RND, TOP RND, LN, 0"FAT, SEL, CKD, BRSD	190	36.12	0	1.37
13724	BEEF, RND, TOP RND, LN, 1/2"FAT, PRIME, CKD, BRLD	215	31.69	0	3.1
13217	BEEF, RND, TOP RND, LN, 1/4" FAT, ALL GRDS, CKD, BRLD	180	31.69	0	1.68
13220	BEEF, RND, TOP RND, LN, 1/4" FAT, CHOIC, CKD, PAN-FRIED	227	35.07	0	2.42
13433	BEEF, RND, TOP RND, LN, 1/4"FAT, ALL GRDS, CKD, BRSD	205	36.12	0	1.92
13216	BEEF, RND, TOP RND, LN, 1/4"FAT, ALL GRDS, RAW	127	22.79	0	1.13
13219	BEEF, RND, TOP RND, LN, 1/4"FAT, CHOIC, CKD, BRLD	189	31.69	0	2.03
13435	BEEF, RND, TOP RND, LN, 1/4"FAT, CHOIC, CKD, BRSD	213	36.12	0	2.23
13218	BEEF, RND, TOP RND, LN, 1/4"FAT, CHOIC, RAW	132	22.79	0	1.34
13224	BEEF, RND, TOP RND, LN, 1/4"FAT, PRIME, CKD, BRLD	215	31.69	0	3.1
13223	BEEF, RND, TOP RND, LN, 1/4"FAT, PRIME, RAW	153	22.79	0	2.27
13222	BEEF, RND, TOP RND, LN, 1/4"FAT, SEL, CKD, BRLD	169	31.69	0	1.27
13437	BEEF, RND, TOP RND, LN, 1/4"FAT, SEL, CKD, BRSD	196	36.12	0	1.58
13221	BEEF, RND, TOP RND, LN, 1/4"FAT, SEL, RAW	120	22.79	0	0.86
13020	BEEF, RTL CUTS, FAT, CKD	680	10.65	0	28.5
13019	BEEF, RTL CUTS, FAT, RAW	674	8.21	0	29.45
13226	BEEF, SHANK CROSSCUTS, LN&FAT, 1/4"FAT, CHOIC, CKD, SIMMRD	263	30.69	0	5.7
13225	BEEF, SHANK CROSSCUTS, LN&FAT, 1/4"FAT, CHOIC, RAW	177	20.53	0	3.81
13228	BEEF, SHANK CROSSCUTS, LN, 1/4"FAT, CHOIC, CKD, SIMMRD	201	33.68	0	2.29
13227	BEEF, SHANK CROSSCUTS, LN, 1/4"FAT, CHOIC, RAW	128	21.75	0	1.28
13457	BEEF, SHRT LOIN, PRTRHS STEAK, LN & FAT, 1/4" FAT, ALL GRDS, RA	238	19.21	0	6.844
13229	BEEF, SHRT LOIN, PRTRHS STEAK, LN & FAT, 1/4" FAT, USDA CHOIC,	250	18.17	0	7.539
13461	BEEF, SHRT LOIN, PRTRHS STEAK, LN & FAT, 1/4" FAT, USDA SEL, RA	222	20.73	0	5.83
13470	BEEF, SHRT LOIN, PRTRHS STEAK, LN ONLY, 0" FAT, USDA SEL, CKD,	194	26.89	0	3.28
13468	BEEF, SHRT LOIN, PRTRHS STEAK, LN ONLY, TO 1/4" FAT, USDA SEL,	149	22.75	0	2.02
23002	BEEF, SHRT LOIN, PRTRHS STEAK, LN&FAT, 1/8"FAT, ALL GRDS, CKD,	297	23.51	0	8.42

NDB #	Food Description (100 gram portions = 3½ ounces = 20 tsp = ½ cup approx.	Calories	Protein	Carbs	Sat Fat
23001	BEEF, SHRT LOIN, PRTRHS STEAK, LN&FAT, 1/8"FAT, ALL GRDS, RAW	247	18.8	0	7.42
13906	BEEF, SHRT LOIN, PRTRHS STEAK, LN&FAT, 1/8"FAT, CHOIC, CKD, BR	299	23.27	0	8.45
13905	BEEF, SHRT LOIN, PRTRHS STEAK, LN&FAT, 1/8"FAT, CHOIC, RAW	258	17.98	0	8.02
23004	BEEF, SHRT LOIN, PRTRHS STEAK, LN&FAT, 1/8"FAT, SEL, CKD, BRLD	294	24.05	0	8.34
23003	BEEF, SHRT LOIN, PRTRHS STEAK, LN&FAT, 1/8"FAT, SEL, RAW	222	20.72	0	6.01
13467	BEEF, SHRT LOIN, PRTRHS STEAK, LN, 0" FAT, USDA CHOIC, CKD, BR	224	25.51	0	4.345
13231	BEEF, SHRT LOIN, PRTRHS STEAK, LN, 1/4" FAT, USDA CHOIC, RAW	160	20.27	0	2.93
13466	BEEF, SHRT LOIN, PRTRHS STEAK, LN, 0" FAT, ALL GRDS, CKD, BRLD	212	26.07	0	3.912
13465	BEEF, SHRT LOIN, PRTRHS STEAK, LN, 1/4" FAT, ALL GRDS, CKD, BRL	210	26.51	0	3.944
13464	BEEF, SHRT LOIN, PRTRHS STEAK, LN, 1/4" FAT, ALL GRDS, RAW	156	21.28	0	2.56
13232	BEEF, SHRT LOIN, PRTRHS STEAK, LN, 1/4" FAT, USDA CHOIC, CKD, B	215	26.04	0	3.96
13469	BEEF, SHRT LOIN, PRTRHS STEAK, LN, 1/4" FAT, USDA SEL, CKD, BRL	203	27.2	0	3.92
13459	BEEF, SHRT LOIN, PRTRHS STK, LN & FAT, 0" FAT, ALL GRDS, CKD, B	276	23.96	0	7.271
13463	BEEF, SHRT LOIN, PRTRHS STK, LN & FAT, 0" FAT, USDA SEL, CKD, B	267	24.47	0	7.04
13471	BEEF, SHRT LOIN, T-BONE STEAK, LN & FAT, 1/4" FAT, ALL GRDS, RA	212	19.39	0	5.566
13233	BEEF, SHRT LOIN, T-BONE STEAK, LN & FAT, 1/4" FAT, USDA CHOIC, R	221	19.17	0	5.838
13475	BEEF, SHRT LOIN, T-BONE STEAK, LN & FAT, 1/4" FAT, USDA SEL, RA	199	19.71	0	5.169
13482	BEEF, SHRT LOIN, T-BONE STEAK, LN ONLY, TO 1/4" FAT, USDA SEL,	132	21.33	0	1.76
23006	BEEF, SHRT LOIN, T-BONE STEAK, LN&FAT, 1/8"FAT, ALL GRDS, CKD,	280	24.33	0	7.56
23005	BEEF, SHRT LOIN, T-BONE STEAK, LN&FAT, 1/8"FAT, ALL GRDS, RAW	220	19.19	0	6.14
13908	BEEF, SHRT LOIN, T-BONE STEAK, LN&FAT, 1/8"FAT, CHOIC, CKD, BR	286	24.04	0	7.83
13907	BEEF, SHRT LOIN, T-BONE STEAK, LN&FAT, 1/8"FAT, CHOIC, RAW	232	18.9	0	6.7
23008	BEEF, SHRT LOIN, T-BONE STEAK, LN&FAT, 1/8"FAT, SEL, CKD, BRLD	265	25.01	0	6.91
23007	BEEF, SHRT LOIN, T-BONE STEAK, LN&FAT, 1/8"FAT, SEL, RAW	192	19.89	0	4.81
13484	BEEF, SHRT LOIN, T-BONE STEAK, LN, 0" FAT, USDA SEL, CKD, BRLD	177	26	0	2.82
13480	BEEF, SHRT LOIN, T-BONE STEAK, LN, 0" FAT, ALL GRDS, CKD, BRLD	189	25.99	0	3.087
13481	BEEF, SHRT LOIN, T-BONE STEAK, LN, 0" FAT, USDA CHOIC, CKD, BR	198	25.98	0	3.27
13479	BEEF, SHRT LOIN, T-BONE STEAK, LN, 1/4" FAT, ALL GRDS, CKD, BRL	202	27.01	0	3.488
13478	BEEF, SHRT LOIN, T-BONE STEAK, LN, 1/4" FAT, ALL GRDS, RAW	145	21	0	2.125
13236	BEEF, SHRT LOIN, T-BONE STEAK, LN, 1/4" FAT, USDA CHOIC, CKD, B	205	26.78	0	3.59
13235	BEEF, SHRT LOIN, T-BONE STEAK, LN, 1/4" FAT, USDA CHOIC, RAW	154	20.78	0	2.375
13483	BEEF, SHRT LOIN, T-BONE STEAK, LN, 1/4" FAT, USDA SEL, CKD, BRL	198	27.35	0	3.34
13473	BEEF, SHRT LOIN, T-BONE STK, LN & FAT, 0" FAT, ALL GRDS, CKD, BR	247	24.18	0	6.074
13477	BEEF, SHRT LOIN, T-BONE STK, LN & FAT, 0" FAT, USDA SEL, CKD, BR	230	24.38	0	5.527
13747	BEEF, SHRT LOIN, TENDERLOIN, LN&FAT, 1/2"FAT, PRIME, CKD, BRLD	318	24.89	0	9.59

NDB #	Food Description (100 gram portions = 3½ ounces = 20 tsp = ½ cup approx.	Calories	Protein	Carbs	Sat Fat
13748	BEEF, SHRT LOIN, TENDERLOIN, LN&FAT, 1/2"FAT, PRIME, CKD, RSTD	358	23.44	0	11.74
13746	BEEF, SHRT LOIN, TENDERLOIN, LN&FAT, 1/2"FAT, PRIME, RAW	288	17.8	0	10.04
13759	BEEF, SHRT LOIN, TENDERLOIN, LN, 1/2"FAT, PRIME, CKD, BRLD	232	28.25	0	4.83
13760	BEEF, SHRT LOIN, TENDERLOIN, LN, 1/2"FAT, PRIME, CKD, RSTD	255	27.54	0	5.97
13445	BEEF, SHRT LOIN, TOP LOIN, LN&FAT, 0"FAT, ALL GRDS, CKD, BRLD	212	28.08	0	3.96
13446	BEEF, SHRT LOIN, TOP LOIN, LN&FAT, 0"FAT, CHOIC, CKD, BRLD	228	27.9	0	4.66
13447	BEEF, SHRT LOIN, TOP LOIN, LN&FAT, 0"FAT, SEL, CKD, BRLD	199	28.08	0	3.41
13768	BEEF, SHRT LOIN, TOP LOIN, LN&FAT, 1/2"FAT, PRIME, CKD, BRLD	339	24.72	0	10.72
13767	BEEF, SHRT LOIN, TOP LOIN, LN&FAT, 1/2"FAT, PRIME, RAW	322	17.87	0	11.69
13262	BEEF, SHRT LOIN, TOP LOIN, LN&FAT, 1/4"FAT, ALL GRDS, CKD, BRLD	287	25.56	0	7.82
13264	BEEF, SHRT LOIN, TOP LOIN, LN&FAT, 1/4"FAT, CHOIC, CKD, BRLD	298	25.38	0	8.31
13263	BEEF, SHRT LOIN, TOP LOIN, LN&FAT, 1/4"FAT, CHOIC, RAW	260	18.73	0	8.1
13268	BEEF, SHRT LOIN, TOP LOIN, LN&FAT, 1/4"FAT, PRIME, CKD, BRLD	323	25.38	0	9.6
13267	BEEF, SHRT LOIN, TOP LOIN, LN&FAT, 1/4"FAT, PRIME, RAW	305	18.33	0	10.33
13266	BEEF, SHRT LOIN, TOP LOIN, LN&FAT, 1/4"FAT, SEL, CKD, BRLD	266	25.92	0	6.8
13265	BEEF, SHRT LOIN, TOP LOIN, LN&FAT, 1/4"FAT, SEL, RAW	230	19.13	0	6.7
13910	BEEF, SHRT LOIN, TOP LOIN, LN&FAT, 1/8"FAT, ALL GRDS, CKD, BRLD	268	26.28	0	6.83
13909	BEEF, SHRT LOIN, TOP LOIN, LN&FAT, 1/8"FAT, ALL GRDS, RAW	224	19.46	0	6.34
13912	BEEF, SHRT LOIN, TOP LOIN, LN&FAT, 1/8"FAT, CHOIC, CKD, BRLD	284	25.92	0	7.57
13911	BEEF, SHRT LOIN, TOP LOIN, LN&FAT, 1/8"FAT, CHOIC, RAW	237	19.32	0	6.91
13916	BEEF, SHRT LOIN, TOP LOIN, LN&FAT, 1/8"FAT, PRIME, CKD, BRLD	310	25.92	0	8.91
13915	BEEF, SHRT LOIN, TOP LOIN, LN&FAT, 1/8"FAT, PRIME, RAW	281	19	0	9.08
13914	BEEF, SHRT LOIN, TOP LOIN, LN&FAT, 1/8"FAT, SEL, CKD, BRLD	253	26.39	0	6.14
13913	BEEF, SHRT LOIN, TOP LOIN, LN&FAT, 1/8"FAT, SEL, RAW	211	19.61	0	5.72
13448	BEEF, SHRT LOIN, TOP LOIN, LN, 0"FAT, ALL GRDS, CKD, BRLD	198	28.62	0	3.2
13449	BEEF, SHRT LOIN, TOP LOIN, LN, 0"FAT, CHOIC, CKD, BRLD	209	28.62	0	3.66
13450	BEEF, SHRT LOIN, TOP LOIN, LN, 0"FAT, SEL, CKD, BRLD	184	28.62	0	2.63
13776	BEEF, SHRT LOIN, TOP LOIN, LN, 1/2"FAT, PRIME, CKD, BRLD	245	28.62	0	5.45
13270	BEEF, SHRT LOIN, TOP LOIN, LN, 1/4"FAT, ALL GRDS, CKD, BRLD	207	28.62	0	3.59
13269	BEEF, SHRT LOIN, TOP LOIN, LN, 1/4"FAT, ALL GRDS, RAW	142	21.53	0	2.09
13272	BEEF, SHRT LOIN, TOP LOIN, LN, 1/4"FAT, CHOIC, CKD, BRLD	214	28.62	0	3.87
13271	BEEF, SHRT LOIN, TOP LOIN, LN, 1/4"FAT, CHOIC, RAW	150	21.53	0	2.43
13276	BEEF, SHRT LOIN, TOP LOIN, LN, 1/4"FAT, PRIME, CKD, BRLD	245	28.62	0	5.45
13275	BEEF, SHRT LOIN, TOP LOIN, LN, 1/4"FAT, PRIME, RAW	189	21.53	0	4.29
13274	BEEF, SHRT LOIN, TOP LOIN, LN, 1/4"FAT, SEL, CKD, BRLD	193	28.62	0	2.98

NDB #	Food Description (100 gram portions = 3½ ounces = 20 tsp = ½ cup approx.	Calories	Protein	Carbs	Sat Fat
13273	BEEF, SHRT LOIN, TOP LOIN, LN, 1/4"FAT, SEL, RAW	133	21.53	0	1.71
23545	BEEF, SIRLOIN, TRI-TIP STK, LN & FAT, 0" FAT, ALL GRDS, CKD, BRLD	265	29.97	0	5.707
13342	BEEF, SNDWCH STEAKS, FLAKED, CHOPD, FORMED & THINLY SLICE	309	16.5	0	11.538
13439	BEEF, TENDERLOIN, LN&FAT, 0"FAT, ALL GRDS, CKD, BRLD	235	27.19	0	5.05
13440	BEEF, TENDERLOIN, LN&FAT, 0"FAT, CHOIC, CKD, BRLD	244	27.02	0	5.51
13441	BEEF, TENDERLOIN, LN&FAT, 0"FAT, SEL, CKD, BRLD	229	27.19	0	4.8
13238	BEEF, TENDERLOIN, LN&FAT, 1/4"FAT, ALL GRDS, CKD, BRLD	291	25.26	0	7.95
13239	BEEF, TENDERLOIN, LN&FAT, 1/4"FAT, ALL GRDS, CKD, RSTD	332	23.61	0	10.13
13237	BEEF, TENDERLOIN, LN&FAT, 1/4"FAT, ALL GRDS, RAW	283	17.76	0	9.31
13241	BEEF, TENDERLOIN, LN&FAT, 1/4"FAT, CHOIC, CKD, BRLD	304	25.08	0	8.56
13242	BEEF, TENDERLOIN, LN&FAT, 1/4"FAT, CHOIC, CKD, RSTD	339	23.61	0	10.42
13240	BEEF, TENDERLOIN, LN&FAT, 1/4"FAT, CHOIC, RAW	288	17.76	0	9.51
13247	BEEF, TENDERLOIN, LN&FAT, 1/4"FAT, PRIME, CKD, BRLD	317	24.91	0	9.33
13248	BEEF, TENDERLOIN, LN&FAT, 1/4"FAT, PRIME, CKD, RSTD	353	23.67	0	11.13
13246	BEEF, TENDERLOIN, LN&FAT, 1/4"FAT, PRIME, RAW	284	17.9	0	9.47
13244	BEEF, TENDERLOIN, LN&FAT, 1/4"FAT, SEL, CKD, BRLD	271	25.61	0	7.04
13245	BEEF, TENDERLOIN, LN&FAT, 1/4"FAT, SEL, CKD, RSTD	324	23.61	0	9.8
13243	BEEF, TENDERLOIN, LN&FAT, 1/4"FAT, SEL, RAW	278	17.76	0	9.09
13918	BEEF, TENDERLOIN, LN&FAT, 1/8"FAT, ALL GRDS, CKD, BRLD	281	25.61	0	7.45
13919	BEEF, TENDERLOIN, LN&FAT, 1/8"FAT, ALL GRDS, CKD, RSTD	324	23.9	0	9.72
13917	BEEF, TENDERLOIN, LN&FAT, 1/8"FAT, ALL GRDS, RAW	273	18.03	0	8.76
13921	BEEF, TENDERLOIN, LN&FAT, 1/8"FAT, CHOIC, CKD, BRLD	295	25.43	0	8.08
13922	BEEF, TENDERLOIN, LN&FAT, 1/8"FAT, CHOIC, CKD, RSTD	331	23.9	0	10.02
13920	BEEF, TENDERLOIN, LN&FAT, 1/8"FAT, CHOIC, RAW	277	18.03	0	8.96
13927	BEEF, TENDERLOIN, LN&FAT, 1/8"FAT, PRIME, CKD, BRLD	308	25.26	0	8.85
13928	BEEF, TENDERLOIN, LN&FAT, 1/8"FAT, PRIME, CKD, RSTD	343	24.04	0	10.63
13926	BEEF, TENDERLOIN, LN&FAT, 1/8"FAT, PRIME, RAW	274	18.15	0	8.96
13924	BEEF, TENDERLOIN, LN&FAT, 1/8"FAT, SEL, CKD, BRLD	266	25.79	0	6.79
13925	BEEF, TENDERLOIN, LN&FAT, 1/8"FAT, SEL, CKD, RSTD	316	23.9	0	9.38
13923	BEEF, TENDERLOIN, LN&FAT, 1/8"FAT, SEL, RAW	267	18.02	0	8.54
13442	BEEF, TENDERLOIN, LN, 0"FAT, ALL GRDS, CKD, BRLD	206	28.25	0	3.55
13443	BEEF, TENDERLOIN, LN, 0"FAT, CHOIC, CKD, BRLD	212	28.25	0	3.78
13444	BEEF, TENDERLOIN, LN, 0"FAT, SEL, CKD, BRLD	200	28.25	0	3.29
13251	BEEF, TENDERLOIN, LN, 1/4" FAT, ALL GRDS, CKD, RSTD	222	27.71	0	4.33
13250	BEEF, TENDERLOIN, LN, 1/4"FAT, ALL GRDS, CKD, BRLD	211	28.25	0	3.74

NDB #	Food Description (100 gram portions = 3½ ounces = 20 tsp = ½ cup approx.	Calories	Protein	Carbs	Sat Fat
13249	BEEF, TENDERLOIN, LN, 1/4"FAT, ALL GRDS, RAW	160	20.78	0	2.95
13253	BEEF, TENDERLOIN, LN, 1/4"FAT, CHOIC, CKD, BRLD	222	28.25	0	4.19
13254	BEEF, TENDERLOIN, LN, 1/4"FAT, CHOIC, CKD, RSTD	231	27.71	0	4.72
13252	BEEF, TENDERLOIN, LN, 1/4"FAT, CHOIC, RAW	166	20.78	0	3.22
13259	BEEF, TENDERLOIN, LN, 1/4"FAT, PRIME, CKD, BRLD	232	28.25	0	4.83
13260	BEEF, TENDERLOIN, LN, 1/4"FAT, PRIME, CKD, RSTD	255	27.54	0	5.97
13258	BEEF, TENDERLOIN, LN, 1/4"FAT, PRIME, RAW	169	20.78	0	3.54
13256	BEEF, TENDERLOIN, LN, 1/4"FAT, SEL, CKD, BRLD	199	28.25	0	3.25
13257	BEEF, TENDERLOIN, LN, 1/4"FAT, SEL, CKD, RSTD	211	27.71	0	3.89
13255	BEEF, TENDERLOIN, LN, 1/4"FAT, SEL, RAW	153	20.78	0	2.65
13261	BEEF, TOP LOIN, LN&FAT, 1/4"FAT, ALL GRDS, RAW	243	19	0	7.29
13451	BEEF, TOP SIRLOIN, LN&FAT, 0"FAT, ALL GRDS, CKD, BRLD	215	29.38	0	3.94
13452	BEEF, TOP SIRLOIN, LN&FAT, 0"FAT, CHOIC, CKD, BRLD	229	29.19	0	4.56
13453	BEEF, TOP SIRLOIN, LN&FAT, 0"FAT, SEL, CKD, BRLD	195	29.7	0	3
13278	BEEF, TOP SIRLOIN, LN&FAT, 1/4"FAT, ALL GRDS, CKD, BRLD	258	27.81	0	6.14
13277	BEEF, TOP SIRLOIN, LN&FAT, 1/4"FAT, ALL GRDS, RAW	217	19.15	0	6.01
13280	BEEF, TOP SIRLOIN, LN&FAT, 1/4"FAT, CHOIC, CKD, BRLD	269	27.61	0	6.67
13281	BEEF, TOP SIRLOIN, LN&FAT, 1/4"FAT, CHOIC, CKD, PAN-FRIED	326	28.11	0	8.91
13279	BEEF, TOP SIRLOIN, LN&FAT, 1/4"FAT, CHOIC, RAW	227	19.02	0	6.46
13283	BEEF, TOP SIRLOIN, LN&FAT, 1/4"FAT, SEL, CKD, BRLD	245	28	0	5.54
13282	BEEF, TOP SIRLOIN, LN&FAT, 1/4"FAT, SEL, RAW	207	19.28	0	5.52
13930	BEEF, TOP SIRLOIN, LN&FAT, 1/8"FAT, ALL GRDS, CKD, BRLD	248	28.2	0	5.63
13929	BEEF, TOP SIRLOIN, LN&FAT, 1/8"FAT, ALL GRDS, RAW	204	19.47	0	5.32
13932	BEEF, TOP SIRLOIN, LN&FAT, 1/8"FAT, CHOIC, CKD, BRLD	259	28	0	6.16
13933	BEEF, TOP SIRLOIN, LN&FAT, 1/8"FAT, CHOIC, CKD, PAN-FRIED	313	28.77	0	8.18
13931	BEEF, TOP SIRLOIN, LN&FAT, 1/8"FAT, CHOIC, RAW	213	19.37	0	5.73
13935	BEEF, TOP SIRLOIN, LN&FAT, 1/8"FAT, SEL, CKD, BRLD	240	28.2	0	5.28
13934	BEEF, TOP SIRLOIN, LN&FAT, 1/8"FAT, SEL, RAW	193	19.6	0	4.85
13454	BEEF, TOP SIRLOIN, LN, 0"FAT, ALL GRDS, CKD, BRLD	191	30.37	0	2.65
13455	BEEF, TOP SIRLOIN, LN, 0"FAT, CHOIC, CKD, BRLD	200	30.37	0	3.04
13456	BEEF, TOP SIRLOIN, LN, 0"FAT, SEL, CKD, BRLD	180	30.37	0	2.18
13287	BEEF, TOP SIRLOIN, LN, 1/4"FAT, ALL GRDS, CKD, BRLD	195	30.37	0	2.8
13286	BEEF, TOP SIRLOIN, LN, 1/4"FAT, ALL GRDS, RAW	130	21.24	0	1.54
13289	BEEF, TOP SIRLOIN, LN, 1/4"FAT, CHOIC, CKD, BRLD	202	30.37	0	3.11
13290	BEEF, TOP SIRLOIN, LN, 1/4"FAT, CHOIC, CKD, PAN-FRIED	238	32.48	0	4.02

NDB #	Food Description (100 gram portions = 3½ ounces = 20 tsp = ½ cup approx.	Calories	Protein	Carbs	Sat Fat
13288	BEEF, TOP SIRLOIN, LN, 1/4"FAT, CHOIC, RAW	136	21.24	0	1.76
13292	BEEF, TOP SIRLOIN, LN, 1/4"FAT, SEL, CKD, BRLD	186	30.37	0	2.41
13291	BEEF, TOP SIRLOIN, LN, 1/4"FAT, SEL, RAW	124	21.24	0	1.3
13319	BEEF, VAR MEATS&BY-PRODUCTS, BRAIN, CKD, PAN-FRIED	196	12.57	0	3.74
13320	BEEF, VAR MEATS&BY-PRODUCTS, BRAIN, CKD, SIMMRD	160	11.07	0	2.92
13318	BEEF, VAR MEATS&BY-PRODUCTS, BRAIN, RAW	126	9.8	0	2.16
13322	BEEF, VAR MEATS&BY-PRODUCTS, HEART, CKD, SIMMRD	175	28.79	0.42	1.68
13321	BEEF, VAR MEATS&BY-PRODUCTS, HEART, RAW	117	17.05	2.58	1.13
13324	BEEF, VAR MEATS&BY-PRODUCTS, KIDNEYS, CKD, SIMMRD	144	25.48	0.96	1.09
13323	BEEF, VAR MEATS&BY-PRODUCTS, KIDNEYS, RAW	107	16.59	2.18	0.97
13326	BEEF, VAR MEATS&BY-PRODUCTS, LIVER, CKD, BRSD	161	24.38	3.41	1.9
13327	BEEF, VAR MEATS&BY-PRODUCTS, LIVER, CKD, PAN-FRIED	217	26.72	7.85	2.67
13325	BEEF, VAR MEATS&BY-PRODUCTS, LIVER, RAW	143	20	5.82	1.5
13329	BEEF, VAR MEATS&BY-PRODUCTS, LUNGS, CKD, BRSD	120	20.4	0	1.27
13328	BEEF, VAR MEATS&BY-PRODUCTS, LUNGS, RAW	92	16.2	0	0.86
13330	BEEF, VAR MEATS&BY-PRODUCTS, MECHANICALLY SEPARATED BF,	276	14.97	0	11.78
13332	BEEF, VAR MEATS&BY-PRODUCTS, PANCREAS, CKD, BRSD	271	27.1	0	5.9
13331	BEEF, VAR MEATS&BY-PRODUCTS, PANCREAS, RAW	235	15.7	0	6.41
13334	BEEF, VAR MEATS&BY-PRODUCTS, SPLEEN, CKD, BRSD	145	25.1	0	1.39
13333	BEEF, VAR MEATS&BY-PRODUCTS, SPLEEN, RAW	105	18.3	0	1
13335	BEEF, VAR MEATS&BY-PRODUCTS, SUET, RAW	854	1.5	0	52.3
13338	BEEF, VAR MEATS&BY-PRODUCTS, THYMUS, CKD, BRSD	319	21.85	0	8.61
13337	BEEF, VAR MEATS&BY-PRODUCTS, THYMUS, RAW	236	12.18	0	7.01
13340	BEEF, VAR MEATS&BY-PRODUCTS, TONGUE, CKD, SIMMRD	283	22.11	0.33	8.93
13339	BEEF, VAR MEATS&BY-PRODUCTS, TONGUE, RAW	224	14.9	3.68	7
13341	BEEF, VAR MEATS&BY-PRODUCTS, TRIPE, RAW	98	14.56	0	2.03
07931	BEERWURST PORK & BF	276	14	3.76	8.438
07002	BEERWURST, BEER SALAMI, BF	329	12.4	1.7	13.03
07003	BEERWURST, BEER SALAMI, PORK	238	14.24	2.06	6.28
11086	BEET GREENS, RAW	19	1.82	3.97	0.009
11736	BEET GRNS, CKD, BLD, DRND, W/SALT	27	2.57	5.46	0.031
11087	BEET GRNS, CKD, BLD, DRND, WO/SALT	27	2.57	5.46	0.031
11081	BEETS, CKD, BLD, DRND	44	1.68	9.96	0.028
11734	BEETS, CKD, BOILED. DRND, W/SALT	44	1.68	9.96	0.028
11084	BEETS, CND, DRND SOL	31	0.91	7.2	0.023

NDB #	Food Description (100 gram portions = 3½ ounces = 20 tsp = ½ cup approx.	Calories	Protein	Carbs	Sat Fat
11735	BEETS, CND, NO SALT, SOL&LIQUIDS	28	0.8	6.58	0.011
11082	BEETS, CND, REG PK, SOL&LIQUIDS	28	0.8	6.58	0.011
11605	BEETS, HARVARD, CND, SOL&LIQUIDS	73	0.84	18.18	0.009
11609	BEETS, PICKLED, CND, SOL&LIQUIDS	65	0.8	16.28	0.013
11080	BEETS, RAW	43	1.61	9.56	0.027
18603	BEST FOODS, BROWNBERRY SAGE&ONION STUFFING MIX, DRY	381	13.3	70.5	0.932
18639	BEST FOODS, THOMAS' ENG MUFFINS, PLN	231	8.7	45.6	1.222
22700	BETTY CROCKER, HAMBURGER HELPER, CHEESEBURGER MACARO	395	11	64.3	2.82
18017	BISCUITS, MXD GRAIN, REFR DOUGH	263	6.1	47.4	1.366
18009	BISCUITS, PLN OR BTTRMLK, COMMLY BKD	364	6.2	48.5	2.49
18010	BISCUITS, PLN OR BTTRMLK, DRY MIX	428	8	63.3	3.965
18011	BISCUITS, PLN OR BTTRMLK, DRY MIX, PREP	335	7.3	48.4	2.789
18016	BISCUITS, PLN OR BTTRMLK, PREP FROM RECIPE	354	7	44.6	4.324
18014	BISCUITS, PLN OR BTTRMLK, REFR DOUGH, HIGHER FAT	318	6.2	43.7	3.396
18015	BISCUITS, PLN OR BTTRMLK, REFR DOUGH, HIGHER FAT, BKD	346	6.7	47.5	3.702
18012	BISCUITS, PLN OR BTTRMLK, REFR DOUGH, LOWER FAT	257	6.7	47.6	1.113
18013	BISCUITS, PLN OR BTTRMLK, REFR DOUGH, LOWER FAT, BKD	299	7.8	55.4	1.294
09046	BLACKBERRIES, CND, HVY SYRUP, SOL&LIQUIDS	92	1.31	23.1	0.005
09048	BLACKBERRIES, FRZ, UNSWTND	64	1.18	15.67	0.015
09042	BLACKBERRIES, RAW	52	0.72	12.76	0.014
07005	BLOOD SAUSAGE	378	14.61	1.27	13.36
09052	BLUEBERRIES, CND, HVY SYRUP, SOL&LIQUIDS	88	0.65	22.06	0.027
09055	BLUEBERRIES, FRZ, SWTND	81	0.4	21.95	0.011
09054	BLUEBERRIES, FRZ, UNSWTND	51	0.42	12.17	0.053
09050	BLUEBERRIES, RAW	56	0.67	14.13	0.032
15189	BLUEFISH, COOKED, DRY HEAT	159	25.69	0	1.172
15005	BLUEFISH, RAW	124	20.04	0	0.915
07006	BOCKWURST PORK VEAL RAW	278	10.91	0.5	9.92
07937	BOLOGNA PORK TURKEY & BF	333	11.56	6.66	11.7
07008	BOLOGNA PORK & BF	312	11.69	2.78	10.69
07936	BOLOGNA PORK & TURKEY LITE	211	13.06	3.45	5.46
07007	BOLOGNA, BEEF	312	12.2	0.8	12.07
07010	BOLOGNA, PORK	247	15.3	0.73	6.88
07011	BOLOGNA, TURKEY	199	13.73	0.97	5.06
11737	BORAGE, CKD, BLD, DRND, W/SALT	25	2.09	3.55	0.197

NDB #	Food Description (100 gram portions = 3½ ounces = 20 tsp = ½ cup approx.	Calories	Protein	Carbs	Sat Fat
11614	BORAGE, CKD, BLD, DRND, WO/SALT	25	2.09	3.55	0.197
11613	BORAGE, RAW	21	1.8	3.06	0.17
09056	BOYSENBERRIES, CND, HVY SYRUP	88	0.99	22.31	0.004
09057	BOYSENBERRIES, FRZ, UNSWTND	50	1.1	12.19	0.009
07922	BRATWURST BF & PORK SMOKED	296	12.2	2.56	6.08
07924	BRATWURST PORK BF & TURKEY LITE SMOKED	195	14.45	3.98	4.788
07910	BRATWURST VEAL CKD	343	13.99	0	14.94
07923	BRATWURST, CHICK, CKD	176	19.44	0	2.952
07013	BRATWURST, PORK, CKD	301	14.08	2.07	9.32
07014	BRAUNSCHWEIGER (A LIVER SAUSAGE), PORK	359	13.5	3.13	10.9
12078	BRAZILNUTS, DRIED, UNBLANCHED	656	14.34	12.8	16.154
18079	BREAD CRUMBS, DRY, GRATED, PLN	395	12.5	72.5	1.212
18376	BREAD CRUMBS, DRY, GRATED, SEASONED	367	14.2	70.4	0.726
18080	BREAD STICKS, PLAIN	412	12	68.4	1.41
18081	BREAD STUFFING, BREAD, DRY MIX	386	11	76.2	0.845
18082	BREAD STUFFING, BREAD, DRY MIX, PREP	178	3.2	21.7	1.734
18084	BREAD STUFFING, CORNBREAD, DRY MIX	389	10	76.7	0.922
18085	BREAD STUFFING, CORNBREAD, DRY MIX, PREP	179	2.9	21.9	1.755
18019	BREAD, BANANA, PREP FROM RECIPE, MADE W/MARGARINE	326	4.3	54.6	2.237
18021	BREAD, BOSTON BROWN, CANNED	195	5.2	43.3	0.282
18022	BREAD, CORNBREAD, DRY MIX, ENR (INCL CORN MUFFIN MIX)	418	7	69.5	3.091
18023	BREAD, CORNBREAD, DRY MIX, PREP	314	7.2	48.1	2.739
18412	BREAD, CORNBREAD, DRY MIX, UNENR (INCL CORN MUFFIN MIX)	418	7	69.5	3.091
18024	BREAD, CORNBREAD, PREP FROM RECIPE, MADE W/LOFAT (2%) MIL	266	6.7	43.5	1.555
18025	BREAD, CRACKED-WHEAT	260	8.7	49.5	0.916
18027	BREAD, EGG	287	9.5	47.8	1.593
18028	BREAD, EGG, TOASTED	315	10.5	52.6	1.616
18029	BREAD, FRENCH OR VIENNA (INCLUDES SOURDOUGH)	274	8.8	51.9	0.641
18030	BREAD, FRENCH OR VIENNA, TSTD (INCLUDES SOURDOUGH)	298	9.6	56.4	0.696
18031	BREAD, INDIAN (NAVAJO) FRY	329	7.1	53.3	2.313
18032	BREAD, IRISH SODA, PREP FROM RECIPE	290	6.6	56	1.111
18033	BREAD, ITALIAN	271	8.8	50	0.855
18035	BREAD, MIXED-GRAIN (INCL WHOLE-GRAIN, 7-GRAIN)	250	10	46.4	0.807
18036	BREAD, MIXED-GRAIN, TSTD (INCL WHOLE-GRAIN, 7-GRAIN)	272	10.9	50.4	0.878
18037	BREAD, OAT BRAN	236	10.4	39.8	0.697

NDB #	Food Description (100 gram portions = 3½ ounces = 20 tsp = ½ cup approx.	Calories	Protein	Carbs	Sat Fat
18038	BREAD, OAT BRAN, TOASTED	259	11.4	43.7	0.766
18039	BREAD, OATMEAL	269	8.4	48.5	0.703
18040	BREAD, OATMEAL, TOASTED	292	9.2	52.7	0.764
18041	BREAD, PITA, WHITE, ENRICHED	275	9.1	55.7	0.166
18413	BREAD, PITA, WHITE, UNENR	275	9.1	55.7	0.166
18042	BREAD, PITA, WHOLE-WHEAT	266	9.8	55	0.41
18043	BREAD, PROT (INCL GLUTEN)	245	12.1	43.8	0.332
18383	BREAD, PROT, TSTD (INCL GLUTEN)	270	13.2	48.1	0.364
18044	BREAD, PUMPERNICKEL	250	8.7	47.5	0.437
18045	BREAD, PUMPERNICKEL, TSTD	275	9.5	52.2	0.481
18047	BREAD, RAISIN, ENRICHED	274	7.9	52.3	1.081
18048	BREAD, RAISIN, TSTD, ENR	297	8.6	56.9	1.175
18414	BREAD, RAISIN, UNENRICHED	274	7.9	52.3	1.081
18049	BREAD, RED-CAL, OAT BRAN	201	8	41.3	0.445
18050	BREAD, RED-CAL, OAT BRAN, TSTD	239	9.5	49.2	0.53
18051	BREAD, RED-CAL, OATMEAL	210	7.6	43.3	0.599
18055	BREAD, RED-CAL, WHEAT	198	9.1	43.6	0.344
18057	BREAD, RED-CAL, WHITE	207	8.7	44.3	0.549
18053	BREAD, REDUCED-CALORIE, RYE	203	9.1	40.5	0.368
18059	BREAD, RICE BRAN	243	8.9	43.5	0.709
18384	BREAD, RICE BRAN, TOASTED	264	9.7	47.3	0.771
18060	BREAD, RYE	259	8.5	48.3	0.626
18061	BREAD, RYE, TOASTED	284	9.4	53.1	0.688
18064	BREAD, WHEAT (INCL WHEAT BERRY)	260	9.1	47.2	0.894
18066	BREAD, WHEAT BRAN	248	8.8	47.8	0.779
18068	BREAD, WHEAT GERM	261	9.6	48.3	0.657
18385	BREAD, WHEAT GERM, TOASTED	293	10.7	54.3	0.738
18065	BREAD, WHEAT, TSTD (INCL WHEAT BERRY)	282	9.9	51.3	0.972
18069	BREAD, WHITE, COMMLY PREP (INCL SOFT BREAD CRUMBS)	267	8.2	49.5	0.526
18416	BREAD, WHITE, COMMLY PREP, LO NA NO SALT	267	8.2	49.5	0.811
18070	BREAD, WHITE, COMMLY PREP, TSTD	293	9	54.4	0.578
18432	BREAD, WHITE, COMMLY PREP, TSTD, LO NA NO SALT	293	9	54.4	0.892
18073	BREAD, WHITE, PREP FROM RECIPE, MADE W/LOFAT (2%) MILK	285	7.9	49.6	1.178
18071	BREAD, WHITE, PREP FROM RECIPE, MADE W/NONFAT DRY MILK	274	7.7	53.6	0.391
18075	BREAD, WHOLE-WHEAT, COMMLY PREP	246	9.7	46.1	0.917

NDB #	Food Description (100 gram portions = 3½ ounces = 20 tsp = ½ cup approx.	Calories	Protein	Carbs	Sat Fat
18076	BREAD, WHOLE-WHEAT, COMMLY PREP, TSTD	277	10.9	51.7	1.03
18077	BREAD, WHOLE-WHEAT, PREP FROM RECIPE	278	8.4	51.4	0.796
18078	BREAD, WHOLE-WHEAT, PREP FROM RECIPE, TSTD	305	9.2	56.4	0.874
12003	BREADFRUIT SEEDS, BOILED	168	5.3	32	0.621
12001	BREADFRUIT SEEDS, RAW	191	7.4	29.24	1.509
12158	BREADFRUIT SEEDS, ROASTED	207	6.2	40.1	0.729
09059	BREADFRUIT, RAW	103	1.07	27.12	0.048
12005	BREADNUTTREE SEEDS, DRIED	367	8.62	79.39	0.454
12004	BREADNUTTREE SEEDS, RAW	217	5.97	46.28	0.267
22679	BREAKFAST BURRITO, HAM&CHS FLAVOR, FRZ ENTREE	214	9.7	28.1	2.01
21005	BREAKFAST ITEMS, BISCUIT W/EGG&SAUSAGE	323	10.64	22.86	8.32
21006	BREAKFAST ITEMS, BISCUIT W/EGG&STEAK	277	12.12	14.37	5.81
21023	BREAKFAST ITEMS, FRENCH TOAST W/BUTTER	264	7.66	26.7	5.74
16353	BROADBEANS (FAVA BNS), MATURE SEEDS, CKD, BLD, W/SALT	110	7.6	19.65	0.066
16053	BROADBEANS (FAVA BNS), MATURE SEEDS, CKD, BLD, WO/SALT	110	7.6	19.65	0.066
16054	BROADBEANS (FAVA BNS), MATURE SEEDS, CND	71	5.47	12.41	0.037
16052	BROADBEANS (FAVA BNS), MATURE SEEDS, RAW	341	26.12	58.3	0.254
11738	BROADBEANS, IMMAT SEEDS, CKD, BLD, DRND, W/SALT	62	4.8	10.1	0.142
11089	BROADBEANS, IMMAT SEEDS, CKD, BLD, DRND, WO/SALT	62	4.8	10.1	0.142
11088	BROADBEANS, IMMAT SEEDS, RAW	72	5.6	11.7	0.138
11969	BROCCOLI, CHINESE, COOKED	22	1.14	3.79	0.11
11742	BROCCOLI, CKD, BLD, DRND, W/SALT	28	2.98	5.06	0.054
11091	BROCCOLI, CKD, BLD, DRND, WO/SALT	28	2.98	5.06	0.054
11740	BROCCOLI, FLOWER CLUSTERS, RAW	28	2.98	5.24	0.054
11743	BROCCOLI, FRZ, CHOPD, CKD, BLD, DRND, W/SALT	28	3.1	5.35	0.018
11093	BROCCOLI, FRZ, CHOPD, CKD, BLD, DRND, WO/SALT	28	3.1	5.35	0.018
11092	BROCCOLI, FRZ, CHOPD, UNPREP	26	2.81	4.79	0.044
11744	BROCCOLI, FRZ, SPEARS, CKD, BLD, DRND, W/SALT	28	3.1	5.35	0.018
11095	BROCCOLI, FRZ, SPEARS, CKD, BLD, DRND, WO/SALT	28	3.1	5.35	0.018
11094	BROCCOLI, FRZ, SPEARS, UNPREP	29	3.06	5.35	0.052
11739	BROCCOLI, LEAVES, RAW	28	2.98	5.24	0.054
11090	BROCCOLI, RAW	28	2.98	5.24	0.054
11741	BROCCOLI, STALKS, RAW	28	2.98	5.24	0.054
07015	BROTWURST PORK & BF LINK	323	14.27	2.96	9.92
11745	BRUSSELS SPROUTS, CKD, BLD, DRND, W/SALT	41	2.55	8.67	0.105

NDB #	Food Description (100 gram portions = 3½ ounces = 20 tsp = ½ cup approx.	Calories	Protein	Carbs	Sat Fat
11099	BRUSSELS SPROUTS, CKD, BLD, DRND, WO/SALT	39	2.55	8.67	0.105
11746	BRUSSELS SPROUTS, FRZ, CKD, BLD, DRND, W/SALT	42	3.64	8.32	0.081
11101	BRUSSELS SPROUTS, FRZ, CKD, BLD, DRND, WO/SALT	42	3.64	8.32	0.081
11100	BRUSSELS SPROUTS, FRZ, UNPREP	41	3.78	7.87	0.084
11098	BRUSSELS SPROUTS, RAW	43	3.38	8.96	0.062
20008	BUCKWHEAT	343	13.25	71.5	0.741
20011	BUCKWHEAT FLR, WHOLE-GROAT	335	12.62	70.59	0.677
20010	BUCKWHEAT GROATS, RSTD, CKD	92	3.38	19.94	0.134
20009	BUCKWHEAT GROATS, RSTD, DRY	346	11.73	74.95	0.591
22617	BUDGET GOURMET LT FR REC CHCK;VEG, CHCK&POT, WINE SAU, F	70	9	3.6	0.567
22616	BUDGET GOURMET LT&HLTHY BF SRLN SALS STK, RED POT&VEG, F	84	5.9	10.9	0.649
22683	BUDGET GOURMET LT&HLTHY TERYAKI CHICK, ORNTL STY VEG, FR	102	6	16.8	0.199
20013	BULGUR, COOKED	83	3.08	18.58	0.042
20012	BULGUR, DRY	342	12.29	75.87	0.232
15190	BURBOT, COOKED, DRY HEAT	115	24.76	0	0.209
15006	BURBOT, RAW	90	19.31	0	0.163
11747	BURDOCK ROOT, CKD, BLD, DRND, W/SALT	88	2.09	21.15	
11105	BURDOCK ROOT, CKD, BLD, DRND, WO/SALT	88	2.09	21.15	0.023
11104	BURDOCK ROOT, RAW	72	1.53	17.35	0.025
07269	BUTCHER BOY MEATS, INC., TURKEY FRANKS	239	13.45	4.66	5.86
01003	BUTTER OIL, ANHYDROUS	876	0.28	0	61.924
01002	BUTTER, WHIPPED, WITH SALT	717	0.85	0.06	50.489
01001	BUTTER, WITH SALT	717	0.85	0.06	50.489
01145	BUTTER, WITHOUT SALT	717	0.85	0.06	50.489
11106	BUTTERBUR, (FUKI), RAW	14	0.39	3.61	
11108	BUTTERBUR, CANNED	3	0.11	0.38	
11748	BUTTERBUR, CKD, BLD, DRND, W/SALT	8	0.23	2.16	
11107	BUTTERBUR, CKD, BLD, DRND, WO/SALT	8	0.23	2.16	
15191	BUTTERFISH, CKD, DRY HEAT	187	22.15	0	
15007	BUTTERFISH, RAW	146	17.28	0	3.38
12084	BUTTERNUTS, DRIED	612	24.9	12.05	1.306
11754	CABBAGE, CHINESE (PAK-CHOI), CKD, BLD, DRND, W/SALT	12	1.56	1.78	0.021
11117	CABBAGE, CHINESE (PAK-CHOI), CKD, BLD, DRND, WO/SALT	12	1.56	1.78	0.021
11116	CABBAGE, CHINESE (PAK-CHOI), RAW	13	1.5	2.18	0.026
11755	CABBAGE, CHINESE (PE-TSAI), CKD, BLD, DRND, W/SALT	14	1.5	2.41	0.036

NDB #	Food Description (100 gram portions = 3½ ounces = 20 tsp = ½ cup approx.	Calories	Protein	Carbs	Sat Fat
11120	CABBAGE, CHINESE (PE-TSAI), CKD, BLD, DRND, WO/SALT	14	1.5	2.41	0.036
11119	CABBAGE, CHINESE (PE-TSAI), RAW	16	1.2	3.23	0.043
11110	CABBAGE, CKD, BLD, DRND, WO/SALT	22	1.02	4.46	0.053
11750	CABBAGE, COMMON (DANISH, DOMESTIC, &POINTED TYPES), STOR	24	1.21	5.37	0.023
11751	CABBAGE, COMMON, CKD, BLD, DRND, W/SALT	22	1.02	4.46	0.053
11749	CABBAGE, COMMON, FRESHLY HARVEST, RAW	24	1.21	5.37	0.023
11970	CABBAGE, NAPA, COOKED	12	1.1	2.23	
11109	CABBAGE, RAW	25	1.44	5.43	0.033
11752	CABBAGE, RED, CKD, BLD, DRND, W/SALT	21	1.05	4.64	0.026
11113	CABBAGE, RED, CKD, BLD, DRND, WO/SALT	21	1.05	4.64	0.026
11112	CABBAGE, RED, RAW	27	1.39	6.12	0.034
11753	CABBAGE, SAVOY, CKD, BLD, DRND, W/SALT	24	1.8	5.41	0.012
11115	CABBAGE, SAVOY, CKD, BLD, DRND, WO/SALT	24	1.8	5.41	0.012
11114	CABBAGE, SAVOY, RAW	27	2	6.1	0.013
18086	CAKE, ANGELFOOD, COMMLY PREP	258	5.9	57.8	0.121
18087	CAKE, ANGELFOOD, DRY MIX	373	8.9	85.1	0.063
18088	CAKE, ANGELFOOD, DRY MIX, PREP	257	6.1	58.7	0.043
18602	CAKE, BETTY CROCKER, SUPERMOIST PARTY CAKE SWIRL, DRY MIX	414	3.9	82.5	2.26
18090	CAKE, BOSTON CRM PIE, COMMLY PREP	252	2.4	42.9	2.445
18092	CAKE, CARROT, DRY MIX, PUDDING-TYPE	415	5.1	79.2	1.472
18095	CAKE, CHERRY FUDGE W/CHOC FRSTNG	264	2.4	38	5.066
18096	CAKE, CHOC, COMMLY PREP W/CHOC FRSTNG	367	4.1	54.6	4.771
18097	CAKE, CHOC, DRY MIX, PUDDING-TYPE	396	4.6	78.7	1.923
18099	CAKE, CHOC, DRY MIX, REG	428	5.9	73	3.264
18101	CAKE, CHOC, PREP FROM RECIPE WO/FRSTNG	358	5.3	53.4	5.43
18110	CAKE, FRUITCAKE, COMMLY PREP	324	2.9	61.6	1.048
18112	CAKE, GERMAN CHOC, DRY MIX, PUDDING-TYPE	401	4	80.1	3.205
18114	CAKE, GINGERBREAD, DRY MIX	437	4.4	74.6	3.46
18116	CAKE, GINGERBREAD, PREP FROM RECIPE	356	3.9	49.2	4.122
18117	CAKE, MARBLE, DRY MIX, PUDDING-TYPE	416	3.4	79.3	2.45
18119	CAKE, PNAPPL UPSIDE-DOWN, PREP FROM RECIPE	319	3.5	50.5	2.915
18120	CAKE, POUND, COMMLY PREP, BUTTER	388	5.5	48.8	11.559
18451	CAKE, POUND, COMMLY PREP, FAT-FREE	283	5.4	61	0.259
18121	CAKE, POUND, COMMLY PREP, OTHER THAN ALL BUTTER, ENR	389	5.2	52.5	4.647
18418	CAKE, POUND, COMMLY PREP, OTHER THAN ALL BUTTER, UNENR	389	5.2	52.5	4.647

NDB #	Food Description (100 gram portions = 3½ ounces = 20 tsp = ½ cup approx.	Calories	Protein	Carbs	Sat Fat
18126	CAKE, SHORTCAKE, BISCUIT-TYPE, PREP FROM RECIPE	346	6.1	48.5	3.772
18127	CAKE, SNACK CAKES, CREME-FILLED, CHOC W/FRSTNG	376	3.4	60.3	2.858
18128	CAKE, SNACK CAKES, CREME-FILLED, SPONGE	364	3.1	63.9	2.561
18452	CAKE, SNACK CAKES, CUPCAKES, CHOC, W/FRSTNG, LOW-FAT	305	4.3	67.2	1.084
18133	CAKE, SPONGE, COMMLY PREP	289	5.4	61.1	0.802
18134	CAKE, SPONGE, PREP FROM RECIPE	297	7.3	57.7	1.301
18135	CAKE, WHITE, DRY MIX, PUDDING-TYPE, ENR	423	3.9	81	2.34
18419	CAKE, WHITE, DRY MIX, PUDDING-TYPE, UNENR	423	3.9	81	2.34
18137	CAKE, WHITE, DRY MIX, REG	426	4.5	78	1.643
18131	CAKE, WHITE, DRY MIX, SPL DIETARY (INCL LEMON-FLAVORED)	397	3	79.6	1.251
18102	CAKE, WHITE, PREP FROM RECIPE W/COCNT FRSTNG	356	4.4	63.2	3.897
18139	CAKE, WHITE, PREP FROM RECIPE WO/FRSTNG	357	5.4	57.2	3.269
18140	CAKE, YEL, COMMLY PREP, W/CHOC FRSTNG	379	3.8	55.4	4.656
18141	CAKE, YEL, COMMLY PREP, W/VANILLA FRSTNG	373	3.5	58.8	2.371
18142	CAKE, YEL, DRY MIX, PUDDING-TYPE	423	4	79.9	2.472
18144	CAKE, YEL, DRY MIX, REG, ENR	432	4.4	78.1	1.738
18420	CAKE, YEL, DRY MIX, REG, UNENR	432	4.4	78.1	1.738
18146	CAKE, YEL, PREP FROM RECIPE WO/FRSTNG	361	5.3	53	3.924
18453	CAKE, YELLOW, DRY MIX, LIGHT	404	4.7	84.1	1.367
18604	CAMPIONE D'ITALIA FOODS, CAMPIONE GARLIC BREAD, FRZ	362	8.5	44.3	2.7
19098	CANDIES, 5TH AVENUE CANDY BAR	482	8.78	62.68	6.65
19248	CANDIES, ALMOND JOY BITES	545	5.58	57.48	20.6
19065	CANDIES, ALMOND JOY CANDY BAR	479	4.13	59.51	17.59
19070	CANDIES, BUTTERSCOTCH	391	0.03	90.4	1.981
19075	CANDIES, CARAMELLO CANDY BAR	462	6.19	63.81	12.72
19074	CANDIES, CARAMELS	382	4.6	77	6.58
19076	CANDIES, CARAMELS, CHOCOLATE-FLAVOR ROLL	405	3.1	84	1.232
19071	CANDIES, CAROB	540	8.15	56.29	29.018
19085	CANDIES, CONFECTIONER'S COATING, BUTTERSCOTCH	539	2.2	67.1	24.1
19086	CANDIES, CONFECTIONER'S COATING, PNUT BUTTER	497	18.3	44.9	13.12
19087	CANDIES, CONFECTIONER'S COATING, WHITE	539	5.87	59.25	19.412
19079	CANDIES, CONFECTIONER'S COATING, YOGURT	522	5.87	63.94	24.113
19179	CANDIES, E.J. BRACH'S, BRACH'S STAR BRITES PEPPERMINT MINTS	393	0	97.7	
19099	CANDIES, FONDANT, PREPARED-FROM-RECIPE	372	0	93.03	0
19301	CANDIES, FUDGE, CHOC MARSHMLLW, W/ NUTS, PREPARED-BY-RE	472	3.23	67.12	9.984

NDB #	Food Description (100 gram portions = 3½ ounces = 20 tsp = ½ cup approx.	Calories	Protein	Carbs	Sat Fat
19100	CANDIES, FUDGE, CHOC, PREPARED-FROM-RECIPE	412	2.15	76.33	6.348
19101	CANDIES, FUDGE, CHOC, W/ NUTS, PREPARED-FROM-RECIPE	466	4.21	68.35	6.453
19104	CANDIES, FUDGE, VANILLA W/ NUTS, PREPARED-FROM-RECIPE	437	3.03	74.9	3.755
19103	CANDIES, FUDGE, VANILLA, PREPARED-FROM-RECIPE	385	1.07	82.58	3.241
19106	CANDIES, GUMDROPS, STARCH JELLY PIECES	386	0	98.9	0
19117	CANDIES, HALAVAH, PLAIN	469	12.49	60.49	4.127
19107	CANDIES, HARD	394	0	98	0
19243	CANDIES, HEATH BITES	530	3.94	63.39	15.62
19084	CANDIES, HERSHEY'S GOLDEN ALMOND SOLITAIRES	570	11.97	46.91	15.23
19236	CANDIES, HERSHEY'S MILK CHOC W/ ALMOND BITES	550	9.76	51	17.39
19130	CANDIES, HERSHEY'S POT OF GOLD ALMOND BAR	577	12.82	46.15	16.667
19108	CANDIES, JELLYBEANS	367	0	93.1	0.14
19237	CANDIES, KIT KAT BITES	511	6.5	64.55	17.1
19109	CANDIES, KIT KAT WAFER BAR	517	6.41	64.17	17.49
19110	CANDIES, KRACKEL CHOC BAR	512	6.62	63.96	15.92
19157	CANDIES, M&M MARS, "M&M'S"MINI MILK CHOC CANDIES	498	4.78	67.12	14.452
19141	CANDIES, M&M MARS, "M&M'S"PLN CHOC CANDIES	492	4.33	71.21	13.08
19140	CANDIES, M&M MARS, "M&M'S"PNUT CHOC CANDIES	516	9.47	60.46	10.331
19159	CANDIES, M&M MARS, 3 MUSKETEERS BAR	416	3.2	76.8	6.5
19115	CANDIES, M&M MARS, MARS ALMOND BAR	467	8.1	62.7	7.268
19135	CANDIES, M&M MARS, MARS MILKY WAY BAR	423	4.5	71.7	7.79
19370	CANDIES, M&M MARS, SKITTLES ORIGINAL BITE SIZE CANDIES	405	0.19	90.64	0.868
19155	CANDIES, M&M MARS, SNICKERS BAR	479	8	59.21	8.994
19156	CANDIES, M&M MARS, STARBURST FRUIT CHEWS	396	0.4	84.5	1.237
19160	CANDIES, M&M MARS, TWIX CARAMEL COOKIE BARS	499	4.6	65.58	8.899
19161	CANDIES, M&M MARS, TWIX PNUT BUTTER COOKIE BARS	530	10.12	52.67	11.392
19116	CANDIES, MARSHMALLOWS	318	1.8	81.3	0.056
19126	CANDIES, MILK CHOC COATD PNUTS	519	13.1	49.4	14.6
19127	CANDIES, MILK CHOC COATD RAISINS	390	4.1	68.3	8.8
19132	CANDIES, MILK CHOC, W/ALMONDS	526	9	53.2	16.98
19134	CANDIES, MILK CHOC, W/RICE CRL	496	6.3	63.4	15.89
19120	CANDIES, MILK CHOCOLATE	513	6.9	59.2	18.48
19142	CANDIES, MOUNDS CANDY BAR	486	4.6	58.59	20.58
19143	CANDIES, MR. GOODBAR CHOC BAR	538	10.22	54.34	14.13
19144	CANDIES, NESTLE, 100 GRAND BAR	466	4.89	70.71	11.16

NDB #	Food Description (100 gram portions = 3½ ounces = 20 tsp = ½ cup approx.	Calories	Protein	Carbs	Sat Fat
19153	CANDIES, NESTLE, AFTER EIGHT MINTS	358	2.2	76.8	8.18
19111	CANDIES, NESTLE, BABY RUTH BAR	481	7.49	65.23	12.3
19069	CANDIES, NESTLE, BUTTERFINGER BAR&DSSRT TOPPING	480	12.45	65.56	10.36
19119	CANDIES, NESTLE, CHUNKY BAR	495	9	57.1	23.22
19145	CANDIES, NESTLE, CRUNCH BAR&DSSRT TOPPING	522	6	65.21	15.19
19158	CANDIES, NESTLE, DEMET'S TURTLES CANDY	485	6.4	58	10.84
19105	CANDIES, NESTLE, GOOBERS CHOC COVERED PNUTS	513	13.7	48.7	12.21
19118	CANDIES, NESTLE, OH HENRY! BAR	431	10.9	64.7	6.72
19149	CANDIES, NESTLE, RAISINETS CHOC COVERED RAISINS	412	4.7	71.2	7.34
19147	CANDIES, PEANUT BAR	522	15.5	47.4	4.678
19148	CANDIES, PNUT BRITTLE, PREPARED-FROM-RECIPE	479	7.57	69.65	4.591
19238	CANDIES, REESE'S BITES	521	11.34	55.18	18
19242	CANDIES, REESE'S CRUNCHY COOKIE CUPS	507	8.47	59.6	11.56
19239	CANDIES, REESE'S NUTRAGEOUS CANDY BAR	517	11.28	52.8	8.86
19151	CANDIES, REESE'S PIECES CANDY	497	12.46	59.86	16.42
19150	CANDIES, REESE'S PNUT BUTTER CUPS	515	10.24	55.36	10.73
19152	CANDIES, ROLO CARAMELS IN MILK CHOC	474	5.08	67.95	14.42
19080	CANDIES, SEMISWEET CHOC	479	4.2	63.1	17.75
19701	CANDIES, SEMISWEET CHOC, MADE W/BUTTER	477	4.2	63.4	17.53
19154	CANDIES, SESAME CRUNCH	517	11.6	50.3	4.46
19136	CANDIES, SKOR TOFFEE BAR	535	3.13	61.72	18.78
19164	CANDIES, SPL DK CHOC BAR	531	5.54	59.41	19.19
19858	CANDIES, SUGAR-COATED ALMONDS	456	7.8	70.2	1.763
19081	CANDIES, SWEET CHOCOLATE	505	3.9	59.6	20.08
19083	CANDIES, SWT CHOC COATD FONDANT	366	2.2	80.2	5.46
19093	CANDIES, SYMPHONY MILK CHOC BAR	531	8.51	58.01	18.34
19067	CANDIES, TWIZZLERS CHERRY BITES	338	2.97	79.38	0.25
19092	CANDIES, TWIZZLERS NIBS CHERRY BITS	347	2.3	79.37	0.54
19112	CANDIES, TWIZZLERS STRAWBERRY TWISTS CANDY	350	2.56	79.74	0
19162	CANDIES, WHATCHAMACALLIT CANDY BAR	494	8.04	63.23	17.04
19180	CANDIES, WILLY WONKA'S EVERLASTING GOBSTOPPERS JAWBREA	369	0	92.3	
19181	CANDIES, YORK BITES	394	1.78	81.64	4.43
19091	CANDIES, YORK PEPPERMINT PATTIE	384	2.19	80.99	4.34
02054	CAPERS, CANNED	23	2.36	4.89	0.233
09060	CARAMBOLA, (STARFRUIT), RAW	33	0.54	7.83	0.023

NDB #	Food Description (100 gram portions = 3½ ounces = 20 tsp = ½ cup approx.	Calories	Protein	Carbs	Sat Fat
02005	CARAWAY SEED	333	19.77	49.9	0.62
14151	CARBON BEV, LO CAL, OTHER THAN COLA OR PEPPER, W/ASPRT, W	0	0.1	0	0
14552	CARBONATED BEV, CHOCOLATE-FLAVORED SODA	42	0	10.7	0
14121	CARBONATED BEV, CLUB SODA	0	0	0	0
14400	CARBONATED BEV, COLA, CONTAINS CAFFEINE	41	0	10.4	0
14148	CARBONATED BEV, COLA, W/HIGHER CAFFEINE	41	0	10.4	0
14147	CARBONATED BEV, COLA, WO/CAFFEINE	41	0	10.4	0
14130	CARBONATED BEV, CRM SODA	51	0	13.3	0
14136	CARBONATED BEV, GINGER ALE	34	0	8.7	0
14142	CARBONATED BEV, GRAPE SODA	43	0	11.2	0
14145	CARBONATED BEV, LEMON-LIME SODA	40	0	10.4	0
14144	CARBONATED BEV, LEMON-LIME SODA, CONTAINS CAFFEINE	40	0	10.4	0
14166	CARBONATED BEV, LO CAL, COLA OR PEP-TYPE, W/NA SACHRN, CN	0	0	0.1	0
14416	CARBONATED BEV, LO CAL, COLA, W/ASPRT, CONTAINS CAFFEINE	1	0.1	0.1	0
14146	CARBONATED BEV, LO CAL, COLA, W/ASPRT, WO/CAFFEINE	1	0.1	0.1	0
14143	CARBONATED BEV, LO CAL, OTHER THN COLA OR PPPR, W/ASPRT,	0	0.1	0	0
14537	CARBONATED BEV, LOCAL, OTHR THAN COLA OR PEP, W/ NA SAC,	0	0	0.1	0
14150	CARBONATED BEV, ORANGE	48	0	12.3	0
14153	CARBONATED BEV, PEPPER-TYPE, CONTAINS CAFFEINE	41	0	10.4	0.07
14157	CARBONATED BEV, ROOT BEER	41	0	10.6	0
14155	CARBONATED BEV, TONIC H2O	34	0	8.8	0
11756	CARDOON, CKD, BLD, DRND, W/SALT	22	0.76	5.33	0.012
11123	CARDOON, CKD, BLD, DRND, WO/SALT	22	0.76	5.33	0.012
11122	CARDOON, RAW	20	0.7	4.89	0.011
09061	CARISSA, (NATAL-PLUM), RAW	62	0.5	13.63	
07270	CARL BUDDIG, CKD CORNED BF, CHOPD, PRESSED	142	19.3	1	2.8
07272	CARL BUDDIG, SMOKED SLICED BF	139	19.3	0.6	2.6
07271	CARL BUDDIG, SMOKED SLICED CHICK, LT&DK MEAT	165	17.9	0.7	2.6
07275	CARL BUDDIG, SMOKED SLICED HAM	163	18.5	1.1	3.1
07273	CARL BUDDIG, SMOKED SLICED TURKEY, LT&DK MEAT	160	17.5	1.8	3.1
07274	CARL BUDDIG. CKD SMOKED BF PASTRAMI, CHOPD, PRESSED	141	19.6	1	3
16055	CAROB FLOUR	222	4.62	88.88	0.09
14168	CAROB-FLAVOR BEV MIX, PDR	372	1.8	93.3	0.03
14169	CAROB-FLAVOR BEV MIX, PDR, PREP W/ WHL MILK	76	3.2	8.8	1.983
15009	CARP, COOKED, DRY HEAT	162	22.86	0	1.388

NDB #	Food Description (100 gram portions = 3½ ounces = 20 tsp = ½ cup approx.	Calories	Protein	Carbs	Sat Fat
15008	CARP, RAW	127	17.83	0	1.083
11655	CARROT JUICE, CANNED	40	0.95	9.29	0.027
11960	CARROTS, BABY, RAW	38	0.84	8.16	0.092
11757	CARROTS, CKD, BLD, DRND, W/SALT	45	1.09	10.48	0.034
11125	CARROTS, CKD, BLD, DRND, WO/SALT	45	1.09	10.48	0.034
11759	CARROTS, CND, NO SALT , DRND SOL	25	0.64	5.54	0.036
11758	CARROTS, CND, NO SALT, SOL&LIQUIDS	23	0.59	5.37	0.025
11128	CARROTS, CND, REG PK, DRND SOL	25	0.64	5.54	0.036
11126	CARROTS, CND, REG PK, SOL&LIQUIDS	23	0.58	5.37	0.025
11130	CARROTS, FROZEN, UNPREPARED	39	1.09	8.99	0.039
11760	CARROTS, FRZ, CKD, BLD, DRND, W/SALT	36	1.19	8.25	0.021
11131	CARROTS, FRZ, CKD, BLD, DRND, WO/SALT	36	1.19	8.25	0.021
11124	CARROTS, RAW	43	1.03	10.14	0.03
12588	CASHEW BUTTER, PLN, W/SALT	587	17.56	27.57	9.763
12088	CASHEW BUTTER, PLN, WO/SALT	587	17.56	27.57	9.763
12585	CASHEW NUTS, DRY RSTD, W/SALT	574	15.31	32.69	9.157
12085	CASHEW NUTS, DRY RSTD, WO/SALT	574	15.31	32.69	9.157
12586	CASHEW NUTS, OIL RSTD, W/SALT	581	16.84	30.16	8.478
12086	CASHEW NUTS, OIL RSTD, WO/SALT	580	16.84	29.87	8.478
11134	CASSAVA, RAW	160	1.36	38.05	0.074
22693	CASTLEBERRY PREMIUM BF STEW, CND ENTREE	135	6.2	8.3	3.24
15011	CATFISH, CHANNEL, CKD, BREADED&FRIED	229	18.09	8.04	3.288
15235	CATFISH, CHANNEL, FARMED, CKD, DRY HEAT	152	18.72	0	1.789
15234	CATFISH, CHANNEL, FARMED, RAW	135	15.55	0	1.768
15233	CATFISH, CHANNEL, WILD, CKD, DRY HEAT	105	18.47	0	0.744
15010	CATFISH, CHANNEL, WILD, RAW	95	16.38	0	0.722
11935	CATSUP	104	1.52	27.29	0.049
11949	CATSUP, LOW SODIUM	104	1.52	27.29	0.049
11761	CAULIFLOWER, CKD, BLD, DRND, W/SALT	23	1.84	4.11	0.07
11136	CAULIFLOWER, CKD, BLD, DRND, WO/SALT	23	1.84	4.11	0.07
11762	CAULIFLOWER, FRZ, CKD, BLD, DRND, W/SALT	19	1.61	3.75	0.033
11138	CAULIFLOWER, FRZ, CKD, BLD, DRND, WO/SALT	19	1.61	3.75	0.033
11137	CAULIFLOWER, FRZ, UNPREP	24	2.01	4.68	0.041
11965	CAULIFLOWER, GREEN, RAW	31	2.95	6.09	0.047
11967	CAULIFLOWER, GRN, CKD, NO SALT	32	3.04	6.28	0.049

NDB #	Food Description (100 gram portions = 3½ ounces = 20 tsp = ½ cup approx.	Calories	Protein	Carbs	Sat Fat
11968	CAULIFLOWER, GRN, CKD, SALT	32	3.04	6.28	0.049
11135	CAULIFLOWER, RAW	25	1.98	5.2	0.032
15012	CAVIAR, BLACK&RED, GRANULAR	252	24.6	4	4.06
11763	CELERIAC, CKD, BLD, DRND, W/SALT	27	0.96	5.9	
11142	CELERIAC, CKD, BLD, DRND, WO/SALT	27	0.96	5.9	
11141	CELERIAC, RAW	42	1.5	9.2	0.079
02007	CELERY SEED	392	18.07	41.35	2.19
11764	CELERY, CKD, BLD, DRND, W/SALT	18	0.83	4.01	0.04
11144	CELERY, CKD, BLD, DRND, WO/SALT	18	0.83	4.01	0.04
11143	CELERY, RAW	16	0.75	3.65	0.037
22542	CELESTE DELUXE PIZZA W/SAUSAGE, GRN&RED PEPPERS&MUSHR	231	10	19.9	4.86
11145	CELTUCE, RAW	18	0.85	3.65	
08025	CEREALS RTE, CRISPY RICE	396	6.4	88.6	0.109
08263	CEREALS RTE, GENERAL MILLS, APPL CINN CHEERIOS	392	6	84	0.99
08262	CEREALS RTE, GENERAL MILLS, BASIC 4	367	8	77	0.8
08274	CEREALS RTE, GENERAL MILLS, BERRY BERRY KIX	393	4	87	0.7
08273	CEREALS RTE, GENERAL MILLS, BOO BERRY	393	3	90	0.4
08013	CEREALS RTE, GENERAL MILLS, CHEERIOS	369	11	74	1.2
08139	CEREALS RTE, GENERAL MILLS, CINN GRAHAMS	378	5	86	0.5
08272	CEREALS RTE, GENERAL MILLS, CINN TOAST CRUNCH	422	5	79	1.8
08271	CEREALS RTE, GENERAL MILLS, COCOA PUFFS	390	4	88	0.7
08017	CEREALS RTE, GENERAL MILLS, COOKIE CRISP	389	4	88	0.6
08019	CEREALS RTE, GENERAL MILLS, CORN CHEX	373	7	86	0.2
08270	CEREALS RTE, GENERAL MILLS, COUNT CHOCULA	395	4	88	0.7
08269	CEREALS RTE, GENERAL MILLS, COUNTRY CORN FLAKES	371	6	85	0.4
08244	CEREALS RTE, GENERAL MILLS, FIBER ONE	197	8	81	0.4
08268	CEREALS RTE, GENERAL MILLS, FRANKENBERRY	392	3	90	0.4
08086	CEREALS RTE, GENERAL MILLS, FRENCH TOAST CRUNCH	390	4	88	0.6
08267	CEREALS RTE, GENERAL MILLS, FRSTD CHEERIOS	382	5	86	0.7
08397	CEREALS RTE, GENERAL MILLS, FRSTD CORN FLAKES	392	4	92	0.2
08266	CEREALS RTE, GENERAL MILLS, FRSTD WHEATIES	373	5	89	0.2
08035	CEREALS RTE, GENERAL MILLS, GOLDEN GRAHAMS	372	5	83	0.6
08398	CEREALS RTE, GENERAL MILLS, HARMONY	365	11	79	0.5
08045	CEREALS RTE, GENERAL MILLS, HONEY NUT CHEERIOS	373	9	80	0.8
08057	CEREALS RTE, GENERAL MILLS, HONEY NUT CHEX	381	5	87	0.4

NDB #	Food Description (100 gram portions = 3½ ounces = 20 tsp = ½ cup approx.	Calories	Protein	Carbs	Sat Fat
08243	CEREALS RTE, GENERAL MILLS, HONEY NUT CLUSTERS	389	8	83	0.6
08278	CEREALS RTE, GENERAL MILLS, KABOOM	383	9	81	0.9
08048	CEREALS RTE, GENERAL MILLS, KIX	377	6	86	0.5
08050	CEREALS RTE, GENERAL MILLS, LUCKY CHARMS	380	7	83	0.8
08345	CEREALS RTE, GENERAL MILLS, MULTI-BRAN CHEX	338	7	84	0.5
08087	CEREALS RTE, GENERAL MILLS, MULTI-GRAIN CHEERIOS	361	8	81	0.9
08277	CEREALS RTE, GENERAL MILLS, NATURE VALLEY LOFAT FRUIT GRA	42	8	80	0.85
08372	CEREALS RTE, GENERAL MILLS, NESQUICK CHOC	407	5	85	1.3
08202	CEREALS RTE, GENERAL MILLS, OATMEAL CRISP W/ ALMONDS	397	10	76	1.1
08190	CEREALS RTE, GENERAL MILLS, OATMEAL CRISP W/ APPLS	377	9	82	0.8
08245	CEREALS RTE, GENERAL MILLS, OATMEAL RAISIN CRISP	370	9	81	0.8
08368	CEREALS RTE, GENERAL MILLS, PARA SU FAMILIA CINN CORN STAR	386	5	87	0.5
08371	CEREALS RTE, GENERAL MILLS, PARA SU FAMILIA RAISIN BRAN	309	9	74	0.5
08261	CEREALS RTE, GENERAL MILLS, RAISIN NUT BRAN	380	9.39	75.37	1.4
08194	CEREALS RTE, GENERAL MILLS, REESE'S PUFFS	425	6	78	1.9
08064	CEREALS RTE, GENERAL MILLS, RICE CHEX	377	6	86	0.4
08370	CEREALS RTE, GENERAL MILLS, RICE CRUNCHINS	381	7	86	0.4
08367	CEREALS RTE, GENERAL MILLS, SUNRISE	380	6	87	0.4
08399	CEREALS RTE, GENERAL MILLS, TOTAL BROWN SUGAR & OAT	339	6.4	76.3	0.5
08246	CEREALS RTE, GENERAL MILLS, TOTAL CORN FLAKES	373	6.05	85.55	0.4
08247	CEREALS RTE, GENERAL MILLS, TOTAL RAISIN BRAN	311	7	75	0.4
08078	CEREALS RTE, GENERAL MILLS, TRIX	391	3	89	0.6
08082	CEREALS RTE, GENERAL MILLS, WHEAT CHEX	345	10	81	0.4
08089	CEREALS RTE, GENERAL MILLS, WHEATIES	355	10	81	0.6
08026	CEREALS RTE, GENERAL MILLS, WHEATIES RAISIN BRAN	333	7	81	0.4
08077	CEREALS RTE, GENERAL MILLS, WHL GRAIN TOTAL	324	8	75	0.6
08037	CEREALS RTE, GRANOLA, HOMEMADE	467	14.7	53	4.75
08040	CEREALS RTE, HEARTLAND NATURAL CEREAL, PLAIN	434	10.1	68.3	3.93
08041	CEREALS RTE, HEARTLAND NATURAL CEREAL, WITH COCONUT	441	10.4	67.9	5.931
08042	CEREALS RTE, HEARTLAND NATURAL CEREAL, WITH RAISINS	425	9.7	69	3.623
08389	CEREALS RTE, HONEY PUFFED KASHI BY KELLOGG	379	10	83.3	
08393	CEREALS RTE, KASHI GOLEAN BY KELLOGG	314	21	71	
08386	CEREALS RTE, KASHI GOLEAN CRUNCH BY KELLOGG	377	17.5	67.9	0.47
08390	CEREALS RTE, KASHI GOOD FRIENDS BY KELLOGG	309	10	81.3	
08387	CEREALS RTE, KASHI HEART TO HEART BY KELLOGG	356	13.4	76.7	

NDB #	Food Description (100 gram portions = 3½ ounces = 20 tsp = ½ cup approx.	Calories	Protein	Carbs	Sat Fat
08392	CEREALS RTE, KASHI MEDLEY BY KELLOGG	378	14	77	
08391	CEREALS RTE, KASHI PILLOWS BY KELLOGG, ASSORTED FLAVORS	370	5.9	84.5	
08005	CEREALS RTE, KELLOGG, KELLOGG'S ALL-BRAN BRAN BUDS	250	7	80	0.4
08253	CEREALS RTE, KELLOGG, KELLOGG'S ALL-BRAN W/ EX FIBER	192	11.3	77	0.6
08254	CEREALS RTE, KELLOGG, KELLOGG'S APPL CINN SQUARES MINI-WH	331	7.2	80.1	0.4
08003	CEREALS RTE, KELLOGG, KELLOGG'S APPL JACKS	390	3	91	0.4
08014	CEREALS RTE, KELLOGG, KELLOGG'S COCOA KRISPIES	381	3.4	87.1	1.7
08258	CEREALS RTE, KELLOGG, KELLOGG'S COMPLETE OAT BRAN FLAKE	350	11	77	0.8
08028	CEREALS RTE, KELLOGG, KELLOGG'S COMPLETE WHEAT BRAN FLA	318	10	79	0.4
08020	CEREALS RTE, KELLOGG, KELLOGG'S CORN FLAKES	361	7	86	0.2
08068	CEREALS RTE, KELLOGG, KELLOGG'S CORN POPS	380	3.7	90	0.23
08023	CEREALS RTE, KELLOGG, KELLOGG'S CRACKLIN' OAT BRAN	409	8.3	71.4	4.2
08259	CEREALS RTE, KELLOGG, KELLOGG'S CRISPIX	377	6.8	86	0.2
08375	CEREALS RTE, KELLOGG, KELLOGG'S CRUNCHEROOS	361	10.1	77	1
08030	CEREALS RTE, KELLOGG, KELLOGG'S FROOT LOOPS	393	3.4	87.5	1.9
08069	CEREALS RTE, KELLOGG, KELLOGG'S FRSTD FLAKES	367	3.3	90.3	0.17
08319	CEREALS RTE, KELLOGG, KELLOGG'S FRSTD MINI-WHEATS, BITE SIZ	344	10.1	81	0.36
08032	CEREALS RTE, KELLOGG, KELLOGG'S FRSTD RICE KRISPIES	379	3.4	89.9	0.2
08309	CEREALS RTE, KELLOGG, KELLOGG'S HONEY CRUNCH CORN FLAK	390	6.8	87	0.55
08377	CEREALS RTE, KELLOGG, KELLOGG'S HONEY FRSTD MINI-WHEATS	340	8.7	81.4	0.36
08283	CEREALS RTE, KELLOGG, KELLOGG'S JUST RIGHT FRUIT & NUT	366	7	81.7	0.5
08284	CEREALS RTE, KELLOGG, KELLOGG'S LOFAT GRANOLA W/ RAISINS	383	8	80	1.5
08189	CEREALS RTE, KELLOGG, KELLOGG'S LOFAT GRANOLA WO/ RAISIN	380	8.2	79.6	1.1
08376	CEREALS RTE, KELLOGG, KELLOGG'S MARSHMLLW BLASTED FROO	383	3.4	90.1	1
08286	CEREALS RTE, KELLOGG, KELLOGG'S MUESLIX	357	9.1	73	0.8
08058	CEREALS RTE, KELLOGG, KELLOGG'S PRODUCT 19	364	7.7	83	0.3
08378	CEREALS RTE, KELLOGG, KELLOGG'S PUFFED RICE	412	8.4	87.2	0.4
08379	CEREALS RTE, KELLOGG, KELLOGG'S PUFFED WHEAT	332	9.1	81.8	0.3
08060	CEREALS RTE, KELLOGG, KELLOGG'S RAISIN BRAN	319	8.5	76.3	0.55
08287	CEREALS RTE, KELLOGG, KELLOGG'S RAISIN SQUARES MINI-WHEAT	336	9.4	79.2	0.35
08065	CEREALS RTE, KELLOGG, KELLOGG'S RICE KRISPIES	387	6.2	88	0.37
08288	CEREALS RTE, KELLOGG, KELLOGG'S RICE KRISPIES TREATS CRL	408	4	87	1.4
08384	CEREALS RTE, KELLOGG, KELLOGG'S SHREDDED WHEAT MINIATUR	332	11.2	80	0.4
08071	CEREALS RTE, KELLOGG, KELLOGG'S SMACKS	387	6.4	89	0.3
08318	CEREALS RTE, KELLOGG, KELLOGG'S SMART START CRL	364	6.2	86	0.4

NDB #	Food Description (100 gram portions = 3½ ounces = 20 tsp = ½ cup approx.	Calories	Protein	Carbs	Sat Fat
08067	CEREALS RTE, KELLOGG, KELLOGG'S SPL K	379	22.5	71	0.35
08383	CEREALS RTE, KELLOGG, KELLOGG'S SPL K RED BERRIES	369	12.4	80.6	0.24
08289	CEREALS RTE, KELLOGG, KELLOGG'S STRAWBERRY MINI-WHEATS	335	7.9	80	0.4
08001	CEREALS RTE, KELLOGG, KELLOGG'S, ALL-BRAN ORIGINAL	260	12.5	74	0.54
08374	CEREALS RTE, KELLOGG, KELLOGG'S, CRISPIX CINN CRUNCH	399	4.8	87	0.5
08381	CEREALS RTE, KELLOGG, KELLOGG'S, CRUNCHIN' RICE KRISPIES	388	6.3	84.4	1.5
08380	CEREALS RTE, KELLOGG, KELLOGG'S, RAISIN BRAN CRUNCH	354	6.1	84.9	0.38
08373	CEREALS RTE, KELLOGG'S COUNTRY INN-GREYFIELD BLEND	414	6.3	74.5	1.4
08031	CEREALS RTE, KELLOGG'S FRSTD MINI-WHEATS, ORIGINAL	340	9.8	80.4	0.36
08385	CEREALS RTE, KELLOGG'S, SMART START SOY PROT	367	19	73	0.6
08343	CEREALS RTE, KRAFT, POST 100% BRAN CRL	287	12.7	78.2	0.3
08320	CEREALS RTE, KRAFT, POST BANANA NUT CRUNCH CRL	422	8.5	74	1.4
08321	CEREALS RTE, KRAFT, POST BLUEBERRY MORNING CRL	383	6.6	78.9	0.6
08322	CEREALS RTE, KRAFT, POST BRAN FLAKES	320	9.4	80.4	0.4
08323	CEREALS RTE, KRAFT, POST COCOA PEBBLES CRL	398	3.5	87.9	3.7
08325	CEREALS RTE, KRAFT, POST FRSTD ALPHA-BITS CRL	405	8.5	83.5	0.8
08339	CEREALS RTE, KRAFT, POST FRSTD SHREDDED WHEAT BITE SIZE C	352	7.8	83.8	0.3
08327	CEREALS RTE, KRAFT, POST FRUIT&FIBRE DATES, RAISINS&WALNUT	385	7.1	76.2	0.8
08324	CEREALS RTE, KRAFT, POST FRUITY PEBBLES CRL	401	3.6	87.9	0.9
08328	CEREALS RTE, KRAFT, POST GOLDEN CRISP CRL	398	5.5	90.9	0.2
08329	CEREALS RTE, KRAFT, POST GRAPE-NUTS CRL	359	10.8	81.3	0.4
08330	CEREALS RTE, KRAFT, POST GRAPE-NUTS FLAKES	365	10	81.5	0.6
08331	CEREALS RTE, KRAFT, POST GREAT GRAINS CRUNCHY PECAN CRL	408	9.3	71.4	1.4
08332	CEREALS RTE, KRAFT, POST GREAT GRAINS RAISIN, DATE&PECAN C	377	8	73.2	1.1
08333	CEREALS RTE, KRAFT, POST HONEY BUNCHES OF OATS HONEY RST	394	7.1	81.9	0.8
08334	CEREALS RTE, KRAFT, POST HONEY BUNCHES OF OATS W/ALMOND	407	7.8	78	1.1
08335	CEREALS RTE, KRAFT, POST HONEYCOMB CRL	395	5.2	88.9	0.6
08326	CEREALS RTE, KRAFT, POST MARSHMLLW ALPHA-BITS CRL	398	5.9	86.7	0.6
08336	CEREALS RTE, KRAFT, POST OREO O'S CRL	415	4.8	79.7	1.6
08337	CEREALS RTE, KRAFT, POST RAISIN BRAN CRL	317	7.9	78.1	0.3
08342	CEREALS RTE, KRAFT, POST THE ORIGIN SHREDDED WHEAT SPOO	340	10.3	83	0.2
08340	CEREALS RTE, KRAFT, POST THE ORIGINAL SHREDDED WHEAT CER	340	10.4	82.9	0.2
08341	CEREALS RTE, KRAFT, POST THE ORIGINAL SHREDDED WHEAT 'N B	334	12.5	79.9	0.2
08338	CEREALS RTE, KRAFT, POST TOASTIES CORN FLAKES	360	6.7	86.7	0
08344	CEREALS RTE, KRAFT, POST WAFFLE CRISP CRL	430	6	79.1	1.4

NDB #	Food Description (100 gram portions = 3½ ounces = 20 tsp = ½ cup approx.	Calories	Protein	Carbs	Sat Fat
08347	CEREALS RTE, MALT-O-MEAL, BERRY COLOSSAL CRUNCH	401	4	85.73	1.23
08346	CEREALS RTE, MALT-O-MEAL, COLOSSAL CRUNCH	401	3.73	85.63	1.33
08083	CEREALS RTE, MALT-O-MEAL, CORN BURSTS	382	3.37	92.47	0.2
08348	CEREALS RTE, MALT-O-MEAL, CRISPY RICE	379	6.2	86.89	0.37
08138	CEREALS RTE, MALT-O-MEAL, MARSHMLLW MATEYS	384	7.57	83.73	0.68
08349	CEREALS RTE, MALT-O-MEAL, TOOTIE FRUITIES	392	4.96	87.7	0.82
08152	CEREALS RTE, NUTRI-GRAIN, WHEAT, SEE NEW PRODUCT 08292	360	8.7	84.6	0.185
08388	CEREALS RTE, PUFFED KASHI BY KELLOGG	365	12.4	81.2	
08218	CEREALS RTE, QUAKER, 100% NAT CRL W/ OATS, HONEY, & RAISINS	441	9.61	68.46	7.24
08054	CEREALS RTE, QUAKER, 100% NAT GRANOLA OATS & HONEY	455	10.6	66.43	8.25
08010	CEREALS RTE, QUAKER, CAP'N CRUNCH	401	4.35	84.82	1.5
08011	CEREALS RTE, QUAKER, CAP'N CRUNCH W/ CRUNCHBERRIES	401	4.45	85.07	1.43
08012	CEREALS RTE, QUAKER, CAP'N CRUNCH'S PNUT BUTTER CRUNCH	416	7.05	78.73	2.09
08364	CEREALS RTE, QUAKER, CINN CRUNCH BAGGED CRL	397	5.07	83.67	1.52
08400	CEREALS RTE, QUAKER, CRANBERRY MACADAMIA NUT CRL	408	6.64	76.98	1.65
08358	CEREALS RTE, QUAKER, CRISPY CORN PUFFS CRL	376	7.23	83.5	0.52
08359	CEREALS RTE, QUAKER, FRSTD OATS	396	6.06	81.96	1.29
08357	CEREALS RTE, QUAKER, FRUITY BRONTOSAURUS BLASTS, BAGGED	376	3.75	89.27	0.23
08401	CEREALS RTE, QUAKER, FRUITY OCEAN ADVENTURE BAGGED CRL	394	4.86	87.24	0.9
08396	CEREALS RTE, QUAKER, HONEY CRISP CORN FLAKES	374	5.68	88.82	0.1
08361	CEREALS RTE, QUAKER, HONEY GRAHAM BAGGED CRL	395	5.6	83.64	1.31
08211	CEREALS RTE, QUAKER, HONEY GRAHAM OH!S	411	3.97	83.78	2
08219	CEREALS RTE, QUAKER, HONEY NUT HEAVEN	392	9.15	77.4	1.09
08395	CEREALS RTE, QUAKER, HONEY NUT OATS	385	6.04	84.53	0.63
08047	CEREALS RTE, QUAKER, KING VITAMAN	386	6.45	84.9	0.79
08085	CEREALS RTE, QUAKER, KRETSCHMER HONEY CRUNCH WHEAT GE	372	26.55	58.11	1.36
08363	CEREALS RTE, QUAKER, KRETSCHMER TSTD WHEAT BRAN	200	17.56	59.51	0.77
08366	CEREALS RTE, QUAKER, KRETSCHMER WHEAT GERM, REG	366	31.43	49.38	1.66
08220	CEREALS RTE, QUAKER, LOFAT 100% NAT GRANOLA W/ RAISINS	390	7.95	81.18	1.39
08353	CEREALS RTE, QUAKER, MOTHER'S CINN OAT CRUNCH	380	10.49	79.21	0.79
08355	CEREALS RTE, QUAKER, MOTHER'S COCOA BUMPERS	376	5.08	87.64	0.31
08354	CEREALS RTE, QUAKER, MOTHER'S GROOVY GRAHAMS	372	5.44	86.38	0.28
08394	CEREALS RTE, QUAKER, MOTHER'S HONEY ROUNDUP	382	5.44	87.77	0.38
08351	CEREALS RTE, QUAKER, MOTHER'S PNUT BUTTER BUMPERS CRL	403	8.28	78.27	1.44
08352	CEREALS RTE, QUAKER, MOTHER'S TSTD OAT BRAN CRL, BROWN S	373	11.9	74.92	0.89

NDB #	Food Description (100 gram portions = 3½ ounces = 20 tsp = ½ cup approx.	Calories	Protein	Carbs	Sat Fat
08360	CEREALS RTE, QUAKER, OATMEAL CRL, BROWN SUGAR BLISS	384	8.78	79.69	1.16
08293	CEREALS RTE, QUAKER, QUAKER APPL ZAPS	393	3.68	88.74	0.87
08215	CEREALS RTE, QUAKER, QUAKER CINN OATMEAL SQUARES	378	10.11	79.83	0.84
08294	CEREALS RTE, QUAKER, QUAKER COCOA BLASTS	394	3.67	88.7	0.95
08018	CEREALS RTE, QUAKER, QUAKER CRUNCHY BRAN	335	5.44	86.34	0.746
08216	CEREALS RTE, QUAKER, QUAKER OAT BRAN CRL	372	12.38	74.89	0.91
08210	CEREALS RTE, QUAKER, QUAKER OAT CINN LIFE	375	8.91	79.64	0.73
08049	CEREALS RTE, QUAKER, QUAKER OAT LIFE, PLN	375	9.92	78.1	0.81
08214	CEREALS RTE, QUAKER, QUAKER OATMEAL SQUARES	378	11.04	78.34	0.9
08066	CEREALS RTE, QUAKER, QUAKER PUFFED RICE	383	7	87.77	0.32
08146	CEREALS RTE, QUAKER, QUAKER PUFFED WHEAT	366	16.26	76.39	0.41
08299	CEREALS RTE, QUAKER, QUAKER SWT PUFFS	391	6.76	87.99	0.36
08212	CEREALS RTE, QUAKER, SUN COUNTRY GRANOLA W/ ALMONDS	467	11.77	67.2	2.22
08059	CEREALS RTE, QUAKER, SWT CRUNCH/QUISP	405	4.44	85	1.58
08362	CEREALS RTE, QUAKER, TSTD OATS/OATMMM'S	380	9.23	77.91	0.91
08156	CEREALS RTE, RICE, PUFFED, FORT	402	6.3	89.8	0.13
08079	CEREALS RTE, WAFFELOS	405	5.6	86.3	
08084	CEREALS RTE, WHEAT GERM, TSTD, PLN	382	29.1	49.6	1.83
08157	CEREALS RTE, WHEAT, PUFFED, FORT	364	14.7	79.6	0.2
08147	CEREALS RTE, WHEAT, SHREDDED, PLN, SUGAR&SALT FREE, SINGL	340	10.98	82.46	0.2
08161	CEREALS, CORN GRITS, WHITE, REG, QUICK, ENR, CKD W/ H2O, W/ S	60	1.4	13	0.03
08091	CEREALS, CORN GRITS, WHITE, REG, QUICK, ENR, CKD W/ H2O, WO/	60	1.4	13	0.03
08090	CEREALS, CORN GRITS, WHITE, REG, QUICK, ENR, DRY	371	8.8	79.6	0.16
08163	CEREALS, CORN GRITS, WHITE, REG, QUICK, UNENR, CKD W/ H2O, W	60	1.4	13	0.03
08162	CEREALS, CORN GRITS, WHITE, REG, QUICK, UNENR, CKD W/ H2O, W	60	1.4	13	0.03
08158	CEREALS, CORN GRITS, WHITE, REG, QUICK, UNENR, DRY	371	8.8	79.6	0.16
08165	CEREALS, CORN GRITS, YEL, REG, QUICK, ENR, CKD W/ H2O, W/ SAL	60	1.4	13	0.03
08164	CEREALS, CORN GRITS, YEL, REG, QUICK, ENR, CKD W/ H2O, WO/ SA	60	1.4	13	0.03
08159	CEREALS, CORN GRITS, YEL, REG, QUICK, ENR, DRY	371	8.8	79.6	0.16
08167	CEREALS, CORN GRITS, YEL, REG, QUICK, UNENR, CKD W/ H2O, W/ S	60	1.4	13	0.03
08166	CEREALS, CORN GRITS, YEL, REG, QUICK, UNENR, CKD W/ H2O, WO/	60	1.4	13	0.03
08160	CEREALS, CORN GRITS, YEL, REG, QUICK, UNENR, DRY	371	8.8	79.6	0.16
08168	CEREALS, CREAM OF RICE, CKD W/ H2O, W/ SALT	52	0.9	11.5	0.02
08101	CEREALS, CREAM OF RICE, CKD W/ H2O, WO/ SALT	52	0.9	11.4	0.027
08100	CEREALS, CREAM OF RICE, DRY	370	6.3	82.4	0.136

NDB #	Food Description (100 gram portions = 3½ ounces = 20 tsp = ½ cup approx.	Calories	Protein	Carbs	Sat Fat
08106	CEREALS, CREAM OF WHEAT, INST, DRY	366	10.6	75.5	0.236
08171	CEREALS, CREAM OF WHEAT, INST, PREP W/ H2O, W/ SALT	64	1.8	13.1	0.031
08107	CEREALS, CREAM OF WHEAT, INST, PREP W/ H2O, WO/ SALT	64	1.8	13.1	0.034
08108	CEREALS, CREAM OF WHEAT, MIX'N EAT, PLN, DRY	361	9.7	75.6	0.203
08109	CEREALS, CREAM OF WHEAT, MIX'N EAT, PLN, PREP W/ H2O	72	1.9	15.1	0.034
08170	CEREALS, CREAM OF WHEAT, QUICK, CKD W/ H2O, W/ SALT	54	1.5	11.2	0.031
08105	CEREALS, CREAM OF WHEAT, QUICK, CKD W/ H2O, WO/ SALT	54	1.5	11.2	0.034
08104	CEREALS, CREAM OF WHEAT, QUICK, DRY	361	10.2	75	0.219
08169	CEREALS, CREAM OF WHEAT, REG, CKD W/ H2O, W/ SALT	53	1.5	11	0.031
08103	CEREALS, CREAM OF WHEAT, REG, CKD W/ H2O, WO/ SALT	53	1.5	11	0.034
08102	CEREALS, CREAM OF WHEAT, REG, DRY	370	10.5	76.5	0.253
08110	CEREALS, CRM OF WHEAT, MIX'N EAT, APPL, BANANA&MAPLE FLAV,	373	6.9	81.6	
08111	CEREALS, CRM OF WHEAT, MIX'N EAT, APPL, BANANA&MAPLE FLAV,	88	1.6	19.3	0.044
08173	CEREALS, FARINA, ENR, CKD W/ H2O, W/ SALT	50	1.4	10.6	0.01
08113	CEREALS, FARINA, ENR, CKD W/H2O, WO/SALT, (WHEAT)	50	1.4	10.6	0.01
08112	CEREALS, FARINA, ENR, DRY	369	10.6	78	0.08
08175	CEREALS, FARINA, UNENR, CKD W/ H2O, W/ SALT	50	1.4	10.6	0.01
08174	CEREALS, FARINA, UNENR, CKD W/ H2O, WO/ SALT	50	1.4	10.6	0.01
08172	CEREALS, FARINA, UNENR, DRY	369	10.6	78	0.08
08176	CEREALS, MALTEX, CKD W/ H2O, W/ SALT	72	2.3	15.9	0.061
08115	CEREALS, MALTEX, CKD W/ H2O, WO/ SALT	72	2.3	15.9	0.069
08114	CEREALS, MALTEX, DRY	352	11.2	77.3	0.336
08177	CEREALS, MALT-O-MEAL, CHOC, DRY	368	10.5	77.7	
08178	CEREALS, MALT-O-MEAL, PLN & CHOC, CKD W/ H2O, W/ SALT	51	1.5	10.8	0.02
08117	CEREALS, MALT-O-MEAL, PLN & CHOC, CKD W/ H2O, WO/ SALT	51	1.5	10.7	0.042
08116	CEREALS, MALT-O-MEAL, PLN, DRY	368	10.5	77.7	
08179	CEREALS, MAYPO, CKD W/ H2O, W/ SALT	71	2.4	13.3	0.185
08119	CEREALS, MAYPO, CKD W/ H2O, WO/ SALT	71	2.4	13.3	0.175
08118	CEREALS, MAYPO, DRY	385	13.2	72	
08240	CEREALS, OAT BRAN, QKR, QKR/MOTHER'S OAT BRAN, PREP W/H2O	43	2.03	7.49	0.17
08122	CEREALS, OATS, INST, FORT, PLN, DRY	369	15.5	64	1.075
08123	CEREALS, OATS, INST, FORT, PLN, PREP W/ H2O	59	2.5	10.2	0.18
08126	CEREALS, OATS, INST, FORT, W/ BRAN & RAISINS, DRY	371	11.4	71.5	
08127	CEREALS, OATS, INST, FORT, W/ BRAN & RAISINS, PREP W/ H2O	81	2.5	15.6	0.182
08128	CEREALS, OATS, INST, FORT, W/ CINN & SPICE, DRY	373	8.47	77.92	0.86

NDB #	Food Description (100 gram portions = 3½ ounces = 20 tsp = ½ cup approx.	Calories	Protein	Carbs	Sat Fat
08129	CEREALS, OATS, INST, FORT, W/ CINN & SPICE, PREP W/ H2O	110	3	21.8	0.221
08132	CEREALS, OATS, INST, FORT, W/ RAISINS & SPICE, DRY	363	10.52	74.48	0.83
08133	CEREALS, OATS, INST, FORT, W/ RAISINS & SPICE, PREP W/ H2O	102	2.7	20.2	0.209
08180	CEREALS, OATS, REG & QUICK & INST, UNENR, CKD W/ H2O, W/ SALT	62	2.6	10.8	0.18
08121	CEREALS, OATS, REG & QUICK & INST, UNENR, CKD W/ H2O, WO/ SAL	62	2.6	10.8	0.18
08120	CEREALS, OATS, REG & QUICK & INST, UNENR, DRY	384	16	67	1.11
08236	CEREALS, QKR, OAT BRAN, PREP W/H2O, NO SALT	43	2.03	7.49	0.17
08301	CEREALS, QKR, OATMEAL, MICRO, QUICK 'N HEARTY, BROWN SUGA	369	9.37	74.69	0.95
08302	CEREALS, QKR, OATMEAL, MICRO, QUICK 'N HEARTY, CINN DOUBLE	359	8.39	74.43	0.87
08221	CEREALS, QUAKER, CORN GRITS, INST, BUTTER FLAVOR, DRY	359	8.25	74.45	1.02
08094	CEREALS, QUAKER, CORN GRITS, INST, CHEDDAR CHS FLAVOR, DR	364	8.39	73.29	1.72
08095	CEREALS, QUAKER, CORN GRITS, INST, CHEDDAR CHS FLAVOR, PR	70	1.6	14.01	0.33
08092	CEREALS, QUAKER, CORN GRITS, INST, PLN, DRY	342	8.43	78.82	0.1
08093	CEREALS, QUAKER, CORN GRITS, INST, PLN, PREP W/H2O	65	1.61	15.06	0.019
08096	CEREALS, QUAKER, CORN GRITS, INST, W/IMITN BACON BITS, DRY	349	9.85	77.35	0.24
08097	CEREALS, QUAKER, CORN GRITS, INST, W/IMITN BACON BITS, PREP	67	1.88	14.78	0.046
08098	CEREALS, QUAKER, CORN GRITS, INST, W/IMITN HAM BITS, DRY	341	9.95	75.26	0.3
08099	CEREALS, QUAKER, CORN GRITS, INST, W/IMITN HAM BITS, PREP W/	65	1.9	14.29	0.057
08237	CEREALS, QUAKER, CREAMY WHEAT, FARINA, ENR, PREP W/H2O, NO	51	1.53	11.26	0.01
08241	CEREALS, QUAKER, CREAMY WHEAT, FARINA, ENR, PREP W/H2O, SA	51	1.53	11.24	0.01
08230	CEREALS, QUAKER, FARINA, CREAMY WHEAT, ENR, DRY	349	10.82	76.13	0.24
08317	CEREALS, QUAKER, FARINA, ENR CINN FLAVOR, DRY	346	12.11	74.54	0.28
08314	CEREALS, QUAKER, HOMINY GRITS, WHITE, QUICK, DRY	347	8.53	79.16	0.26
08316	CEREALS, QUAKER, HOMINY GRITS, WHITE, REG, DRY	347	8.53	79.16	0.26
08315	CEREALS, QUAKER, HOMINY GRITS, YEL, QUICK, DRY	337	8.26	77.76	0.45
08231	CEREALS, QUAKER, OAT BRAN, QUAKER/MOTHER'S OAT BRAN, DRY	364	17.03	62.94	1.43
08225	CEREALS, QUAKER, OATMEAL, INST, FRUIT&CRM VAR, DRY	385	8.17	75.12	1.56
08227	CEREALS, QUAKER, OATMEAL, INST, FRUIT&CRM VAR, PREP W/H2O	118	2.51	23.06	0.48
08229	CEREALS, QUAKER, OATMEAL, INST, LO NA, DRY	368	14.22	66.07	1.35
08234	CEREALS, QUAKER, OATMEAL, INST, LO NA, PREP W/H2O	93	3.59	16.67	0.341
08130	CEREALS, QUAKER, OATMEAL, INST, MAPLE&BROWN SUGAR, DRY	371	10.12	76.08	0.85
08131	CEREALS, QUAKER, OATMEAL, INST, MAPLE&BROWN SUGAR, PREP	99	2.69	20.26	0.23
08228	CEREALS, QUAKER, OATMEAL, INST, RAISINS, DATES&WALNUTS, DR	365	8.87	73.69	0.94
08235	CEREALS, QUAKER, OATMEAL, INST, RAISINS, DATES&WALNUTS, PR	116	2.83	23.5	0.3
08124	CEREALS, QUAKER, OATMEAL, INST, W/APPLS&CINN, DRY	367	9.4	76.97	0.86

NDB #	Food Description (100 gram portions = 3½ ounces = 20 tsp = ½ cup approx.	Calories	Protein	Carbs	Sat Fat
08125	CEREALS, QUAKER, OATMEAL, INST, W/APPLS&CINN, PREP W/H2O	84	2.14	17.55	0.196
08303	CEREALS, QUAKER, OATMEAL, MICRO, QUICK 'N HEARTY, HONEY BR	368	9.53	74.61	0.95
08300	CEREALS, QUAKER, OATMEAL, MICROWAVE, QUICK 'N HEARTY APPL	368	8.18	77.43	0.83
08304	CEREALS, QUAKER, OATMEAL, MICROWAVE, QUICK 'N HEARTY, REG	365	13.24	65.69	1.36
08200	CEREALS, QUAKER, QUAKER MULTIGRAIN OATMEAL, DRY	333	11.3	73.44	0.52
08249	CEREALS, QUAKER, QUAKER MULTIGRAIN OATMEAL, PREP W/H2O, N	61	2.08	13.49	0.096
08252	CEREALS, QUAKER, QUAKER MULTIGRAIN OATMEAL, PREP W/H2O, S	61	2.07	13.47	0.095
08232	CEREALS, QUAKER, SCOTCH BARLEY, REG&QUICK, DRY	346	10.74	76.38	0.47
08185	CEREALS, RALSTON, CKD W/ H2O, W/ SALT	53	2.2	11.2	0.056
08135	CEREALS, RALSTON, CKD W/ H2O, WO/ SALT	53	2.2	11.2	0.052
08134	CEREALS, RALSTON, DRY	341	14.1	72.1	
08184	CEREALS, ROMAN MEAL WITH OATS, CKD W/ H2O, W/ SALT	71	3	14.2	0.072
08155	CEREALS, ROMAN MEAL WITH OATS, CKD W/ H2O, WO/ SALT	71	3	14.2	0.072
08181	CEREALS, ROMAN MEAL, PLN, CKD W/ H2O, W/ SALT	61	2.7	13.7	0.053
08137	CEREALS, ROMAN MEAL, PLN, CKD W/ H2O, WO/ SALT	61	2.7	13.7	0.053
08136	CEREALS, ROMAN MEAL, PLN, DRY	322	14.4	72	0.326
08350	CEREALS, RTE, MALT-O-MEAL, TOASTY O'S	372	11.07	74.67	1.23
08143	CEREALS, WHEATENA, CKD W/ H2O	56	2	11.8	0.075
08182	CEREALS, WHEATENA, CKD W/ H2O, W/ SALT	56	2	11.8	0.09
08142	CEREALS, WHEATENA, DRY	357	13.1	75.6	0.43
08183	CEREALS, WHL WHEAT HOT NAT CRL, CKD W/ H2O, W/ SALT	62	2	13.7	0.06
08145	CEREALS, WHL WHEAT HOT NAT CRL, CKD W/ H2O, WO/ SALT	62	2	13.7	0.06
08144	CEREALS, WHL WHEAT HOT NAT CRL, DRY	342	11.2	75.2	0.3
11765	CHARD, SWISS, CKD, BLD, DRND, W/SALT	20	1.88	4.14	
11148	CHARD, SWISS, CKD, BLD, DRND, WO/SALT	20	1.88	4.14	0.012
11147	CHARD, SWISS, RAW	19	1.8	3.74	0.03
11766	CHAYOTE, FRUIT, CKD, BLD, DRND, W/SALT	24	0.62	5.09	0.086
11150	CHAYOTE, FRUIT, CKD, BLD, DRND, WO/SALT	24	0.62	5.09	0.086
11149	CHAYOTE, FRUIT, RAW	19	0.82	4.5	0.028
01045	CHEESE FD, COLD PK, AMERICAN	331	19.66	8.32	15.355
01149	CHEESE FD, PAST PROCESS, AMERICAN, W/DI NA PO4	328	19.61	7.29	15.443
01046	CHEESE FD, PAST PROCESS, AMERICAN, WO/DI NA PO4	328	19.61	7.29	15.443
01047	CHEESE FD, PAST PROCESS, SWISS	323	21.92	4.5	15.487
01163	CHEESE FONDUE	229	14.23	3.77	8.721
01164	CHEESE SAU, PREP FROM RECIPE	197	10.33	5.48	8.034

NDB #	Food Description (100 gram portions = 3½ ounces = 20 tsp = ½ cup approx.	Calories	Protein	Carbs	Sat Fat
01150	CHEESE SPRD, PAST PROCESS, AMERICAN, W/DI NA PO4	290	16.41	8.73	13.327
01048	CHEESE SPRD, PAST PROCESS, AMERICAN, WO/DI NA PO4	290	16.41	8.73	13.327
01161	CHEESE SUB, MOZZARELLA	248	11.47	23.67	3.711
01004	CHEESE, BLUE	353	21.4	2.34	18.669
01005	CHEESE, BRICK	371	23.24	2.79	18.764
01006	CHEESE, BRIE	334	20.75	0.45	17.41
01007	CHEESE, CAMEMBERT	300	19.8	0.46	15.259
01008	CHEESE, CARAWAY	376	25.18	3.06	18.584
01009	CHEESE, CHEDDAR	403	24.9	1.28	21.092
01010	CHEESE, CHESHIRE	387	23.37	4.78	19.475
01011	CHEESE, COLBY	394	23.76	2.57	20.218
01012	CHEESE, COTTAGE, CRMD, LRG OR SML CURD	103	12.49	2.68	2.853
01013	CHEESE, COTTAGE, CRMD, W/FRUIT	124	9.9	13.3	2.151
01016	CHEESE, COTTAGE, LOWFAT, 1% MILKFAT	72	12.39	2.72	0.645
01015	CHEESE, COTTAGE, LOWFAT, 2% MILKFAT	90	13.74	3.63	1.221
01014	CHEESE, COTTAGE, NONFAT, UNCRMD, DRY, LRG OR SML CURD	85	17.27	1.85	0.273
01017	CHEESE, CREAM	349	7.55	2.66	21.966
01186	CHEESE, CREAM, FAT FREE	96	14.41	5.8	0.899
01018	CHEESE, EDAM	357	24.99	1.43	17.572
01019	CHEESE, FETA	264	14.21	4.09	14.946
01020	CHEESE, FONTINA	389	25.6	1.55	19.196
01021	CHEESE, GJETOST	466	9.65	42.65	19.16
01156	CHEESE, GOAT, HARD TYPE	452	30.52	2.17	24.609
01157	CHEESE, GOAT, SEMISOFT TYPE	364	21.58	2.54	20.639
01159	CHEESE, GOAT, SOFT TYPE	268	18.52	0.89	14.575
01022	CHEESE, GOUDA	356	24.94	2.22	17.614
01023	CHEESE, GRUYERE	413	29.81	0.36	18.913
01024	CHEESE, LIMBURGER	327	20.05	0.49	16.746
01168	CHEESE, LOFAT, CHEDDAR OR COLBY	173	24.35	1.91	4.342
01169	CHEESE, LOW-SODIUM, CHEDDAR OR COLBY	398	24.35	1.91	20.768
01165	CHEESE, MEXICAN, QUESO ANEJO	373	21.44	4.63	19.033
01166	CHEESE, MEXICAN, QUESO ASADERO	356	22.6	2.87	17.939
01167	CHEESE, MEXICAN, QUESO CHIHUAHUA	374	21.56	5.56	18.843
01025	CHEESE, MONTEREY	373	24.48	0.68	19.066
01028	CHEESE, MOZZARELLA, PART SKIM MILK	254	24.26	2.77	10.114

NDB #	Food Description (100 gram portions = 3½ ounces = 20 tsp = ½ cup approx.	Calories	Protein	Carbs	Sat Fat
01029	CHEESE, MOZZARELLA, PART SKIM MILK, LO MOIST	280	27.47	3.14	10.877
01026	CHEESE, MOZZARELLA, WHL MILK	281	19.42	2.22	13.152
01027	CHEESE, MOZZARELLA, WHL MILK, LO MOIST	318	21.6	2.47	15.561
01030	CHEESE, MUENSTER	368	23.41	1.12	19.113
01031	CHEESE, NEUFCHATEL	260	9.96	2.94	14.797
01032	CHEESE, PARMESAN, GRATED	456	41.56	3.74	19.072
01033	CHEESE, PARMESAN, HARD	392	35.75	3.22	16.41
01146	CHEESE, PARMESAN, SHREDDED	415	37.86	3.41	17.37
01042	CHEESE, PAST PROCESS, AMERICAN, W/DI NA PO4	375	22.15	1.6	19.694
01147	CHEESE, PAST PROCESS, AMERICAN, WO/DI NA PO4	375	22.15	1.6	19.694
01043	CHEESE, PAST PROCESS, PIMENTO	375	22.13	1.73	19.663
01044	CHEESE, PAST PROCESS, SWISS, W/DI NA PO4	334	24.73	2.1	16.045
01148	CHEESE, PAST PROCESS, SWISS, WO/DI NA PO4	334	24.73	2.1	16.045
01034	CHEESE, PORT DE SALUT	352	23.78	0.57	16.691
01035	CHEESE, PROVOLONE	351	25.58	2.14	17.078
01037	CHEESE, RICOTTA, PART SKIM MILK	138	11.39	5.14	4.927
01036	CHEESE, RICOTTA, WHOLE MILK	174	11.26	3.04	8.295
01038	CHEESE, ROMANO	387	31.8	3.63	17.115
01039	CHEESE, ROQUEFORT	369	21.54	2	19.263
01040	CHEESE, SWISS	376	28.43	3.38	17.779
01041	CHEESE, TILSIT	340	24.41	1.88	16.775
18147	CHEESECAKE COMMLY PREP	321	5.5	25.5	9.921
18148	CHEESECAKE PREP FROM MIX, NO-BAKE TYPE	274	5.5	35.5	6.691
07016	CHEESEFURTER BF & PORK W/ CHS SMOKED	327	14.05	1.49	10.47
22516	CHEF BOYARDEE BEEFARONI, MACARONI W/BF IN TOM SAU, CND E	87	3.89	14.69	0.56
22515	CHEF BOYARDEE BF RAVIOLI IN TOMATO&MEAT SAU, CND ENTREE	94	3.43	15.12	1.02
22517	CHEF BOYARDEE MINI RAVIOLI, BF RAVIOLI W/TOM&MT SAU, CND EN	95	3.49	16.12	0.7
22518	CHEF BOYARDEE SPAGHETTI&MEATBALLS IN TOMATO SAU, CND EN	104	3.78	14.19	1.61
22520	CHEF BOYARDEE TEEN MUTNT NINJA TURTL PSTA, MTBALL, TOM SA	107	3.85	15.83	1.41
09062	CHERIMOYA, RAW	74	1.65	17.7	
09067	CHERRIES, SOUR, RED, CND, EX HVY SYRUP PK, SOL&LIQUIDS	114	0.71	29.23	0.021
09064	CHERRIES, SOUR, RED, CND, H2O PK, SOL&LIQUIDS (INCL USDA CM	36	0.77	8.94	0.023
09066	CHERRIES, SOUR, RED, CND, HVY SYRUP PK, SOL&LIQUIDS	91	0.73	23.27	0.021
09065	CHERRIES, SOUR, RED, CND, LT SYRUP PK, SOL&LIQUIDS	75	0.74	19.3	0.022
09068	CHERRIES, SOUR, RED, FRZ, UNSWTND	46	0.92	11.02	0.1

NDB #	Food Description (100 gram portions = 3½ ounces = 20 tsp = ½ cup approx.	Calories	Protein	Carbs	Sat Fat
09063	CHERRIES, SOUR, RED, RAW	50	1	12.18	0.068
09070	CHERRIES, SWEET, RAW	72	1.2	16.55	0.216
09075	CHERRIES, SWT, CND, EX HVY SYRUP PK, SOL&LIQUIDS	102	0.59	26.23	0.033
09071	CHERRIES, SWT, CND, H2O PK, SOL&LIQUIDS	46	0.77	11.76	0.028
09074	CHERRIES, SWT, CND, HVY SYRUP PK, SOL&LIQUIDS	83	0.6	21.27	0.034
09072	CHERRIES, SWT, CND, JUC PK, SOL&LIQUIDS	54	0.91	13.81	0.004
09073	CHERRIES, SWT, CND, LT SYRUP PK, SOL&LIQUIDS	67	0.61	17.29	0.034
09076	CHERRIES, SWT, FRZ, SWTND	89	1.15	22.36	0.03
02008	CHERVIL, DRIED	237	23.2	49.1	0.169
12095	CHESTNUTS, CHINESE, BLD&STMD	153	2.88	33.64	0.112
12094	CHESTNUTS, CHINESE, DRIED	363	6.82	79.76	0.266
12093	CHESTNUTS, CHINESE, RAW	224	4.2	49.07	0.164
12096	CHESTNUTS, CHINESE, ROASTED	239	4.48	52.36	0.175
12101	CHESTNUTS, EUROPEAN, BLD&STMD	131	2	27.76	0.26
12100	CHESTNUTS, EUROPEAN, DRIED, PEELED	369	5.01	78.43	0.736
12099	CHESTNUTS, EUROPEAN, DRIED, UNPEELED	374	6.39	77.31	0.837
12098	CHESTNUTS, EUROPEAN, RAW, PEELED	196	1.63	44.17	0.235
12097	CHESTNUTS, EUROPEAN, RAW, UNPEELED	213	2.42	45.54	0.425
12167	CHESTNUTS, EUROPEAN, RSTD	245	3.17	52.96	0.414
12203	CHESTNUTS, JAPANESE, BLD&STMD	56	0.82	12.64	0.028
12175	CHESTNUTS, JAPANESE, DRIED	360	5.25	81.43	0.183
12202	CHESTNUTS, JAPANESE, RAW	154	2.25	34.91	0.078
12204	CHESTNUTS, JAPANESE, RSTD	201	2.97	45.13	0.118
19163	CHEWING GUM	341	0	96.7	0.042
19033	CHEX MIX	425	11	65.1	5.53
12006	CHIA SEEDS, DRIED	472	16.62	47.87	10.536
07932	CHICKEN BREAST FAT-FREE MESQ FLAVOR SLICED	80	16.8	2.25	0.13
07933	CHICKEN BREAST OVEN-ROASTED FAT-FREE SLICED	79	16.79	2.17	0.13
22906	CHICKEN POT PIE, FRZ ENTREE	223	6.01	19.68	4.455
07017	CHICKEN ROLL LT MEAT	154	19.53	2.44	1.97
07018	CHICKEN SPRD	158	18.01	4.05	3.23
05002	CHICKEN, BROILER OR FRYER, MEAT&SKN&GIBLETS&NECK, FRIED,	291	22.84	9.03	4.67
05054	CHICKEN, BROILERS OR FRYERS, BACK, MEAT ONLY, CKD, FRIED	288	29.99	5.68	4.12
05055	CHICKEN, BROILERS OR FRYERS, BACK, MEAT ONLY, CKD, RSTD	239	28.19	0	3.6
05056	CHICKEN, BROILERS OR FRYERS, BACK, MEAT ONLY, CKD, STWD	209	25.31	0	3.04

NDB #	Food Description (100 gram portions = 3½ ounces = 20 tsp = ½ cup approx.	Calories	Protein	Carbs	Sat Fat
05053	CHICKEN, BROILERS OR FRYERS, BACK, MEAT ONLY, RAW	137	19.56	0	1.52
05049	CHICKEN, BROILERS OR FRYERS, BACK, MEAT&SKN, CKD, FRIED, BA	331	21.97	10.25	5.83
05050	CHICKEN, BROILERS OR FRYERS, BACK, MEAT&SKN, CKD, FRIED, FL	331	27.79	6.5	5.61
05051	CHICKEN, BROILERS OR FRYERS, BACK, MEAT&SKN, CKD, RSTD	300	25.95	0	5.82
05052	CHICKEN, BROILERS OR FRYERS, BACK, MEAT&SKN, CKD, STWD	258	22.18	0	5.02
05048	CHICKEN, BROILERS OR FRYERS, BACK, MEAT&SKN, RAW	319	14.05	0	8.34
05063	CHICKEN, BROILERS OR FRYERS, BREAST, MEAT ONLY, CKD, FRIED	187	33.44	0.51	1.29
05064	CHICKEN, BROILERS OR FRYERS, BREAST, MEAT ONLY, CKD, RSTD	165	31.02	0	1.01
05065	CHICKEN, BROILERS OR FRYERS, BREAST, MEAT ONLY, CKD, STWD	151	28.98	0	0.85
05062	CHICKEN, BROILERS OR FRYERS, BREAST, MEAT ONLY, RAW	110	23.09	0	0.33
05058	CHICKEN, BROILERS OR FRYERS, BREAST, MEAT&SKN, CKD, FRIED,	260	24.84	8.99	3.52
05059	CHICKEN, BROILERS OR FRYERS, BREAST, MEAT&SKN, CKD, FRIED,	222	31.84	1.64	2.45
05060	CHICKEN, BROILERS OR FRYERS, BREAST, MEAT&SKN, CKD, RSTD	197	29.8	0	2.19
05061	CHICKEN, BROILERS OR FRYERS, BREAST, MEAT&SKN, CKD, STWD	184	27.39	0	2.08
05057	CHICKEN, BROILERS OR FRYERS, BREAST, MEAT&SKN, RAW	172	20.85	0	2.58
05044	CHICKEN, BROILERS OR FRYERS, DK MEAT, MEAT ONLY, CKD, FRIED	239	28.99	2.59	3.12
05045	CHICKEN, BROILERS OR FRYERS, DK MEAT, MEAT ONLY, CKD, RSTD	205	27.37	0	2.66
05046	CHICKEN, BROILERS OR FRYERS, DK MEAT, MEAT ONLY, CKD, STWD	192	25.97	0	2.45
05043	CHICKEN, BROILERS OR FRYERS, DK MEAT, MEAT ONLY, RAW	125	20.08	0	1.1
05035	CHICKEN, BROILERS OR FRYERS, DK MEAT, MEAT&SKN, CKD, FRIED,	298	21.85	9.38	4.95
05036	CHICKEN, BROILERS OR FRYERS, DK MEAT, MEAT&SKN, CKD, FRIED,	285	27.22	4.08	4.58
05037	CHICKEN, BROILERS OR FRYERS, DK MEAT, MEAT&SKN, CKD, RSTD	253	25.97	0	4.37
05038	CHICKEN, BROILERS OR FRYERS, DK MEAT, MEAT&SKN, CKD, STWD	233	23.5	0	4.06
05034	CHICKEN, BROILERS OR FRYERS, DK MEAT, MEAT&SKN, RAW	237	16.69	0	5.26
05072	CHICKEN, BROILERS OR FRYERS, DRUMSTK, MEAT ONLY, CKD, FRIE	195	28.62	0	2.13
05073	CHICKEN, BROILERS OR FRYERS, DRUMSTK, MEAT ONLY, CKD, RST	172	28.29	0	1.48
05074	CHICKEN, BROILERS OR FRYERS, DRUMSTK, MEAT ONLY, CKD, STW	169	27.5	0	1.51
05071	CHICKEN, BROILERS OR FRYERS, DRUMSTK, MEAT ONLY, RAW	119	20.59	0	0.86
05067	CHICKEN, BROILERS OR FRYERS, DRUMSTK, MEAT&SKN, CKD, FRIE	268	21.95	8.28	4.14
05068	CHICKEN, BROILERS OR FRYERS, DRUMSTK, MEAT&SKN, CKD, FRIE	245	26.96	1.63	3.66
05069	CHICKEN, BROILERS OR FRYERS, DRUMSTK, MEAT&SKN, CKD, RSTD	216	27.03	0	3.05
05070	CHICKEN, BROILERS OR FRYERS, DRUMSTK, MEAT&SKN, CKD, STW	204	25.32	0	2.91
05066	CHICKEN, BROILERS OR FRYERS, DRUMSTK, MEAT&SKN, RAW	161	19.27	0	2.39
05047	CHICKEN, BROILERS OR FRYERS, FAT, RAW	629	3.73	0	19.37
05021	CHICKEN, BROILERS OR FRYERS, GIBLETS, CKD, FRIED	277	32.54	4.35	3.8

NDB #	Food Description (100 gram portions = 3½ ounces = 20 tsp = ½ cup approx.	Calories	Protein	Carbs	Sat Fat
05022	CHICKEN, BROILERS OR FRYERS, GIBLETS, CKD, SIMMRD	157	25.85	0.95	1.49
05020	CHICKEN, BROILERS OR FRYERS, GIBLETS, RAW	124	17.88	1.8	1.36
05081	CHICKEN, BROILERS OR FRYERS, LEG, MEAT ONLY, CKD, FRIED	208	28.38	0.65	2.49
05082	CHICKEN, BROILERS OR FRYERS, LEG, MEAT ONLY, CKD, RSTD	191	27.03	0	2.29
05083	CHICKEN, BROILERS OR FRYERS, LEG, MEAT ONLY, CKD, STWD	185	26.26	0	2.2
05080	CHICKEN, BROILERS OR FRYERS, LEG, MEAT ONLY, RAW	120	20.13	0	0.95
05076	CHICKEN, BROILERS OR FRYERS, LEG, MEAT&SKN, CKD, FRIED, BAT	273	21.77	8.72	4.28
05077	CHICKEN, BROILERS OR FRYERS, LEG, MEAT&SKN, CKD, FRIED, FLR	254	26.84	2.5	3.9
05078	CHICKEN, BROILERS OR FRYERS, LEG, MEAT&SKN, CKD, RSTD	232	25.96	0	3.72
05079	CHICKEN, BROILERS OR FRYERS, LEG, MEAT&SKN, CKD, STWD	220	24.17	0	3.57
05075	CHICKEN, BROILERS OR FRYERS, LEG, MEAT&SKN, RAW	187	18.15	0	3.3
05040	CHICKEN, BROILERS OR FRYERS, LT MEAT, MEAT ONLY, CKD, FRIED	192	32.82	0.42	1.52
05041	CHICKEN, BROILERS OR FRYERS, LT MEAT, MEAT ONLY, CKD, RSTD	173	30.91	0	1.27
05042	CHICKEN, BROILERS OR FRYERS, LT MEAT, MEAT ONLY, CKD, STWD	159	28.88	0	1.12
05039	CHICKEN, BROILERS OR FRYERS, LT MEAT, MEAT ONLY, RAW	114	23.2	0	0.44
05030	CHICKEN, BROILERS OR FRYERS, LT MEAT, MEAT&SKN, CKD, FRIED,	277	23.55	9.5	4.12
05031	CHICKEN, BROILERS OR FRYERS, LT MEAT, MEAT&SKN, CKD, FRIED,	246	30.45	1.82	3.32
05032	CHICKEN, BROILERS OR FRYERS, LT MEAT, MEAT&SKN, CKD, RSTD	222	29.02	0	3.05
05033	CHICKEN, BROILERS OR FRYERS, LT MEAT, MEAT&SKN, CKD, STWD	201	26.14	0	2.8
05029	CHICKEN, BROILERS OR FRYERS, LT MEAT, MEAT&SKN, RAW	186	20.27	0	3.16
05012	CHICKEN, BROILERS OR FRYERS, MEAT ONLY, CKD, FRIED	219	30.57	1.69	2.46
05011	CHICKEN, BROILERS OR FRYERS, MEAT ONLY, RAW	119	21.39	0	0.79
05013	CHICKEN, BROILERS OR FRYERS, MEAT ONLY, RSTD	190	28.93	0	2.04
05014	CHICKEN, BROILERS OR FRYERS, MEAT ONLY, STWD	177	27.29	0	1.84
05003	CHICKEN, BROILERS OR FRYERS, MEAT&SKN&GIBLETS&NECK, FRIE	272	28.57	3.27	4.16
05001	CHICKEN, BROILERS OR FRYERS, MEAT&SKN&GIBLETS&NECK, RAW	213	18.33	0.13	4.24
05004	CHICKEN, BROILERS OR FRYERS, MEAT&SKN&GIBLETS&NECK, RST	234	26.78	0.06	3.7
05005	CHICKEN, BROILERS OR FRYERS, MEAT&SKN&GIBLETS&NECK, STW	216	24.49	0.06	3.45
05007	CHICKEN, BROILERS OR FRYERS, MEAT&SKN, CKD, FRIED, BATTER	289	22.54	9.42	4.61
05008	CHICKEN, BROILERS OR FRYERS, MEAT&SKN, CKD, FRIED, FLR	269	28.56	3.15	4.06
05009	CHICKEN, BROILERS OR FRYERS, MEAT&SKN, CKD, RSTD	239	27.3	0	3.79
05010	CHICKEN, BROILERS OR FRYERS, MEAT&SKN, CKD, STWD	219	24.68	0	3.5
05006	CHICKEN, BROILERS OR FRYERS, MEAT&SKN, RAW	215	18.6	0	4.31
05089	CHICKEN, BROILERS OR FRYERS, NECK, MEAT ONLY, CKD, FRIED	229	26.87	1.77	3
05090	CHICKEN, BROILERS OR FRYERS, NECK, MEAT ONLY, CKD, SIMMRD	179	24.56	0	2.1

NDB #	Food Description (100 gram portions = 3½ ounces = 20 tsp = ½ cup approx.	Calories	Protein	Carbs	Sat Fat
05088	CHICKEN, BROILERS OR FRYERS, NECK, MEAT ONLY, RAW	154	17.55	0	2.25
05087	CHICKEN, BROILERS OR FRYERS, NECK, MEAT&SKN, CKD SIMMRD	247	19.61	0	5
05085	CHICKEN, BROILERS OR FRYERS, NECK, MEAT&SKN, CKD, FRIED, BA	330	19.82	8.7	6.22
05086	CHICKEN, BROILERS OR FRYERS, NECK, MEAT&SKN, CKD, FRIED, FL	332	24.01	4.24	6.32
05084	CHICKEN, BROILERS OR FRYERS, NECK, MEAT&SKN, RAW	297	14.07	0	7.27
05016	CHICKEN, BROILERS OR FRYERS, SKN ONLY, CKD, FRIED, BATTER	394	10.32	23.15	7.61
05017	CHICKEN, BROILERS OR FRYERS, SKN ONLY, CKD, FRIED, FLR	502	19.09	9.34	11.67
05018	CHICKEN, BROILERS OR FRYERS, SKN ONLY, CKD, RSTD	454	20.36	0	11.42
05019	CHICKEN, BROILERS OR FRYERS, SKN ONLY, CKD, STWD	363	15.22	0	9.28
05015	CHICKEN, BROILERS OR FRYERS, SKN ONLY, RAW	349	13.33	0	9.08
05097	CHICKEN, BROILERS OR FRYERS, THIGH, MEAT ONLY, CKD, FRIED	218	28.18	1.18	2.78
05098	CHICKEN, BROILERS OR FRYERS, THIGH, MEAT ONLY, CKD, RSTD	209	25.94	0	3.03
05099	CHICKEN, BROILERS OR FRYERS, THIGH, MEAT ONLY, CKD, STWD	195	25	0	2.71
05096	CHICKEN, BROILERS OR FRYERS, THIGH, MEAT ONLY, RAW	119	19.65	0	0.97
05092	CHICKEN, BROILERS OR FRYERS, THIGH, MEAT&SKN, CKD, FRIED, B	277	21.61	9.08	4.41
05093	CHICKEN, BROILERS OR FRYERS, THIGH, MEAT&SKN, CKD, FRIED, FL	262	26.75	3.18	4.09
05094	CHICKEN, BROILERS OR FRYERS, THIGH, MEAT&SKN, CKD, RSTD	247	25.06	0	4.33
05095	CHICKEN, BROILERS OR FRYERS, THIGH, MEAT&SKN, CKD, STWD	232	23.26	0	4.11
05091	CHICKEN, BROILERS OR FRYERS, THIGH, MEAT&SKN, RAW	211	17.27	0	4.34
05106	CHICKEN, BROILERS OR FRYERS, WING, MEAT ONLY, CKD, FRIED	211	30.15	0	2.5
05107	CHICKEN, BROILERS OR FRYERS, WING, MEAT ONLY, CKD, RSTD	203	30.46	0	2.26
05108	CHICKEN, BROILERS OR FRYERS, WING, MEAT ONLY, CKD, STWD	181	27.18	0	2
05105	CHICKEN, BROILERS OR FRYERS, WING, MEAT ONLY, RAW	126	21.97	0	0.94
05101	CHICKEN, BROILERS OR FRYERS, WING, MEAT&SKN, CKD, FRIED, BA	324	19.87	10.94	5.83
05102	CHICKEN, BROILERS OR FRYERS, WING, MEAT&SKN, CKD, FRIED, FL	321	26.11	2.39	6.06
05103	CHICKEN, BROILERS OR FRYERS, WING, MEAT&SKN, CKD, RSTD	290	26.86	0	5.45
05104	CHICKEN, BROILERS OR FRYERS, WING, MEAT&SKN, CKD, STWD	249	22.78	0	4.71
05100	CHICKEN, BROILERS OR FRYERS, WING, MEAT&SKN, RAW	222	18.33	0	4.36
05138	CHICKEN, CAPONS, GIBLETS, CKD, SIMMRD	164	26.39	0.76	1.77
05137	CHICKEN, CAPONS, GIBLETS, RAW	130	18.28	1.42	1.64
05134	CHICKEN, CAPONS, MEAT&SKN&GIBLETS&NECK, CKD, RSTD	226	28.35	0.04	3.28
05133	CHICKEN, CAPONS, MEAT&SKN&GIBLETS&NECK, RAW	232	18.51	0.08	4.89
05136	CHICKEN, CAPONS, MEAT&SKN, CKD, RSTD	229	28.96	0	3.26
05135	CHICKEN, CAPONS, MEAT&SKN, RAW	234	18.77	0	4.95
05277	CHICKEN, CND, MEAT ONLY, W/BROTH	165	21.77	0	2.2

NDB #	Food Description (100 gram portions = 3½ ounces = 20 tsp = ½ cup approx.	Calories	Protein	Carbs	Sat Fat
05310	CHICKEN, CORNISH GAME HENS, MEAT ONLY, CKD, RSTD	134	23.3	0	0.99
05309	CHICKEN, CORNISH GAME HENS, MEAT ONLY, RAW	116	20.04	0	0.85
05308	CHICKEN, CORNISH GAME HENS, MEAT&SKN, CKD, RSTD	260	22.27	0	5.05
05307	CHICKEN, CORNISH GAME HENS, MEAT&SKN, RAW	200	17.15	0	3.89
05024	CHICKEN, GIZZARD, ALL CLASSES, CKD, SIMMRD	153	27.15	1.14	1.04
05023	CHICKEN, GIZZARD, ALL CLASSES, RAW	118	18.19	0.58	1.2
05026	CHICKEN, HEART, ALL CLASSES, CKD, SIMMRD	185	26.41	0.1	2.26
05025	CHICKEN, HEART, ALL CLASSES, RAW	153	15.55	0.71	2.66
05028	CHICKEN, LIVER, ALL CLASSES, CKD, SIMMRD	157	24.36	0.88	1.84
05027	CHICKEN, LIVER, ALL CLASSES, RAW	125	17.97	3.42	1.3
05120	CHICKEN, ROASTING, DK MEAT, MEAT ONLY, CKD, RSTD	178	23.25	0	2.43
05119	CHICKEN, ROASTING, DK MEAT, MEAT ONLY, RAW	113	18.74	0	0.93
05116	CHICKEN, ROASTING, GIBLETS, CKD, SIMMRD	165	26.77	0.86	1.64
05115	CHICKEN, ROASTING, GIBLETS, RAW	127	18.14	1.14	1.54
05118	CHICKEN, ROASTING, LT MEAT, MEAT ONLY, CKD, RSTD	153	27.13	0	1.08
05117	CHICKEN, ROASTING, LT MEAT, MEAT ONLY, RAW	109	22.2	0	0.37
05114	CHICKEN, ROASTING, MEAT ONLY, CKD, RSTD	167	25.01	0	1.81
05113	CHICKEN, ROASTING, MEAT ONLY, RAW	111	20.33	0	0.67
05110	CHICKEN, ROASTING, MEAT&SKN&GIBLETS&NECK, CKD, RSTD	220	23.96	0.05	3.66
05109	CHICKEN, ROASTING, MEAT&SKN&GIBLETS&NECK, RAW	213	17.09	0.09	4.41
05112	CHICKEN, ROASTING, MEAT&SKN, CKD, RSTD	223	23.97	0	3.74
05111	CHICKEN, ROASTING, MEAT&SKN, RAW	216	17.14	0	4.53
05132	CHICKEN, STEWING, DK MEAT, MEAT ONLY, CKD, STWD	258	28.14	0	4.07
05131	CHICKEN, STEWING, DK MEAT, MEAT ONLY, RAW	157	19.7	0	2.08
05128	CHICKEN, STEWING, GIBLETS, CKD, SIMMRD	194	25.73	0.11	2.66
05127	CHICKEN, STEWING, GIBLETS, RAW	168	17.89	2.13	2.63
05130	CHICKEN, STEWING, LT MEAT, MEAT ONLY, CKD, STWD	213	33.04	0	1.98
05129	CHICKEN, STEWING, LT MEAT, MEAT ONLY, RAW	137	23.1	0	0.97
05126	CHICKEN, STEWING, MEAT ONLY, CKD, STWD	237	30.42	0	3.1
05125	CHICKEN, STEWING, MEAT ONLY, RAW	148	21.26	0	
05122	CHICKEN, STEWING, MEAT&SKN, &GIBLETS&NECK, CKD, STWD	276	26.53	0.01	4.9
05121	CHICKEN, STEWING, MEAT&SKN, &GIBLETS&NECK, RAW	251	17.48	0.19	5.48
05124	CHICKEN, STEWING, MEAT&SKN, CKD, STWD	285	26.88	0	5.11
05123	CHICKEN, STEWING, MEAT&SKN, RAW	258	17.55	0	5.71
16157	CHICKPEA FLOUR (BESAN)	369	22.39	57.8	0.693

NDB #	Food Description (100 gram portions = 3½ ounces = 20 tsp = ½ cup approx.	Calories	Protein	Carbs	Sat Fat
16058	CHICKPEAS (GARBANZO BNS, BENGAL GM), MATURE SEEDS, CND	119	4.95	22.62	0.118
16056	CHICKPEAS (GARBANZO BNS, BENGAL GM), MATURE SEEDS, RAW	364	19.3	60.66	0.626
16057	CHICKPEAS , MATURE SEEDS, CKD, BLD, WO/SALT	164	8.86	27.41	0.269
16357	CHICKPEAS, MATURE SEEDS, CKD, BLD, W/SALT	164	8.86	27.41	0.269
11152	CHICORY GREENS, RAW	23	1.7	4.7	0.073
11154	CHICORY ROOTS, RAW	73	1.4	17.51	0.048
11151	CHICORY, WITLOOF, RAW	17	0.9	4	0.024
03860	CHILD FORMULA, ROSS, PEDIASURE, W/IRON, RTF	95	2.86	10.5	1.256
22904	CHILI CON CARNE W/BNS, CND ENTREE	115	9.09	11.03	0.95
02009	CHILI POWDER	314	12.26	54.66	2.953
16059	CHILI WITH BEANS, CANNED	112	5.71	11.91	2.352
11615	CHIVES, FREEZE-DRIED	311	21.2	64.29	0.591
11156	CHIVES, RAW	30	3.27	4.35	0.146
14181	CHOCOLATE SYRUP	279	2.1	65.1	0.519
14182	CHOCOLATE SYRUP, PREP W/ WHL MILK	91	3.13	12.9	1.803
14175	CHOCOLATE-FLAVOR BEV MIX, PDR	349	3.3	90.3	1.834
14177	CHOCOLATE-FLAVOR BEV MIX, PDR, PREP W/ WHL MILK	85	3.3	11.6	2.059
07019	CHORIZO, PORK AND BEEF	455	24.1	1.86	14.38
11698	CHRYSANTHEMUM LEAVES, RAW	24	3.36	3.01	
11767	CHRYSANTHEMUM, GARLAND, CKD, BLD, DRND, W/SALT	20	1.64	4.31	
11158	CHRYSANTHEMUM, GARLAND, CKD, BLD, DRND, WO/SALT	20	1.64	4.31	0.022
11157	CHRYSANTHEMUM, GARLAND, RAW	21	1.56	4.37	
22674	CHUN KING SWT&SOUR VEG FRUIT&SAU W/CHICK, CND ENTREE	65	2.3	12.5	
22592	CINNAMON SWIRL FRENCH TOAST W/SAUSAGE, FRZ BRKFST	266	8.4	24.5	4.68
02010	CINNAMON, GROUND	261	3.89	79.85	0.65
15013	CISCO, RAW	98	18.99	0	0.421
15014	CISCO, SMOKED	177	16.36	0	1.741
14262	CITRUS FRUIT JUC DRK, FRZ CONC	162	1.2	40.3	0.007
14263	CITRUS FRUIT JUC DRK, FRZ CONC, PREP W/H2O	46	0.3	11.5	0.002
14187	CLAM&TOMATO JUC, CND	48	0.6	10.95	0.048
15157	CLAM, MIXED SPECIES, RAW	74	12.77	2.57	0.094
15158	CLAM, MXD SP, CKD, BREADED&FRIED	202	14.24	10.33	2.683
15159	CLAM, MXD SP, CKD, MOIST HEAT	148	25.55	5.13	0.188
15160	CLAM, MXD SP, CND, DRND SOL	148	25.55	5.13	0.188
15162	CLAM, MXD SP, CND, LIQ	2	0.4	0.1	0.002

NDB #	Food Description (100 gram portions = 3½ ounces = 20 tsp = ½ cup approx.	Calories	Protein	Carbs	Sat Fat
02011	CLOVES, GROUND	323	5.98	61.21	5.438
14195	COCOA MIX, NESTLE, CARNATION HOT COCOA MIX W/MARSHMALLO	399	4.81	86.62	1.47
14198	COCOA MIX, NESTLE, CARNATION NO SUGAR HOT COCOA MIX	365	28.69	56.22	1.35
14197	COCOA MIX, NESTLE, CARNATION RICH CHOC HOT COCOA MIX	400	4.63	86.56	1.04
14192	COCOA MIX, PDR	361	10.8	79.1	2.408
14194	COCOA MIX, PDR, PREP W/ H2O	50	1.5	10.9	0.332
14390	COCOA MIX, W/ ASPRT, PDR, PREP FROM ITEM 14196	28	1.16	5.62	0
14196	COCOA MIX, W/ASPRT, PDR, WO/ CA OR P, W/ NA&VIT A	322	14.87	72.06	0
19165	COCOA, DRY PDR, UNSWTND	229	19.6	54.3	8.07
19171	COCOA, DRY PDR, UNSWTND, HERSHEY'S EUROPEAN STYLE COCO	400	20	60	0
19166	COCOA, DRY PDR, UNSWTND, PROC W/ALKALI	222	18.1	54.8	7.76
12116	COCONUT CRM, CND (LIQ EXPRESSED FROM GRATED MEAT)	192	2.69	8.35	15.713
12115	COCONUT CRM, RAW (LIQ EXPRESSED FROM GRATED MEAT)	330	3.63	6.65	30.753
12119	COCONUT H2O (LIQ FROM COCONUTS)	19	0.72	3.71	0.176
12177	COCONUT MEAT, DRIED (DESICCATED), CRMD	684	5.3	21.52	61.257
12108	COCONUT MEAT, DRIED (DESICCATED), NOT SWTND	660	6.88	24.41	57.218
12110	COCONUT MEAT, DRIED (DESICCATED), SWTND, FLAKED, CND	443	3.35	40.91	28.101
12109	COCONUT MEAT, DRIED (DESICCATED), SWTND, FLAKED, PACKAGE	474	3.28	47.59	28.509
12179	COCONUT MEAT, DRIED (DESICCATED), SWTND, SHREDDED	501	2.88	47.67	31.468
12114	COCONUT MEAT, DRIED (DESICCATED), TSTD	592	5.3	44.4	41.678
12104	COCONUT MEAT, RAW	354	3.33	15.23	29.698
12118	COCONUT MILK, CND (LIQ EXPRESSED FROM GRATED MEAT&H2O)	197	2.02	2.81	18.915
12176	COCONUT MILK, FRZ (LIQ EXPRESSED FROM GRATED MEAT&H2O)	202	1.61	5.58	18.445
12117	COCONUT MILK, RAW (LIQ EXPRESSED FROM GRATED MEAT&H2O)	230	2.29	5.54	21.14
15016	COD, ATLANTIC, CKD, DRY HEAT	105	22.83	0	0.168
15017	COD, ATLANTIC, CND, SOL&LIQ	105	22.76	0	0.167
15018	COD, ATLANTIC, DRIED&SALTED	290	62.82	0	0.462
15015	COD, ATLANTIC, RAW	82	17.81	0	0.131
15192	COD, PACIFIC, CKD, DRY HEAT	105	22.95	0	0.104
15019	COD, PACIFIC, RAW	82	17.9	0	0.081
14236	COFFEE SUB, CRL GRAIN BEV, PDR	328	5.5	81	0.633
14421	COFFEE SUB, CRL GRAIN BEV, PDR, PREP W/ WHL MILK	65	3.3	5.6	2.061
14237	COFFEE SUB, CRL GRAIN BEV, PREP W/H2O	5	0.1	1	0.008
14204	COFFEE&COCOA (MOCHA) PDR, W/WHTNR&LO CAL SWTNR, DECAF	528	10.8	50.1	26.26
14210	COFFEE, BREWED, ESPRESSO, REST-PREP	9	0.01	1.53	0.092

NDB #	Food Description (100 gram portions = 3½ ounces = 20 tsp = ½ cup approx.	Calories	Protein	Carbs	Sat Fat
14208	COFFEE, BREWED, PREP W/DISTILLED H2O	2	0.1	0.4	0.002
14209	COFFEE, BREWED, PREP W/TAP H2O	2	0.1	0.4	0.002
14201	COFFEE, BREWED, PREP W/TAP H2O, DECAFFEINATED	2	0.1	0.4	0.002
14218	COFFEE, INST, DECAFFEINATED, PDR	224	11.6	42.6	0.101
14219	COFFEE, INST, DECAFFEINATED, PDR, PREP W/H2O	2	0.1	0.4	0.001
14214	COFFEE, INST, REG, PDR	241	12.2	41.1	0.197
14215	COFFEE, INST, REG, PREP W/H2O	2	0.1	0.4	0.002
14222	COFFEE, INST, W/CHICORY, PDR	351	9.3	74.2	0.071
14223	COFFEE, INST, W/CHICORY, PREP W/H2O	4	0.1	0.7	0.001
14228	COFFEE, INST, W/SUGAR, CAPPUCCINO-FLAVOR PDR	437	3.1	75.4	3.13
14229	COFFEE, INST, W/SUGAR, FRENCH-FLAVOR, PDR	499	4.5	57.5	6.098
14224	COFFEE, INST, W/SUGAR, MOCHA-FLAVOR, PDR	441	4.2	73.4	3.836
18103	COFFEECAKE, CHEESE	339	7	44.3	5.391
18104	COFFEECAKE, CINN W/CRUMB TOPPING, COMMLY PREP, ENR	418	6.8	46.7	5.797
18417	COFFEECAKE, CINN W/CRUMB TOPPING, COMMLY PREP, UNENR	418	6.8	46.7	5.797
18107	COFFEECAKE, CINN W/CRUMB TOPPING, DRY MIX	436	4.8	77.7	2.957
18108	COFFEECAKE, CINN W/CRUMB TOPPING, DRY MIX, PREP	318	5.5	52.8	1.855
18105	COFFEECAKE, CREME-FILLED W/CHOC FRSTNG	331	5	53.8	2.833
18106	COFFEECAKE, FRUIT	311	5.2	51.5	2.495
11159	COLESLAW, HOME-PREPARED	69	1.29	12.41	0.385
11768	COLLARDS, CKD, BLD, DRND, W/SALT	26	2.11	4.9	0.047
11162	COLLARDS, CKD, BLD, DRND, WO/SALT	26	2.11	4.9	0.047
11769	COLLARDS, FRZ, CHOPD, CKD, BLD, DRND, W/SALT	36	2.97	7.11	0.04
11164	COLLARDS, FRZ, CHOPD, CKD, BLD, DRND, WO/SALT	36	2.97	7.11	0.06
11163	COLLARDS, FRZ, CHOPD, UNPREP	33	2.69	6.45	0.048
11161	COLLARDS, RAW	30	2.45	5.69	0.055
18600	CONAGRA, BANQUET APPL PIE, FRZ, READY TO BAKE	261	2.6	36.99	5.11
14115	CONTINENTAL MILLS, ALPINE SPIC CIDR INST APL FLV DRK MIX, PDR	395	0	98.8	
18150	COOKIES, ANIMAL CRACKERS (INCL ARROWROOT, TEA BISCUITS,)	446	6.9	74.1	3.463
18151	COOKIES, BROWNIES, COMMLY PREP	405	4.8	63.9	4.235
18152	COOKIES, BROWNIES, DRY MIX, REG	434	4	76.6	2.519
18196	COOKIES, BROWNIES, DRY MIX, SPL DIETARY	426	2.9	80.4	2.018
18197	COOKIES, BROWNIES, DRY MIX, SPL DIETARY, PREP	384	3.8	71.3	5.096
18154	COOKIES, BROWNIES, PREP FROM RECIPE	466	6.2	50.2	7.319
18155	COOKIES, BUTTER, COMMLY PREP, ENR	467	6.1	68.9	11.051

NDB #	Food Description (100 gram portions = 3½ ounces = 20 tsp = ½ cup approx.	Calories	Protein	Carbs	Sat Fat
18421	COOKIES, BUTTER, COMMLY PREP, UNENR	467	6.1	68.9	11.051
18159	COOKIES, CHOC CHIP, COMMLY PREP, REG, HIGHER FAT, ENR	481	5.4	66.8	7.476
18422	COOKIES, CHOC CHIP, COMMLY PREP, REG, HIGHER FAT, UNENR	481	5.4	66.8	7.476
18158	COOKIES, CHOC CHIP, COMMLY PREP, REG, LOWER FAT	453	5.8	73.3	3.81
18160	COOKIES, CHOC CHIP, COMMLY PREP, SOFT-TYPE	458	3.5	59.1	7.411
18198	COOKIES, CHOC CHIP, COMMLY PREP, SPL DIETARY	450	3.9	73.4	4.183
18161	COOKIES, CHOC CHIP, DRY MIX	497	4.6	66.1	8.316
18378	COOKIES, CHOC CHIP, PREP FROM RECIPE, MADE W/BUTTER	488	5.7	58.2	14.071
18165	COOKIES, CHOC CHIP, PREP FROM RECIPE, MADE W/MARGARINE	488	5.7	58.4	8.074
18163	COOKIES, CHOC CHIP, REFR DOUGH	443	4.4	61.4	6.729
18164	COOKIES, CHOC CHIP, REFR DOUGH, BKD	492	4.9	68.2	7.759
18166	COOKIES, CHOC SNDWCH, W/CREME FILLING, REG	472	4.7	70.3	3.657
18167	COOKIES, CHOC SNDWCH, W/CREME FILLING, REG, CHOCOLATE-C	481	3.6	66.1	7.426
18199	COOKIES, CHOC SNDWCH, W/CREME FILLING, SPL DIETARY	461	4.5	67.7	3.825
18168	COOKIES, CHOC SNDWCH, W/EX CREME FILLING	500	3.6	68.1	3.874
18157	COOKIES, CHOCOLATE WAFERS	433	6.6	72.4	4.241
18169	COOKIES, COCNT MACAROONS, PREP FROM RECIPE	404	3.6	72.2	11.236
18170	COOKIES, FIG BARS	348	3.7	70.9	1.123
18171	COOKIES, FORTUNE	378	4.2	84	0.669
18156	COOKIES, FUDGE, CAKE-TYPE (INCL TROLLEY CAKES)	349	5	78.3	1.112
18172	COOKIES, GINGERSNAPS	416	5.6	76.9	2.451
18174	COOKIES, GRAHAM CRACKERS, CHOCOLATE-COATED	484	5.8	66.5	13.38
18173	COOKIES, GRAHAM CRACKERS, PLN OR HONEY (INCL CINN)	423	6.9	76.8	1.519
18175	COOKIES, LADYFINGERS, W/LEMON JUC&RIND	365	10.6	59.7	3.477
18423	COOKIES, LADYFINGERS, WO/LEMON JUC&RIND	365	10.6	59.7	3.477
18176	COOKIES, MARSHMLLW, CHOCOLATE-COATED (INCL MARSHMLLW	421	4	67.7	4.722
18177	COOKIES, MOLASSES	430	5.6	73.8	3.212
18456	COOKIES, OATMEAL, COMMLY PREP, FAT-FREE	326	5.9	78.6	0.314
18178	COOKIES, OATMEAL, COMMLY PREP, REG	450	6.2	68.7	4.519
18179	COOKIES, OATMEAL, COMMLY PREP, SOFT-TYPE	409	6.1	65.7	3.63
18200	COOKIES, OATMEAL, COMMLY PREP, SPL DIETARY	449	4.8	69.9	2.693
18180	COOKIES, OATMEAL, DRY MIX	462	6.5	67.3	4.755
18184	COOKIES, OATMEAL, PREP FROM RECIPE, W/RAISINS	435	6.5	68.4	3.232
18377	COOKIES, OATMEAL, PREP FROM RECIPE, WO/RAISINS	447	6.8	66.4	3.581
18182	COOKIES, OATMEAL, REFR DOUGH	424	5.4	59.1	4.751

NDB #	Food Description (100 gram portions = 3½ ounces = 20 tsp = ½ cup approx.	Calories	Protein	Carbs	Sat Fat
18183	COOKIES, OATMEAL, REFR DOUGH, BKD	471	6	65.7	5.339
18190	COOKIES, PNUT BUTTER SNDWCH, REG	478	8.8	65.6	4.995
18201	COOKIES, PNUT BUTTER SNDWCH, SPL DIETARY	535	10	50.8	4.937
18185	COOKIES, PNUT BUTTER, COMMLY PREP, REG	477	9.6	58.9	4.485
18186	COOKIES, PNUT BUTTER, COMMLY PREP, SOFT-TYPE	457	5.3	57.7	6.149
18189	COOKIES, PNUT BUTTER, PREP FROM RECIPE	475	9	58.9	4.438
18187	COOKIES, PNUT BUTTER, REFR DOUGH	458	8.2	52.1	5.791
18188	COOKIES, PNUT BUTTER, REFR DOUGH, BKD	503	9.1	57.3	6.199
18191	COOKIES, RAISIN, SOFT-TYPE	401	4.1	68	3.46
18193	COOKIES, SHORTBREAD, COMMLY PREP, PECAN	542	4.9	58.3	8.204
18192	COOKIES, SHORTBREAD, COMMLY PREP, PLN	502	6.1	64.5	6.106
18209	COOKIES, SUGAR WAFERS W/CREME FILLING, REG	511	4.1	70.1	3.622
18202	COOKIES, SUGAR WAFERS W/CREME FILLING, SPL DIETARY	502	3.1	66	3.829
18204	COOKIES, SUGAR, COMMLY PREP, REG (INCL VANILLA)	478	5.1	67.9	5.435
18203	COOKIES, SUGAR, COMMLY PREP, SPL DIETARY	431	4.1	76.8	1.872
18208	COOKIES, SUGAR, PREP FROM RECIPE, MADE W/MARGARINE	472	5.9	60	4.69
18205	COOKIES, SUGAR, REFR DOUGH	436	4.2	59	5.265
18206	COOKIES, SUGAR, REFR DOUGH, BKD	484	4.7	65.6	5.906
18210	COOKIES, VANILLA SNDWCH W/CREME FILLING	483	4.5	72.1	2.979
18213	COOKIES, VANILLA WAFERS, HIGHER FAT	473	4.3	71.1	4.936
18212	COOKIES, VANILLA WAFERS, LOWER FAT	441	5	73.6	3.838
02012	CORIANDER LEAF, DRIED	279	21.93	52.1	0.115
11165	CORIANDER LEAVES, RAW	23	2.13	3.67	0.014
02013	CORIANDER SEED	298	12.37	54.99	0.99
20015	CORN BRAN, CRUDE	224	8.36	85.64	0.13
19419	CORN CAKES	387	8.1	83.4	0.42
19800	CORN CAKES, VERY LO NA	387	8.1	83.4	0.42
20017	CORN FLOUR, MASA, ENRICHED	365	9.34	76.27	0.532
20018	CORN FLR, DEGERMED, UNENR, YEL	375	5.59	82.75	0.171
20317	CORN FLR, MASA, ENR, YEL	365	9.34	76.27	0.532
20316	CORN FLR, WHOLE-GRAIN, WHITE	361	6.93	76.85	0.543
20016	CORN FLR, WHOLE-GRAIN, YEL	361	6.93	76.85	0.543
11656	CORN PUDD, HOME-PREPARED	109	4.39	12.76	2.537
11184	CORN W/RED&GRN PEPPERS, CND, SOL&LIQUIDS	75	2.33	18.17	0.085
11900	CORN, SWEET, WHITE, RAW	86	3.22	19.02	0.182

NDB #	Food Description (100 gram portions = 3½ ounces = 20 tsp = ½ cup approx.	Calories	Protein	Carbs	Sat Fat
11167	CORN, SWEET, YELLOW, RAW	86	3.22	19.02	0.182
11902	CORN, SWT, WHITE, CKD, BLD, DRND, W/SALT	108	3.32	25.11	0.197
11901	CORN, SWT, WHITE, CKD, BLD, DRND, WO/SALT	108	3.32	25.11	0.197
11907	CORN, SWT, WHITE, CND, CRM STYLE, NO SALT	72	1.74	18.13	0.065
11906	CORN, SWT, WHITE, CND, CRM STYLE, REG PK	72	1.74	18.13	0.065
11909	CORN, SWT, WHITE, CND, VACUUM PK, NO SALT	79	2.41	19.44	0.077
11908	CORN, SWT, WHITE, CND, VACUUM PK, REG PK	79	2.41	19.44	0.077
11905	CORN, SWT, WHITE, CND, WHL KERNEL, DRND SOL	81	2.62	18.59	0.154
11904	CORN, SWT, WHITE, CND, WHL KERNEL, NO SALT, SOL&LIQUIDS	64	1.95	15.4	0.077
11903	CORN, SWT, WHITE, CND, WHL KERNEL, REG PK, SOL&LIQUIDS	64	1.95	15.4	0.077
11912	CORN, SWT, WHITE, FRZ, KRNLS CUT OFF COB, BLD, DRND, W/SALT	80	2.75	19.56	0.066
11911	CORN, SWT, WHITE, FRZ, KRNLS CUT OFF COB, BLD, DRND, WO/SAL	80	2.75	19.56	0.066
11910	CORN, SWT, WHITE, FRZ, KRNLS CUT OFF COB, UNPREP	88	3.02	20.8	0.119
11915	CORN, SWT, WHITE, FRZ, KRNLS ON COB, CKD, BLD, DRND, W/SALT	93	3.11	22.33	0.114
11914	CORN, SWT, WHITE, FRZ, KRNLS ON COB, CKD, BLD, DRND, WO/SAL	93	3.11	22.33	0.114
11913	CORN, SWT, WHITE, FRZ, KRNLS ON COB, UNPREP	98	3.28	23.5	0.12
11770	CORN, SWT, YEL, CKD, BLD, DRND, W/SALT	108	3.32	25.11	0.197
11168	CORN, SWT, YEL, CKD, BLD, DRND, WO/SALT	108	3.32	25.11	0.197
11170	CORN, SWT, YEL, CND, BRINE PK, REG PK, SOL&LIQUIDS	64	1.95	15.4	0.077
11772	CORN, SWT, YEL, CND, CRM STYLE, NO SALT	72	1.74	18.13	0.065
11174	CORN, SWT, YEL, CND, CRM STYLE, REG PK	72	1.74	18.13	0.065
11771	CORN, SWT, YEL, CND, NO SALT, SOL&LIQUIDS	64	1.95	15.4	0.077
11773	CORN, SWT, YEL, CND, VACUUM PK, NO SALT	79	2.41	19.44	0.077
11176	CORN, SWT, YEL, CND, VACUUM PK, REG PK	79	2.41	19.44	0.077
11172	CORN, SWT, YEL, CND, WHL KERNEL, DRND SOL	81	2.62	18.59	0.154
11179	CORN, SWT, YEL, FRZ, KRNLS CUT OFF COB, BLD, DRND, WO/SALT	80	2.75	19.56	0.066
11178	CORN, SWT, YEL, FRZ, KRNLS CUT OFF COB, UNPREP	88	3.02	20.8	0.119
11775	CORN, SWT, YEL, FRZ, KRNLS ON COB, CKD, BLD, DRND, W/SALT	93	3.11	22.33	0.114
11181	CORN, SWT, YEL, FRZ, KRNLS ON COB, CKD, BLD, DRND, WO/SALT	93	3.11	22.33	0.114
11180	CORN, SWT, YEL, FRZ, KRNLS ON COB, UNPREP	98	3.28	23.5	0.12
11774	CORN, SWT, YEL, FRZ, KRNLS, CUT OFF COB, BLD, DRND, W/SALT	80	2.75	19.56	0.066
20314	CORN, WHITE	365	9.42	74.26	0.667
20014	CORN, YELLOW	365	9.42	74.26	0.667
19004	CORN-BASED, EXTRUDED, CHIPS, BARBECUE-FLAVOR	523	7	56.2	4.46
19003	CORN-BASED, EXTRUDED, CHIPS, PLN	539	6.6	56.9	4.55

NDB #	Food Description (100 gram portions = 3½ ounces = 20 tsp = ½ cup approx.	Calories	Protein	Carbs	Sat Fat
19006	CORN-BASED, EXTRUDED, CONES, NACHO-FLAVOR	536	6.5	57.3	26.79
19005	CORN-BASED, EXTRUDED, CONES, PLN	510	5.8	62.9	22.75
19007	CORN-BASED, EXTRUDED, ONION-FLAVOR	500	7.7	65.1	4.34
19008	CORN-BASED, EXTRUDED, PUFFS OR TWISTS, CHEESE-FLAVOR	554	7.6	53.8	6.59
07020	CORNED BEEF LOAF, JELLIED	153	22.9	0	2.6
20322	CORNMEAL, DEGERMED, ENR, WHITE	366	8.48	77.68	0.225
20022	CORNMEAL, DEGERMED, ENR, YEL	366	8.48	77.68	0.225
20522	CORNMEAL, DEGERMED, UNENR, WHITE	366	8.48	77.68	0.225
20422	CORNMEAL, DEGERMED, UNENR, YEL	366	8.48	77.68	0.225
20323	CORNMEAL, SELF-RISING, BOLTED, PLN, ENR, WHITE	334	8.28	70.28	0.478
20023	CORNMEAL, SELF-RISING, BOLTED, PLN, ENR, YEL	334	8.28	70.28	0.478
20324	CORNMEAL, SELF-RISING, BOLTED, W/WHEAT FLR, ENR, WHITE	348	8.41	73.43	0.4
20024	CORNMEAL, SELF-RISING, BOLTED, W/WHEAT FLR, ENR, YEL	348	8.41	73.43	0.4
20325	CORNMEAL, SELF-RISING, DEGERMED, ENR, WHITE	355	8.41	74.79	0.234
20025	CORNMEAL, SELF-RISING, DEGERMED, ENR, YEL	355	8.41	74.79	0.234
20320	CORNMEAL, WHOLE-GRAIN, WHITE	362	8.12	76.89	0.505
20020	CORNMEAL, WHOLE-GRAIN, YEL	362	8.12	76.89	0.505
19401	CORNNUTS, BARBECUE-FLAVOR	436	9	71.7	2.58
19402	CORNNUTS, NACHO-FLAVOR	438	9.4	71.6	2.56
19009	CORNNUTS, PLAIN	439	8.5	73.3	2.54
11190	CORNSALAD, RAW	21	2	3.6	
20027	CORNSTARCH	381	0.26	91.27	0.009
12008	COTTONSEED FLR, LOFAT (GLANDLESS)	332	49.83	36.1	0.31
12007	COTTONSEED FLR, PART DEFATTED (GLANDLESS)	359	40.96	40.54	1.588
12160	COTTONSEED KRNLS, RSTD (GLANDLESS)	506	32.59	21.9	9.699
12011	COTTONSEED MEAL, PART DEFATTED (GLANDLESS)	367	49.1	38.43	1.207
20029	COUSCOUS, COOKED	112	3.79	23.22	0.029
20028	COUSCOUS, DRY	376	12.76	77.43	0.117
11777	COWPEAS (BLACKEYES), IMMAT SEEDS, CKD, BLD, DRND, W/SALT	97	3.17	20.33	0.096
11192	COWPEAS (BLACKEYES), IMMAT SEEDS, CKD, BLD, DRND, WO/SALT	97	3.17	20.33	0.096
11778	COWPEAS (BLACKEYES), IMMAT SEEDS, FRZ, CKD, BLD, DRND, W/SA	132	8.49	23.76	0.175
11195	COWPEAS (BLACKEYES), IMMAT SEEDS, FRZ, UNPREP	139	8.98	25.13	0.185
11191	COWPEAS (BLACKEYES), IMMAT SEEDS, RAW	90	2.95	18.9	0.09
11196	COWPEAS (BLACKEYES), IMMTRE SEEDS, FRZ, CKD, BLD, DRND, WO	132	8.49	23.76	0.175
16361	COWPEAS, CATJANG, MATURE SEEDS, CKD, BLD, W/SALT	117	8.13	20.32	0.185

NDB #	Food Description (100 gram portions = 3½ ounces = 20 tsp = ½ cup approx.	Calories	Protein	Carbs	Sat Fat
16061	COWPEAS, CATJANG, MATURE SEEDS, CKD, BLD, WO/SALT	117	8.13	20.32	0.185
16060	COWPEAS, CATJANG, MATURE SEEDS, RAW	343	23.85	59.64	0.542
16062	COWPEAS, COMMON (BLACKEYES, CROWDER, SOUTHERN), MTRE S	336	23.52	60.03	0.331
16063	COWPEAS, COMMON (BLKEYES, CRWDR, STHRN), MTURE, CKD, BLD	116	7.73	20.77	0.138
16363	COWPEAS, COMMON, MATURE SEEDS, CKD, BLD, W/SALT	116	7.73	20.77	0.138
16065	COWPEAS, COMMON, MATURE SEEDS, CND W/PORK	83	2.74	16.53	0.605
16064	COWPEAS, COMMON, MATURE SEEDS, CND, PLN	77	4.74	13.63	0.144
11780	COWPEAS, LEAFY TIPS, CKD, BLD, DRND, W/SALT	22	4.67	2.8	0.026
11202	COWPEAS, LEAFY TIPS, CKD, BLD, DRND, WO/SALT	22	4.67	2.8	0.026
11201	COWPEAS, LEAFY TIPS, RAW	29	4.1	4.82	0.066
11779	COWPEAS, YOUNG PODS W/SEEDS, CKD, BLD, DRND, W/SALT	34	2.6	7	0.079
11198	COWPEAS, YOUNG PODS W/SEEDS, CKD, BLD, DRND, WO/SALT	34	2.6	7	0.079
11197	COWPEAS, YOUNG PODS W/SEEDS, RAW	44	3.3	9.5	0.079
18625	CPC FD SERVICE, OROWEAT SEASONED DRSNG MIX, DRY	357	13.4	71.9	0.344
15137	CRAB, ALASKA KING, CKD, MOIST HEAT	97	19.35	0	0.133
15138	CRAB, ALASKA KING, IMITN, MADE FROM SURIMI	102	12.02	10.22	0.26
15136	CRAB, ALASKA KING, RAW	84	18.29	0	0.09
15141	CRAB, BLUE, CANNED	99	20.52	0	0.252
15140	CRAB, BLUE, CKD, MOIST HEAT	102	20.2	0	0.228
15142	CRAB, BLUE, CRAB CAKES	155	20.21	0.48	1.483
15139	CRAB, BLUE, RAW	87	18.06	0.04	0.222
15226	CRAB, DUNGENESS, CKD, MOIST HEAT	110	22.32	0.95	0.168
15143	CRAB, DUNGENESS, RAW	86	17.41	0.74	0.132
15227	CRAB, QUEEN, CKD, MOIST HEAT	115	23.72	0	0.183
15144	CRAB, QUEEN, RAW	90	18.5	0	0.143
09077	CRABAPPLES, RAW	76	0.4	19.95	0.048
18236	CRACKER MEAL	383	9.3	80.9	0.271
18214	CRACKERS, CHEESE, REGULAR	503	10.1	58.2	9.371
18434	CRACKERS, CHS, LO NA	503	10.1	58.2	9.638
18215	CRACKERS, CHS, SANDWICH-TYPE W/PNUT BUTTER FILLING	482	12.6	57	5.447
18216	CRACKERS, CRISPBREAD, RYE	366	7.9	82.2	0.145
18218	CRACKERS, MATZO, EGG	391	12.3	78.6	0.548
18400	CRACKERS, MATZO, EGG&ONION	391	10	77.1	0.936
18217	CRACKERS, MATZO, PLN	395	10	83.7	0.226
18219	CRACKERS, MATZO, WHOLE-WHEAT	351	13.1	78.9	0.243

NDB #	Food Description (100 gram portions = 3½ ounces = 20 tsp = ½ cup approx.	Calories	Protein	Carbs	Sat Fat
18220	CRACKERS, MELBA TOAST, PLN	390	12.1	76.6	0.445
18424	CRACKERS, MELBA TOAST, PLN, WO/SALT	390	12.1	76.6	0.445
18221	CRACKERS, MELBA TOAST, RYE (INCL PUMPERNICKEL)	389	11.6	77.3	0.453
18222	CRACKERS, MELBA TOAST, WHEAT	374	12.9	76.4	0.337
18223	CRACKERS, MILK	455	7.6	69.7	2.633
18224	CRACKERS, RUSK TOAST	407	13.5	72.3	1.376
18225	CRACKERS, RYE, SANDWICH-TYPE W/CHS FILLING	481	9.2	60.8	5.987
18226	CRACKERS, RYE, WAFERS, PLAIN	334	9.6	80.4	0.108
18227	CRACKERS, RYE, WAFERS, SEASONED	381	9	73.8	1.287
18228	CRACKERS, SALTINES (INCL OYSTER, SODA, SOUP)	434	9.2	71.5	2.932
18457	CRACKERS, SALTINES, FAT-FREE, LOW-SODIUM	393	10.5	82.3	0.244
18425	CRACKERS, SALTINES, LO SALT (INCL OYSTER, SODA, SOUP)	434	9.2	71.5	2.932
18426	CRACKERS, SALTINES, UNSALTED TOPS (INCL OYSTER, SODA, SOUP	434	9.2	71.5	2.932
18229	CRACKERS, STD SNACK-TYPE, REG	502	7.4	61	3.776
18427	CRACKERS, STD SNACK-TYPE, REG, LO SALT	502	7.4	61	3.776
18230	CRACKERS, STD SNACK-TYPE, SNDWCH, W/CHS FILLING	477	9.3	61.7	6.125
18231	CRACKERS, STD SNACK-TYPE, SNDWCH, W/PNUT BUTTER FILLING	488	11.1	58.7	5.596
18428	CRACKERS, WHEAT, LOW SALT	473	8.6	64.9	5.178
18232	CRACKERS, WHEAT, REGULAR	473	8.6	64.9	5.178
18233	CRACKERS, WHEAT, SNDWCH, W/CHS FILLING	497	9.8	58.2	4.129
18234	CRACKERS, WHEAT, SNDWCH, W/PNUT BUTTER FILLING	495	13.5	53.8	4.602
18235	CRACKERS, WHOLE-WHEAT	443	8.8	68.6	3.393
18429	CRACKERS, WHOLE-WHEAT, LO SALT	443	8.8	68.6	3.393
09078	CRANBERRIES, RAW	49	0.39	12.68	0.017
14242	CRANBERRY JUC COCKTAIL, BTLD	57	0	14.4	0.009
14243	CRANBERRY JUC COCKTAIL, BTLD, LO CAL, W/CA, SACCHARIN&COR	19	0	4.7	0
14430	CRANBERRY JUC COCKTAIL, FRZ CONC	201	0.05	51.45	0
14431	CRANBERRY JUC COCKTAIL, FRZ CONC, PREP W/H2O	55	0	14	0
09081	CRANBERRY SAU, CND, SWTND	151	0.2	38.9	0.013
14238	CRANBERRY-APPLE JUC DRK, BTLD	67	0.1	17.1	0
14240	CRANBERRY-APRICOT JUC DRK, BTLD	64	0.2	16.2	0
14241	CRANBERRY-GRAPE JUC DRK, BTLD	56	0.2	14	0.033
09082	CRANBERRY-ORANGE RELISH, CND	178	0.3	46.2	0.012
15243	CRAYFISH, MXD SP, FARMED, CKD, MOIST HEAT	87	17.52	0	0.216
15242	CRAYFISH, MXD SP, FARMED, RAW	72	14.85	0	0.163

NDB #	Food Description (100 gram portions = 3½ ounces = 20 tsp = ½ cup approx.	Calories	Protein	Carbs	Sat Fat
15146	CRAYFISH, MXD SP, WILD, CKD, MOIST HEAT	82	16.77	0	0.181
15145	CRAYFISH, MXD SP, WILD, RAW	77	15.97	0	0.159
18237	CREAM PUFFS, PREP FROM RECIPE, SHELL (INCL ECLAIR)	362	9	22.8	5.599
18238	CREAM PUFFS, PREP FROM RECIPE, SHELL, W/CUSTARD FILLING	258	6.7	22.9	3.679
01067	CREAM SUB, LIQ, W/HYDR VEG OIL&SOY PROT	136	1	11.38	1.937
01068	CREAM SUB, LIQ, W/LAURIC ACID OIL&NA CASEINATE	136	1	11.38	9.304
01069	CREAM SUBSTITUTE, POWDERED	546	4.79	54.88	32.525
01049	CREAM, FLUID, HALF AND HALF	130	2.96	4.3	7.158
01053	CREAM, FLUID, HVY WHIPPING	345	2.05	2.79	23.032
01050	CREAM, FLUID, LT (COFFEE CRM OR TABLE CRM)	195	2.7	3.66	12.02
01052	CREAM, FLUID, LT WHIPPING	292	2.17	2.96	19.337
01056	CREAM, SOUR, CULTURED	214	3.16	4.27	13.047
01055	CREAM, SOUR, RED FAT, CULTURED	135	2.94	4.26	7.47
01054	CREAM, WHIPPED, CRM TOPPING, PRESSURIZED	257	3.2	12.49	13.831
11781	CRESS, GARDEN, CKD, BLD, DRND, W/SALT	23	1.9	3.8	0.02
11204	CRESS, GARDEN, CKD, BLD, DRND, WO/SALT	23	1.9	3.8	0.02
11203	CRESS, GARDEN, RAW	32	2.6	5.5	0.023
19010	CRISPED RICE BAR, CHOC CHIP	404	5.1	73	5.24
15021	CROAKER, ATLANTIC, CKD, BREADED&FRIED	221	18.2	7.54	3.476
15020	CROAKER, ATLANTIC, RAW	104	17.78	0	1.088
18240	CROISSANTS, APPLE	254	7.4	37.1	4.994
18239	CROISSANTS, BUTTER	406	8.2	45.8	11.659
18241	CROISSANTS, CHEESE	414	9.2	47	10.628
18242	CROUTONS, PLAIN	407	11.9	73.5	1.51
18243	CROUTONS, SEASONED	465	10.8	63.5	5.247
11206	CUCUMBER, PEELED, RAW	12	0.57	2.5	0.042
11205	CUCUMBER, WITH PEEL, RAW	13	0.69	2.76	0.034
02014	CUMIN SEED	375	17.81	44.24	1.535
09083	CURRANTS, EUROPEAN BLACK, RAW	63	1.4	15.38	0.034
09084	CURRANTS, RED&WHITE, RAW	56	1.4	13.8	0.017
09085	CURRANTS, ZANTE, DRIED	283	4.08	74.08	0.028
02015	CURRY POWDER	325	12.66	58.15	2.237
15193	CUSK, COOKED, DRY HEAT	112	24.35	0	
15022	CUSK, RAW	87	18.99	0	0.13
09086	CUSTARD-APPLE, (BULLOCK'S-HEART), RAW	101	1.7	25.2	0.231

NDB #	Food Description (100 gram portions = 3½ ounces = 20 tsp = ½ cup approx.	Calories	Protein	Carbs	Sat Fat
15229	CUTTLEFISH, MXD SP, CKD, MOIST HEAT	158	32.48	1.64	0.236
15163	CUTTLEFISH, MXD SP, RAW	79	16.24	0.82	0.118
14422	DAIRY DRK MIX, CHOC, RED CAL, W/ASPRT, PDR	298	25	50.2	1.871
14423	DAIRY DRK MIX, CHOC, RED CAL, W/ASPRT, PDR, PREP W/H2O	31	2.6	5.2	0.196
11207	DANDELION GREENS, RAW	45	2.7	9.2	0.17
11782	DANDELION GRNS, CKD, BLD, DRND, W/SALT	33	2	6.4	
11208	DANDELION GRNS, CKD, BLD, DRND, WO/SALT	33	2	6.4	0.146
18245	DANISH PASTRY, CHEESE	374	8	37.2	6.794
18244	DANISH PASTRY, CINN, ENR	403	7	44.6	5.681
18430	DANISH PASTRY, CINN, UNENR	403	7	44.6	5.681
18246	DANISH PASTRY, FRUIT, ENR	371	5.4	47.8	4.86
18431	DANISH PASTRY, FRUIT, UNENR (INCL APPL, CINN, RAISIN, STRAWBE	371	5.4	47.8	2.826
18433	DANISH PASTRY, LEMON, UNENR	371	5.4	47.8	2.826
18247	DANISH PASTRY, NUT (INCL ALMOND, RAISIN NUT, CINN NUT)	430	7.1	45.7	5.821
18435	DANISH PASTRY, RASPBERRY, UNENR	371	5.4	47.8	2.826
09087	DATES, DOMESTIC, NAT&DRY	275	1.97	73.51	0.191
01071	DESSERT TOPPING, PDR, 1.5 OZ PREP W/1/2 CUP MILK	189	3.6	16.53	10.684
01070	DESSERT TOPPING, POWDERED	577	4.9	52.54	36.723
01072	DESSERT TOPPING, PRESSURIZED	264	0.98	16.07	18.912
01073	DESSERT TOPPING, SEMI SOLID, FRZ	318	1.25	23.05	21.783
19197	DESSERTS, CPC, ALSA MOUSSE MIX, PDR, DK CHOC	501	9.43	61.33	17.16
19220	DESSERTS, RENNIN, CHOC, DRY MIX	363	2.4	91.5	1.94
19225	DESSERTS, RENNIN, TABLETS, UNSWTND	84	1	19.8	0.041
19222	DESSERTS, RENNIN, VANILLA, DRY MIX	383	0	99	
02016	DILL SEED	305	15.98	55.17	0.73
02017	DILL WEED, DRIED	253	19.96	55.82	0.234
02045	DILL WEED, FRESH	43	3.46	7.02	0.06
11925	DOCK, CKD, BLD, DRND, W/SALT	20	1.83	2.93	
11617	DOCK, CKD, BLD, DRND, WO/SALT	20	1.83	2.93	
11616	DOCK, RAW	22	2	3.2	
15194	DOLPHINFISH, CKD, DRY HEAT	109	23.72	0	0.241
15023	DOLPHINFISH, RAW	85	18.5	0	0.188
19032	DOO DADS SNACK MIX, ORIGINAL FLAVOR	456	10.3	64.3	3.53
18251	DOUGHNUTS, CAKE-TYPE, CHOC, SUGARED OR GLAZED	417	4.5	57.4	5.132
18248	DOUGHNUTS, CAKE-TYPE, PLN (INCL UNSUGARED, OLD-FASHIONE	421	5	49.7	3.625

NDB #	Food Description (100 gram portions = 3½ ounces = 20 tsp = ½ cup approx.	Calories	Protein	Carbs	Sat Fat
18249	DOUGHNUTS, CAKE-TYPE, PLN, CHOCOLATE-COATED OR FRSTD	474	5	48	8.107
18250	DOUGHNUTS, CAKE-TYPE, PLN, SUGARED OR GLAZED	426	5.2	50.8	5.926
18252	DOUGHNUTS, CAKE-TYPE, WHEAT, SUGARED OR GLAZED	360	6.3	42.6	3.023
18253	DOUGHNUTS, FRENCH CRULLERS, GLAZED	412	3.1	59.5	4.667
18255	DOUGHNUTS, YEAST-LEAVENED, GLAZED, ENR (INCL HONEY BUNS)	403	6.4	44.3	5.813
18436	DOUGHNUTS, YEAST-LEAVENED, GLAZED, UNENR (INCL HONEY BU	403	6.4	44.3	5.813
18254	DOUGHNUTS, YEAST-LEAVENED, W/CREME FILLING	361	6.4	30	5.43
18256	DOUGHNUTS, YEAST-LEAVENED, W/JELLY FILLING	340	5.9	39	4.843
15195	DRUM, FRESHWATER, CKD, DRY HEAT	153	22.49	0	1.434
15024	DRUM, FRESHWATER, RAW	119	17.54	0	1.119
05143	DUCK, DOMESTICATED, LIVER, RAW	136	18.74	3.53	1.44
05142	DUCK, DOMESTICATED, MEAT ONLY, CKD, RSTD	201	23.48	0	4.17
05141	DUCK, DOMESTICATED, MEAT ONLY, RAW	132	18.28	0	2.32
05140	DUCK, DOMESTICATED, MEAT&SKN, CKD, RSTD	337	18.99	0	9.67
05139	DUCK, DOMESTICATED, MEAT&SKN, RAW	404	11.49	0	13.22
05145	DUCK, WILD, BREAST, MEAT ONLY, RAW	123	19.85	0	1.32
05144	DUCK, WILD, MEAT&SKN, RAW	211	17.42	0	5.04
05316	DUCK, YNG DUCKL, DOM, WH PEKIN, BRST, MEAT, BNLESS, CKD WO/	140	27.6	0	0.578
05318	DUCK, YNG DUCKL, DOM, WH PEKIN, LEG, MEAT, BONE IN, CKD WO/S	178	29.1	0	1.339
05315	DUCK, YNG DUCKLING, DOM, WH PEKIN, BRST, MEAT&SKN, BNLESS,	202	24.5	0	2.922
05317	DUCK, YNG DUCKLING, DOM, WH PEKIN, LEG, MEAT&SKN, BONE IN, C	217	26.75	0	2.975
09422	DURIAN, RAW OR FROZEN	147	1.47	27.09	
07021	DUTCH BRAND LOAF CHICK PORK & BF	283	12	7.26	9.032
18257	ECLAIRS, CUSTARD-FILLED W/CHOC GLAZE, PREP FROM RECIPE	262	6.4	24.2	4.119
15025	EEL, MIXED SPECIES, RAW	184	18.44	0	2.358
15026	EEL, MXD SP, CKD, DRY HEAT	236	23.65	0	3.023
19169	EGG CUSTARDS, DRY MIX	410	6.9	82.8	2.03
19205	EGG CUSTARDS, DRY MIX, PREP W/ 2% MILK	111	4.08	17.42	1.357
19170	EGG CUSTARDS, DRY MIX, PREP W/ WHL MILK	121	4.04	17.29	2.122
01142	EGG SUBSTITUTE, FROZEN	160	11.29	3.2	1.93
01143	EGG SUBSTITUTE, LIQUID	84	12	0.64	0.659
01144	EGG SUBSTITUTE, POWDER	444	55.5	21.8	3.766
01138	EGG, DUCK, WHOLE, FRESH, RAW	185	12.81	1.45	3.681
01139	EGG, GOOSE, WHOLE, FRESH, RAW	185	13.87	1.35	3.595
01140	EGG, QUAIL, WHOLE, FRESH, RAW	158	13.05	0.41	3.557

NDB #	Food Description (100 gram portions = 3½ ounces = 20 tsp = ½ cup approx.	Calories	Protein	Carbs	Sat Fat
01141	EGG, TURKEY, WHL, FRSH, RAW	171	13.68	1.15	3.632
01173	EGG, WHITE, DRIED	382	81.1	7.8	0
01135	EGG, WHITE, DRIED, FLAKES, GLUCOSE RED	351	76.92	4.17	0
01136	EGG, WHITE, DRIED, PDR, GLUCOSE RED	376	82.4	4.47	0
01124	EGG, WHITE, RAW, FRESH	50	10.52	1.03	0
01172	EGG, WHITE, RAW, FROZEN	47	9.8	1.05	0
01129	EGG, WHL, CKD, HARD-BOILED	155	12.58	1.12	3.267
01132	EGG, WHL, CKD, SCRMBLD	166	11.09	2.2	3.679
01134	EGG, WHL, DRIED, STABILIZED, GLUCOSE RED	615	48.17	2.38	13.198
01128	EGG, WHOLE, COOKED, FRIED	199	13.54	1.36	4.167
01130	EGG, WHOLE, COOKED, OMELET	152	10.33	1.04	3.18
01131	EGG, WHOLE, COOKED, POACHED	149	12.44	1.22	3.087
01133	EGG, WHOLE, DRIED	594	47.35	4.95	12.727
01123	EGG, WHOLE, RAW, FRESH	149	12.49	1.22	3.1
01171	EGG, WHOLE, RAW, FROZEN	148	11.95	1.05	3.147
01137	EGG, YOLK, DRIED	666	34.25	3.6	17.154
01125	EGG, YOLK, RAW, FRESH	358	16.76	1.78	9.552
01126	EGG, YOLK, RAW, FROZEN	303	15.5	1.15	7.82
01160	EGG, YOLK, RAW, FRZ, SALTED	274	14	1.6	7.028
01127	EGG, YOLK, RAW, FRZ, SUGARED	307	13.8	10.8	6.97
01057	EGGNOG	135	3.81	13.54	4.443
14245	EGGNOG-FLAVOR MIX, PDR, PREP W/ WHL MILK	96	3	14.3	1.893
14244	EGGNOG-FLAVOR MIX, POWDER	390	0.4	97.4	0.291
11783	EGGPLANT, CKD, BLD, DRND, W/SALT	28	0.83	6.64	0.044
11210	EGGPLANT, CKD, BLD, DRND, WO/SALT	28	0.83	6.64	0.044
11209	EGGPLANT, RAW	26	1.02	6.07	0.034
22704	EL RIO CHILI CON CARNE, NO BNS, CND ENTREE	117	5.8	6.2	2.86
09088	ELDERBERRIES, RAW	73	0.66	18.4	0.023
05624	EMU, FAN FILLET, CKD, BRLD	154	31.27	0	0.583
05623	EMU, FAN FILLET, RAW	103	22.5	0	0.201
05625	EMU, FLAT FILLET, RAW	102	22.25	0	0.187
05627	EMU, FULL RUMP, CKD, BRLD	168	33.67	0	0.87
05626	EMU, FULL RUMP, RAW	112	22.83	0	0.672
05622	EMU, GROUND, CKD, PAN-BROILED	163	28.43	0	1.242
05621	EMU, GROUND, RAW	134	22.77	0	1.022

NDB #	Food Description (100 gram portions = 3½ ounces = 20 tsp = ½ cup approx.	Calories	Protein	Carbs	Sat Fat
05628	EMU, INSIDE DRUM, RAW	108	22.22	0	0.574
05629	EMU, INSIDE DRUMS, CKD, BRLD	156	32.38	0	0.654
05630	EMU, OUTSIDE DRUM, RAW	103	23.08	0	0.122
05631	EMU, OYSTER, RAW	141	22.81	0	1.231
05632	EMU, TOP LOIN, CKD, BRLD	152	29.07	0	0.794
11213	ENDIVE, RAW	17	1.25	3.35	0.048
18260	ENGLISH MUFFINS, MIXED-GRAIN (INCL GRANOLA)	235	9.1	46.3	0.23
18261	ENGLISH MUFFINS, MIXED-GRAIN, TSTD (INCL GRANOLA)	255	9.9	50.3	0.25
18258	ENGLISH MUFFINS, PLN, ENR, W/CA PROP (INCL SOURDOUGH)	235	7.7	46	0.259
18437	ENGLISH MUFFINS, PLN, ENR, WO/CA PROP (INCL SOURDOUGH)	235	7.7	46	0.259
18259	ENGLISH MUFFINS, PLN, TSTD, ENR, W/CA PROP (INCL SOURDOUGH	255	8.4	50	0.281
18438	ENGLISH MUFFINS, PLN, UNENR, W/CA PROP (INCL SOURDOUGH)	235	7.7	46	0.259
18439	ENGLISH MUFFINS, PLN, UNENR, WO/CA PROP (INCL SOURDOUGH)	235	7.7	46	0.259
18262	ENGLISH MUFFINS, RAISIN-CINNAMON (INCL APPLE-CINNAMON)	243	7.5	48.7	0.394
18263	ENGLISH MUFFINS, RAISIN-CINNAMON, TSTD (INCL APPLE-CINNAMO	264	8.2	53	0.428
18264	ENGLISH MUFFINS, WHEAT	223	8.7	44.8	0.287
18265	ENGLISH MUFFINS, WHEAT, TSTD	243	9.4	48.7	0.312
18266	ENGLISH MUFFINS, WHOLE-WHEAT	203	8.8	40.4	0.334
18267	ENGLISH MUFFINS, WHOLE-WHEAT, TSTD	221	9.6	44.1	0.363
21046	ENTREES, CRAB CAKE	266	18.75	8.52	3.74
21047	ENTREES, FISH FILLET, BATTERED OR BREADED, &FRIED	232	14.66	16.97	2.82
21050	ENTREES, PIZZA W/CHS, MEAT, &VEG	233	16.47	26.95	1.943
21051	ENTREES, PIZZA W/PEPPERONI	255	14.26	27.98	3.149
21049	ENTREES, PIZZA WITH CHEESE	223	12.19	32.54	2.445
11984	EPAZOTE, RAW	32	0.33	7.44	
11618	EPPAW, RAW	150	4.6	31.68	
16138	FALAFEL, HOME-PREPARED	333	13.31	31.84	2.383
21002	FAST FOODS BISCUIT W/ EGG	274	8.53	23.46	3.477
21003	FAST FOODS, BISCUIT, W/EGG&BACON	305	11.33	19.06	5.3
21004	FAST FOODS, BISCUIT, W/EGG&HAM	230	10.64	15.79	3.08
21007	FAST FOODS, BISCUIT, W/EGG, CHS, &BACON	331	11.29	23.21	7.915
21008	FAST FOODS, BISCUIT, W/HAM	342	11.85	38.75	10.096
21009	FAST FOODS, BISCUIT, W/SAUSAGE	391	9.77	32.29	11.468
21027	FAST FOODS, BROWNIE	405	4.57	64.95	5.22
21066	FAST FOODS, BURRITO, W/BF	238	12.09	26.6	4.754

NDB #	Food Description (100 gram portions = 3½ ounces = 20 tsp = ½ cup approx.	Calories	Protein	Carbs	Sat Fat
21067	FAST FOODS, BURRITO, W/BF&CHILI PEPPERS	212	10.7	24.6	3.98
21068	FAST FOODS, BURRITO, W/BF, CHS, &CHILI PEPPERS	208	13.46	20.96	3.42
21060	FAST FOODS, BURRITO, W/BNS	206	6.48	32.92	3.174
21062	FAST FOODS, BURRITO, W/BNS&CHILI PEPPERS	202	8.03	28.47	3.729
21061	FAST FOODS, BURRITO, W/BNS&CHS	203	8.1	29.55	3.682
21063	FAST FOODS, BURRITO, W/BNS&MEAT	220	9.73	28.58	3.6
21064	FAST FOODS, BURRITO, W/BNS, CHS, &BF	163	7.18	19.55	3.522
21065	FAST FOODS, BURRITO, W/BNS, CHS, &CHILI PEPPERS	197	9.91	25.35	3.332
21069	FAST FOODS, BURRITO, W/FRUIT (APPL OR CHERRY)	312	3.38	47.27	6.175
21100	FAST FOODS, CHEESEBURGER, LRG, DOUBLE PATTY, W/CONDMNT	273	14.72	15.37	6.85
21098	FAST FOODS, CHEESEBURGER, LRG, SINGLE PATTY, W/CONDMNT&	257	12.87	17.53	6.867
21099	FAST FOODS, CHEESEBURGER, LRG, SINGLE PATTY, W/HAM, COND	293	15.55	14.83	8.317
21094	FAST FOODS, CHEESEBURGER, REG, DOUBLE PATTY&BUN, PLN	288	13.83	27.66	5.943
21095	FAST FOODS, CHEESEBURGER, REG, DOUBLE PATTY&BUN, W/CON	285	13.04	23.3	5.6
21092	FAST FOODS, CHEESEBURGER, REG, DOUBLE PATTY, PLN	295	17.85	14.23	8.385
21093	FAST FOODS, CHEESEBURGER, REG, DOUBLE PATTY, W/CONDMNT	251	12.8	21.2	5.251
21090	FAST FOODS, CHEESEBURGER, REG, SINGLE PATTY, W/CONDMNT	261	14.12	23.48	5.582
21091	FAST FOODS, CHEESEBURGER, REG, SINGLE PATTY, W/CONDMNT&	233	11.58	18.27	5.966
21101	FAST FOODS, CHEESEBURGER, TRIPLE PATTY, PLN	262	18.44	8.78	7.14
21102	FAST FOODS, CHICK FILLET SNDWCH, PLN	283	13.25	21.26	4.685
21103	FAST FOODS, CHICK FILLET SNDWCH, W/CHS	277	12.9	18.24	5.46
21037	FAST FOODS, CHICK, BREADED&FRIED, BNLESS PIECES, PLN	301	17	14.41	4.39
21038	FAST FOODS, CHICK, BREADED&FRIED, BNLESS PIECES, W/BARB. S	254	13.19	19.25	4.285
21039	FAST FOODS, CHICK, BREADED&FRIED, BNLESS PIECES, W/HONEY	286	14.58	23.37	4.776
21040	FAST FOODS, CHICK, BREADED&FRIED, BNLESS PIECES, W/MUSTAR	248	13.4	16.04	4.397
21041	FAST FOODS, CHICK, BREADED&FRIED, BNLESS PIECES, W/SWT&S	266	13.04	22.27	4.242
21035	FAST FOODS, CHICK, BREADED&FRIED, DK MEAT (DRUMSTK OR THI	291	20.32	10.61	4.763
21036	FAST FOODS, CHICK, BREADED&FRIED, LT MEAT (BREAST OR WING)	303	21.91	12.01	4.812
21042	FAST FOODS, CHILI CON CARNE	101	9.73	8.67	1.356
21070	FAST FOODS, CHIMICHANGA, W/BF	244	11.27	24.6	4.888
21071	FAST FOODS, CHIMICHANGA, W/BF&CHS	242	10.96	21.49	6.108
21072	FAST FOODS, CHIMICHANGA, W/BF&RED CHILI PEPPERS	223	9.53	24.09	4.354
21073	FAST FOODS, CHIMICHANGA, W/BF, CHS, &RED CHILI PEPPERS	202	8.15	21.26	4.649
21043	FAST FOODS, CLAMS, BREADED&FRIED	392	11.15	33.75	5.742
21127	FAST FOODS, COLESLAW	148	1.47	12.88	1.622

NDB #	Food Description (100 gram portions = 3½ ounces = 20 tsp = ½ cup approx.	Calories	Protein	Carbs	Sat Fat
21029	FAST FOODS, COOKIES, ANIMAL CRACKERS	446	6.18	75.33	5.272
21030	FAST FOODS, COOKIES, CHOC CHIP	423	5.25	65.86	9.709
21128	FAST FOODS, CORN ON THE COB W/BUTTER	106	3.06	21.88	1.125
21011	FAST FOODS, CROISSANT, W/EGG&CHS	290	10.07	19.14	11.075
21012	FAST FOODS, CROISSANT, W/EGG, CHS, &BACON	320	12.58	18.33	11.963
21013	FAST FOODS, CROISSANT, W/EGG, CHS, &HAM	312	12.45	15.92	11.497
21014	FAST FOODS, CROISSANT, W/EGG, CHS, &SAUSAGE	327	12.69	15.45	11.391
21015	FAST FOODS, DANISH PASTRY, CHS	388	6.41	31.53	5.63
21016	FAST FOODS, DANISH PASTRY, CINN	397	5.46	53.24	3.953
21017	FAST FOODS, DANISH PASTRY, FRUIT	356	5.06	47.94	3.527
21104	FAST FOODS, EGG&CHS SNDWCH	233	10.69	17.76	4.538
21018	FAST FOODS, EGG, SCRAMBLED	212	13.84	2.08	6.153
21074	FAST FOODS, ENCHILADA, W/CHS	196	5.91	17.51	6.496
21075	FAST FOODS, ENCHILADA, W/CHS&BF	168	6.21	15.87	4.712
21076	FAST FOODS, ENCHIRITO, W/CHS, BF, &BNS	178	9.27	17.51	4.118
21019	FAST FOODS, ENG MUFFIN, W/BUTTER	300	7.73	48.19	3.857
21020	FAST FOODS, ENG MUFFIN, W/CHS&SAUSAGE	342	13.34	25.36	8.566
21021	FAST FOODS, ENG MUFFIN, W/EGG, CHS, &CANADIAN BACON	211	12.18	19.52	3.405
21022	FAST FOODS, ENG MUFFIN, W/EGG, CHS, &SAUSAGE	295	13.13	18.77	7.525
21105	FAST FOODS, FISH SNDWCH, W/TARTAR SAU	273	10.72	25.96	3.313
21106	FAST FOODS, FISH SNDWCH, W/TARTAR SAU&CHS	286	11.26	26.03	4.448
21024	FAST FOODS, FRENCH TOAST STKS	364	5.87	41.03	3.34
21077	FAST FOODS, FRIJOLES W/CHS	135	6.81	17.19	2.44
21116	FAST FOODS, HAM&CHS SNDWCH	241	14.17	22.84	4.409
21117	FAST FOODS, HAM, EGG, &CHS SNDWCH	243	13.46	21.64	5.175
21114	FAST FOODS, HAMBURGER, LRG, DOUBLE PATTY, W/CONDMNT&VE	239	15.17	17.82	4.654
21202	FAST FOODS, HAMBURGER, LRG, SINGLE PATTY, W/CONDMNT	248	13.43	21.41	4.608
21115	FAST FOODS, HAMBURGER, LRG, TRIPLE PATTY, W/CONDMNT	267	19.3	11.04	6.147
21110	FAST FOODS, HAMBURGER, REG, DOUBLE PATTY, PLN	309	17	24.39	5.896
21111	FAST FOODS, HAMBURGER, REG, DOUBLE PATTY, W/CONDMNT	268	14.8	18.02	5.582
21107	FAST FOODS, HAMBURGER, REG, SINGLE PATTY, PLN	305	13.69	33.9	4.601
21108	FAST FOODS, HAMBURGER, REG, SINGLE PATTY, W/CONDMNT	257	11.62	32.31	3.361
21109	FAST FOODS, HAMBURGER, REG, SINGLE PATTY, W/CONDMNT&VEG	254	11.74	24.81	3.755
21118	FAST FOODS, HOTDOG, PLAIN	247	10.6	18.4	5.213
21119	FAST FOODS, HOTDOG, W/CHILI	260	11.85	27.45	4.258

NDB #	Food Description (100 gram portions = 3½ ounces = 20 tsp = ½ cup approx.	Calories	Protein	Carbs	Sat Fat
21120	FAST FOODS, HOTDOG, W/CORN FLR COATING (CORNDOG)	263	9.6	31.88	2.949
21129	FAST FOODS, HUSH PUPPIES	329	6.25	44.74	3.444
21028	FAST FOODS, ICE MILK, VANILLA, SOFT-SERVE, W/CONE	159	3.78	23.41	3.429
21078	FAST FOODS, NACHOS, W/CHS	306	8.05	32.15	6.885
21079	FAST FOODS, NACHOS, W/CHS&JALAPENO PEPPERS	298	8.24	29.45	6.872
21080	FAST FOODS, NACHOS, W/CHS, BNS, GROUND BF, &PEPPERS	223	7.76	21.89	4.897
21081	FAST FOODS, NACHOS, W/CINN&SUGAR	543	6.6	58.16	16.707
21130	FAST FOODS, ONION RINGS, BREADED&FRIED	332	4.46	37.74	8.377
21048	FAST FOODS, OYSTERS, BATTERED OR BREADED, &FRIED	265	9.02	28.69	3.294
21025	FAST FOODS, PANCAKES W/BUTTER&SYRUP	224	3.56	39.18	2.522
21131	FAST FOODS, POTATO, BKD&TOPPED W/CHS SAU	160	4.94	15.71	3.567
21132	FAST FOODS, POTATO, BKD&TOPPED W/CHS SAU&BACON	151	6.16	14.86	3.389
21133	FAST FOODS, POTATO, BKD&TOPPED W/CHS SAU&BROCCOLI	119	4.03	13.74	2.511
21134	FAST FOODS, POTATO, BKD&TOPPED W/CHS SAU&CHILI	122	5.88	14.14	3.3
21135	FAST FOODS, POTATO, BKD&TOPPED W/SOUR CRM&CHIVES	130	2.21	16.56	3.315
21138	FAST FOODS, POTATO, FRENCH FR IN VEG OIL	342	4.3	39.81	3.85
21139	FAST FOODS, POTATO, MASHED	83	2.31	16.12	0.479
21026	FAST FOODS, POTATOES, HASHED BROWN	210	2.7	22.43	6.005
21121	FAST FOODS, RST BF SNDWCH, PLN	249	15.47	24.06	2.594
21057	FAST FOODS, SALAD, VEG TOSSED, WO/DRSNG, W/TURKEY, HAM&C	82	7.98	1.45	2.508
21052	FAST FOODS, SALAD, VEG, TOSSED, WO/DRSNG	16	1.25	3.22	0.01
21054	FAST FOODS, SALAD, VEG, TOSSED, WO/DRSNG, W/CHICK	48	8	1.71	0.265
21053	FAST FOODS, SALAD, VEG, TOSSED, WO/DRSNG, W/CHS&EGG	47	4.04	2.19	1.371
21055	FAST FOODS, SALAD, VEG, TOSSED, WO/DRSNG, W/PASTA&SEAFOO	91	3.94	7.67	0.616
21056	FAST FOODS, SALAD, VEG, TOSSED, WO/DRSNG, W/SHRIMP	45	6.15	2.8	0.276
21058	FAST FOODS, SCALLOPS, BREADED&FRIED	268	10.94	26.73	3.391
21059	FAST FOODS, SHRIMP, BREADED&FRIED	277	11.51	24.39	3.28
21124	FAST FOODS, SUBMARINE SNDWCH, W/COLD CUTS	200	9.58	22.39	2.986
21125	FAST FOODS, SUBMARINE SNDWCH, W/RST BF	190	13.26	20.51	3.281
21126	FAST FOODS, SUBMARINE SNDWCH, W/TUNA SALAD	228	11.6	21.63	2.082
21032	FAST FOODS, SUNDAE, CARAMEL	196	4.71	31.81	2.91
21033	FAST FOODS, SUNDAE, HOT FUDGE	180	3.57	30.17	3.179
21034	FAST FOODS, SUNDAE, STRAWBERRY	175	4.09	29.18	2.444
21082	FAST FOODS, TACO	216	12.08	15.63	6.648
21083	FAST FOODS, TACO SALAD	141	6.68	11.91	3.446

NDB #	Food Description (100 gram portions = 3½ ounces = 20 tsp = ½ cup approx.	Calories	Protein	Carbs	Sat Fat
21084	FAST FOODS, TACO SALAD W/CHILI CON CARNE	111	6.67	10.18	2.299
21087	FAST FOODS, TOSTADA, W/BF&CHS	193	11.65	13.97	6.377
21085	FAST FOODS, TOSTADA, W/BNS&CHS	155	6.67	18.42	3.727
21086	FAST FOODS, TOSTADA, W/BNS, BF, &CHS	148	7.15	13.18	5.1
04001	FAT, BEEF TALLOW	902	0	0	49.8
04542	FAT, CHICKEN	900	0	0	29.8
04574	FAT, DUCK	900	0	0	33.2
04576	FAT, GOOSE	900	0	0	27.7
04520	FAT, MUTTON TALLOW	902	0	0	47.3
04575	FAT, TURKEY	900	0	0	29.4
09334	FEIJOA, RAW	49	1.24	10.63	
02018	FENNEL SEED	345	15.8	52.29	0.48
11957	FENNEL, BULB, RAW	31	1.24	7.29	
02019	FENUGREEK SEED	323	23	58.35	1.46
11996	FIDDLEHEAD FERNS, FRZ, UNPREP	34	4.31	5.74	
11995	FIDDLEHEAD FERNS, RAW	34	4.55	5.54	
22682	FIESTA CAFE BF&BEAN CHIMICHANGA, FRZ	186	10.6	24.5	0.95
09093	FIGS, CND, EX HVY SYRUP PK, SOL&LIQUIDS	107	0.38	27.86	0.02
09090	FIGS, CND, H2O PK, SOL&LIQUIDS	53	0.4	13.99	0.02
09092	FIGS, CND, HVY SYRUP PK, SOL&LIQUIDS	88	0.38	22.9	0.02
09091	FIGS, CND, LT SYRUP PK, SOL&LIQUIDS	69	0.39	17.95	0.02
09095	FIGS, DRIED, STEWED	108	1.29	27.57	0.099
09094	FIGS, DRIED, UNCOOKED	255	3.05	65.35	0.234
09089	FIGS, RAW	74	0.75	19.18	0.06
11985	FIREWEED, LEAVES, RAW	103	4.71	19.22	
04589	FISH OIL, COD LIVER	902	0	0	22.608
04590	FISH OIL, HERRING	902	0	0	21.29
04591	FISH OIL, MENHADEN	902	0	0	30.427
04592	FISH OIL, MENHADEN, FULLY HYDR	902	0	0	95.6
04593	FISH OIL, SALMON	902	0	0	19.872
04594	FISH OIL, SARDINE	902	0	0	29.892
15027	FISH PORTIONS&STKS, FRZ, PREHTD	272	15.65	23.75	3.149
19187	FLAN, CARAMEL CUSTARD, DRY MIX	348	0	91.6	
19231	FLAN, CARAMEL CUSTARD, DRY MIX, PREP W/ 2% MILK	103	2.99	18.82	1.035
19232	FLAN, CARAMEL CUSTARD, DRY MIX, PREP W/ 2% MILK	113	2.95	18.68	1.8

NDB #	Food Description (100 gram portions = 3½ ounces = 20 tsp = ½ cup approx.	Calories	Protein	Carbs	Sat Fat
15029	FLATFISH (FLOUNDER&SOLE SP), CKD, DRY HEAT	117	24.16	0	0.363
15028	FLATFISH (FLOUNDER&SOLE SP), RAW	91	18.84	0	0.283
12200	FORMULATED, WHEAT-BASED, ALL FLAVORS XCPT MACADAMIA, W	647	13.11	20.79	9.37
12199	FORMULATED, WHEAT-BASED, FLAV, MACADAMIA FLAV, WO/SALT	619	11.19	27.91	8.482
12140	FORMULATED, WHEAT-BASED, UNFLAVORED, W/SALT	622	13.82	23.68	8.701
07022	FRANKFURTER BF	327	11.24	4.06	11.688
07945	FRANKFURTER BF HTD	326	11.54	3.77	11.436
07023	FRANKFURTER BF & PORK	301	11.53	1.52	10.77
07950	FRANKFURTER MEAT	290	10.26	4.17	7.666
07949	FRANKFURTER MEAT HTD	278	9.77	4.9	7.22
07024	FRANKFURTER, CHICK	257	12.93	6.79	5.54
07939	FRANKFURTER, PORK	269	12.81	0.28	8.719
07025	FRANKFURTER, TURKEY	226	14.28	1.49	5.89
22710	FREEZER QUEEN GRAVY&SLICED BF MEAL, MSHD POT&CARROTS, F	81	6	10	0.51
18268	FRENCH TOAST, FRZ, RTH	213	7.4	32.1	1.533
18269	FRENCH TOAST, PREP FROM RECIPE, MADE W/LOFAT (2%) MILK	229	7.7	25	2.723
19240	FROSTINGS, CHOC, CREAMY, DRY MIX	389	1.3	92	
19241	FROSTINGS, CHOC, CREAMY, DRY MIX, PREP W/ BUTTER	404	1.09	70.85	5.36
19372	FROSTINGS, CHOC, CREAMY, DRY MIX, PREP W/ MARGARINE	404	1.1	71.02	1.74
19226	FROSTINGS, CHOC, CREAMY, RTE	397	1.1	63.2	5.526
19227	FROSTINGS, COCONUT-NUT, RTE	412	1.5	52.8	7.03
19228	FROSTINGS, CRM CHEESE-FLAVOR, RTE	415	0.1	67.32	4.545
19375	FROSTINGS, GLAZE, PREPARED-FROM-RECIPE	359	0.6	73.5	1.75
19244	FROSTINGS, VANILLA, CREAMY, DRY MIX	410	0.3	93.8	
19371	FROSTINGS, VANILLA, CREAMY, DRY MIX, PREP W/ MARGARINE	413	0.34	74.28	1.74
19230	FROSTINGS, VANILLA, CREAMY, RTE	419	0.1	69.4	4.89
19246	FROSTINGS, WHITE, FLUFFY, DRY MIX	371	2.3	94.9	
19247	FROSTINGS, WHITE, FLUFFY, DRY MIX, PREP W/H2O	244	1.5	62.6	0
19217	FROZEN ICE NOVELTIES, FRUIT, NO SUGAR ADDED	24	0.5	6.2	0
43450	FROZEN JUC NOVELITES, JUC W/ CRM	133	1.6	29.7	1.235
19263	FROZEN JUC NOVELTIES, FRUIT & JUC BARS	82	1.2	20.2	0
43346	FROZEN JUC NOVELTIES, ORANGE	92	0.5	23.1	0
42185	FROZEN YOGURTS, CHOC, NONFAT MILK, W/ LO CAL SWTNR	107	4.4	19.7	0.505
19393	FROZEN YOGURTS, CHOC, SOFT-SERVE	160	4	24.9	3.63
19293	FROZEN YOGURTS, VANILLA, SOFT-SERVE	159	4	24.2	3.42

NDB #	Food Description (100 gram portions = 3½ ounces = 20 tsp = ½ cup approx.	Calories	Protein	Carbs	Sat Fat
19294	FRUIT BUTTERS, APPLE	173	0.39	42.77	0
09101	FRUIT COCKTAIL, CND, EX HVY SYRUP, SOL&LIQUIDS	88	0.39	22.89	0.01
09098	FRUIT COCKTAIL, CND, EX LT SYRUP, SOL&LIQUIDS	45	0.4	11.63	0.01
09096	FRUIT COCKTAIL, CND, H2O PK, SOL&LIQUIDS	32	0.42	8.51	0.006
09100	FRUIT COCKTAIL, CND, HVY SYRUP, SOL&LIQUIDS	73	0.39	18.91	0.01
09097	FRUIT COCKTAIL, CND, JUC PK, SOL&LIQUIDS	46	0.46	11.86	0.001
09099	FRUIT COCKTAIL, CND, LT SYRUP, SOL&LIQUIDS	57	0.4	14.93	0.01
19011	FRUIT LEATHER, BARS	351	1.8	78.5	4.02
19014	FRUIT LEATHER, ROLLS	350	1	84.3	0.65
14267	FRUIT PUNCH DRINK, CANNED	47	0	11.9	0.002
14268	FRUIT PUNCH DRK, FRZ CONC	162	0.2	41.4	0.003
14269	FRUIT PUNCH DRK, FRZ CONC, PREP W/H2O	46	0	11.7	0.001
14405	FRUIT PUNCH JUC DRK, FRZ CONC	175	0.3	43.1	0.087
14406	FRUIT PUNCH JUC DRK, FRZ CONC, PREP W/H2O	50	0.1	12.2	0.025
14265	FRUIT PUNCH-FLAVOR DRK, PDR, W/ NA	382	0	97.7	0.057
14266	FRUIT PUNCH-FLAVOR DRK, PDR, W/ NA, PREP W/H2O	37	0	9.5	0.006
14540	FRUIT PUNCH-FLAVOR DRK, PDR, WO/ NA	382	0	97.7	0.057
14541	FRUIT PUNCH-FLAVOR DRK, PDR, WO/ NA, PREP W/H2O	37	0	9.5	0.006
09106	FRUIT SALAD, CND, EX HVY SYRUP, SOL&LIQUIDS	88	0.33	22.77	0.009
09102	FRUIT SALAD, CND, H2O PK, SOL&LIQUIDS	30	0.35	7.87	0.009
09105	FRUIT SALAD, CND, HVY SYRUP, SOL&LIQUIDS	73	0.34	19.11	0.01
09103	FRUIT SALAD, CND, JUC PK, SOL&LIQUIDS	50	0.51	13.05	0.004
09104	FRUIT SALAD, CND, LT SYRUP, SOL&LIQUIDS	58	0.34	15.14	0.009
09325	FRUIT SALAD, TROPICAL, CND, HVY SYRUP, SOL&LIQUIDS	86	0.41	22.36	0.019
09189	FRUIT, MXD, (PCH, CHER-SWT & SR, RASPB, GRAPE, BOYS), FRZ, S	98	1.42	24.23	0.025
09187	FRUIT, MXD, (PEACH&PEAR&PNAPPL), CND, HVY SYRUP, SOL&LIQUI	72	0.37	18.76	0.014
09188	FRUIT, MXD, (PRUNE&APRICOT&PEAR), DRIED	243	2.46	64.06	0.04
14383	FRUIT-FLAVORED THIRST QUENCHER BEV, LO CAL	11	0	3	0
11988	FUNGI, CLOUD EARS, DRIED	284	9.25	73	
17330	GAME MEAT BISON, GROUND, RAW	223	18.67	0	6.802
17332	GAME MEAT BISON, TOP SIRLOIN, LN, 1" STEAK, CKD, BRLD	171	28.05	0	2.412
17145	GAME MEAT, ANTELOPE, CKD, RSTD	150	29.45	0	0.97
17144	GAME MEAT, ANTELOPE, RAW	114	22.38	0	0.74
17147	GAME MEAT, BEAR, CKD, SIMMRD	259	32.42	0	3.54
17146	GAME MEAT, BEAR, RAW	161	20.1	0	

NDB #	Food Description (100 gram portions = 3½ ounces = 20 tsp = ½ cup approx.	Calories	Protein	Carbs	Sat Fat
17151	GAME MEAT, BEAVER, CKD, RSTD	212	34.85	0	2.07
17150	GAME MEAT, BEAVER, RAW	146	24.05	0	
17153	GAME MEAT, BEEFALO, COMP OF CUTS, CKD, RSTD	188	30.66	0	2.68
17152	GAME MEAT, BEEFALO, COMP OF CUTS, RAW	143	23.3	0	2.04
17333	GAME MEAT, BISON, CHUCK, SHLDR CLOD, LN, 3-5 LB RST, CKD, BR	193	33.78	0	2.32
17334	GAME MEAT, BISON, CHUCK, SHLDR CLOD, LN, 3-5 LB RST, RAW	119	21.12	0	1.345
17331	GAME MEAT, BISON, GROUND, CKD, PAN-BROILED	238	23.77	0	6.461
17157	GAME MEAT, BISON, LN, CKD, RSTD	143	28.44	0	0.91
17156	GAME MEAT, BISON, LN, RAW	109	21.62	0	0.69
17268	GAME MEAT, BISON, RIBEYE, LN, 0"FAT, RAW	116	22.1	0	0.898
17335	GAME MEAT, BISON, RIBEYE, LN, 1" STEAK, CKD, BRLD	177	29.45	0	2.419
17269	GAME MEAT, BISON, SHLDR CLOD, LN, 0"FAT, RAW	109	21.1	0	0.749
17266	GAME MEAT, BISON, TOP RND, LN, 0"FAT, RAW	110	22.3	0	0.61
17336	GAME MEAT, BISON, TOP RND, LN, 1" STEAK, CKD, BRLD	174	30.18	0	1.957
17337	GAME MEAT, BISON, TOP RND, LN, 1" STEAK, RAW	122	23.32	0	1.039
17267	GAME MEAT, BISON, TOP SIRLOIN, LN, 0"FAT, RAW	113	21.4	0	0.885
17159	GAME MEAT, BOAR, WILD, CKD, RSTD	160	28.3	0	1.3
17158	GAME MEAT, BOAR, WILD, RAW	122	21.51	0	0.99
17161	GAME MEAT, BUFFALO, H2O, CKD, RSTD	131	26.83	0	0.6
17160	GAME MEAT, BUFFALO, H2O, RAW	99	20.39	0	0.46
17163	GAME MEAT, CARIBOU, CKD, RSTD	167	29.77	0	1.7
17162	GAME MEAT, CARIBOU, RAW	127	22.63	0	1.29
17165	GAME MEAT, DEER, CKD, RSTD	158	30.21	0	1.25
17344	GAME MEAT, DEER, GROUND, CKD, PAN-BROILED	187	26.45	0	3.993
17343	GAME MEAT, DEER, GROUND, RAW	157	21.78	0	3.361
17345	GAME MEAT, DEER, LOIN, LN, 1" STEAK, CKD, BRLD	150	30.2	0	0.878
17164	GAME MEAT, DEER, RAW	120	22.96	0	0.95
17346	GAME MEAT, DEER, SHLDR CLOD, LN, 3-5 LB RST, CKD, BRSD	191	36.28	0	1.959
17347	GAME MEAT, DEER, TENDERLOIN, LN, 0.5-1 LB RST, CKD, BRLD	149	29.9	0	1.142
17348	GAME MEAT, DEER, TOP RND, LN, 1" STEAK, CKD, BRLD	152	31.47	0	1.03
17167	GAME MEAT, ELK, CKD, RSTD	146	30.19	0	0.7
17339	GAME MEAT, ELK, GROUND, CKD, PAN-BROILED	193	26.64	0	4.002
17338	GAME MEAT, ELK, GROUND, RAW	172	21.76	0	3.469
17340	GAME MEAT, ELK, LOIN, LN, CKD, BRLD	167	31	0	1.511
17166	GAME MEAT, ELK, RAW	111	22.95	0	0.53

NDB #	Food Description (100 gram portions = 3½ ounces = 20 tsp = ½ cup approx.	Calories	Protein	Carbs	Sat Fat
17341	GAME MEAT, ELK, RND, LN, CKD, BRLD	156	30.94	0	1.037
17342	GAME MEAT, ELK, TENDERLOIN, LN, CKD, BRLD	162	30.76	0	1.342
17169	GAME MEAT, GOAT, CKD, RSTD	143	27.1	0	0.93
17171	GAME MEAT, HORSE, CKD, RSTD	175	28.14	0	1.9
17170	GAME MEAT, HORSE, RAW	133	21.39	0	1.44
17173	GAME MEAT, MOOSE, CKD, RSTD	134	29.27	0	0.29
17172	GAME MEAT, MOOSE, RAW	102	22.24	0	0.22
17175	GAME MEAT, MUSKRAT, CKD, RSTD	234	30.09	0	
17174	GAME MEAT, MUSKRAT, RAW	162	20.76	0	
17176	GAME MEAT, OPOSSUM, CKD, RSTD	221	30.2	0	1.206
17178	GAME MEAT, RABBIT, DOMESTICATED, COMP OF CUTS, CKD, RSTD	197	29.06	0	2.4
17179	GAME MEAT, RABBIT, DOMESTICATED, COMP OF CUTS, CKD, STWD	206	30.38	0	2.51
17177	GAME MEAT, RABBIT, DOMESTICATED, COMP OF CUTS, RAW	136	20.05	0	1.66
17181	GAME MEAT, RABBIT, WILD, CKD, STWD	173	33.02	0	1.05
17180	GAME MEAT, RABBIT, WILD, RAW	114	21.79	0	0.69
17182	GAME MEAT, RACCOON, CKD, RSTD	255	29.2	0	4.07
17184	GAME MEAT, SQUIRREL, CKD, RSTD	173	30.77	0	0.85
17183	GAME MEAT, SQUIRREL, RAW	120	21.23	0	0.38
02020	GARLIC POWDER	332	16.8	72.71	0.135
11215	GARLIC, RAW	149	6.36	33.07	0.089
14131	GATORADE LEMON LIME FLAVOR MIX, PDR	364	0	95.3	
15030	GEFILTEFISH, COMM, SWT RECIPE	84	9.07	7.41	0.412
19172	GELATIN DSSRT, DRY MIX	381	7.8	90.5	0
19173	GELATIN DSSRT, DRY MIX, PREP W/ H2O	59	1.2	14	0
19175	GELATIN DSSRT, DRY MIX, RED CAL, W/ ASPRT	345	55.3	33.3	0
19703	GELATIN DSSRT, DRY MIX, RED CAL, W/ ASPRT, ADDED P, K, NA, VIT	345	55.3	33.3	0
19704	GELATIN DSSRT, DRY MIX, RED CAL, W/ ASPRT, NO ADDED NA	345	55.3	33.3	0
19176	GELATIN DSSRT, DRY MIX, RED CAL, W/ ASPRT, PREP W/ H2O	7	1.1	0.7	0
19702	GELATIN DSSRT, DRY MIX, W/ ADDED VIT C, SODIUM-CITRATE & SAL	381	7.8	90.5	0
14271	GELATIN, DRINKING, ORANGE-FLAVOR, PDR	382	35.3	60.4	0.152
14397	GELATIN, DRINKING, ORANGE-FLAVOR, PDR, PREP W/H2O	49	4.5	7.7	0.019
19177	GELATINS, DRY PDR, UNSWTND	335	85.6	0	0.07
18642	GENERAL MILLS, BETTY CROCKER SUPERMOIST YEL CAKE MIX, DRY	413	3.8	81.3	2.28
18601	GENERAL MILLS, BETTY CROCKER WILD BLUEBERRY MUFFIN MIX, D	321	5.2	64.9	1.022
18605	GENERAL MILLS, GOLD MEDAL IMITATION BLUEBERRY MUFFIN MIX,	410	4.3	78.8	1.638

NDB #	Food Description (100 gram portions = 3½ ounces = 20 tsp = ½ cup approx.	Calories	Protein	Carbs	Sat Fat
11216	GINGER ROOT, RAW	69	1.74	15.09	0.203
02021	GINGER, GROUND	347	9.12	70.79	1.94
12129	GINKGO NUTS, CANNED	111	2.29	22.1	0.309
12128	GINKGO NUTS, DRIED	348	10.35	72.45	0.381
12127	GINKGO NUTS, RAW	182	4.32	37.6	0.319
17168	GOAT, RAW	109	20.6	0	0.71
05149	GOOSE, DOMESTICATED, MEAT ONLY, CKD, RSTD	238	28.97	0	4.56
05148	GOOSE, DOMESTICATED, MEAT ONLY, RAW	161	22.75	0	2.79
05147	GOOSE, DOMESTICATED, MEAT&SKN, CKD, RSTD	305	25.16	0	6.87
05146	GOOSE, DOMESTICATED, MEAT&SKN, RAW	371	15.86	0	9.78
05150	GOOSE, LIVER, RAW	133	16.37	6.32	1.59
09109	GOOSEBERRIES, CND, LT SYRUP PK, SOL&LIQUIDS	73	0.65	18.75	0.013
09107	GOOSEBERRIES, RAW	44	0.88	10.18	0.038
11785	GOURD, DISHCLOTH (TOWELGOURD), CKD, BLD, DRND, W/SALT	56	0.66	14.34	0.027
11221	GOURD, DISHCLOTH (TOWELGOURD), CKD, BLD, DRND, WO/SALT	56	0.66	14.34	0.027
11220	GOURD, DISHCLOTH (TOWELGOURD), RAW	20	1.2	4.36	0.016
11784	GOURD, WHITE-FLOWERED (CALABASH), CKD, BLD, DRND, W/SALT	15	0.6	3.69	0.002
11219	GOURD, WHITE-FLOWERED (CALABASH), CKD, BLD, DRND, WO/SAL	15	0.6	3.69	0.002
11218	GOURD, WHITE-FLOWERED (CALABASH), RAW	14	0.62	3.39	0.002
19016	GRANOLA BARS, HARD, ALMOND	495	7.7	62	12.51
19017	GRANOLA BARS, HARD, CHOC CHIP	438	7.3	72.1	11.41
19019	GRANOLA BARS, HARD, PEANUT	479	11	63.7	2.52
19015	GRANOLA BARS, HARD, PLAIN	471	10.1	64.4	2.37
19420	GRANOLA BARS, HARD, PNUT BUTTER	483	9.8	62.3	3.2
19024	GRANOLA BARS, SOFT, COATD, MILK CHOC COATING, CHOC CHIP	466	5.8	63.8	14.22
19026	GRANOLA BARS, SOFT, COATD, MILK CHOC COATING, PNUT BUTTER	509	10.2	53.4	17.01
19404	GRANOLA BARS, SOFT, UNCOATED, CHOC CHIP	420	7.3	69.1	10.18
19405	GRANOLA BARS, SOFT, UNCOATED, CHOC CHIP, GRAHAM&MARSHM	427	6.1	70.8	9.18
19406	GRANOLA BARS, SOFT, UNCOATED, NUT&RAISIN	454	8	63.6	9.54
19020	GRANOLA BARS, SOFT, UNCOATED, PLN	443	7.4	67.3	7.24
19021	GRANOLA BARS, SOFT, UNCOATED, PNUT BUTTER	426	10.5	64.4	3.65
19027	GRANOLA BARS, SOFT, UNCOATED, PNUT BUTTER&CHOC CHIP	432	9.8	62.2	5.59
19022	GRANOLA BARS, SOFT, UNCOATED, RAISIN	448	7.6	66.4	9.57
14277	GRAPE DRINK, CANNED	45	0	11.5	0.003
09135	GRAPE JUC, CND OR BTLD, UNSWTND, WO/ VIT C	61	0.56	14.96	0.025

NDB #	Food Description (100 gram portions = 3½ ounces = 20 tsp = ½ cup approx.	Calories	Protein	Carbs	Sat Fat
09137	GRAPE JUC, FRZ CONC, SWTND, DIL W/3 VOLUME H2O, W/ VIT C	51	0.19	12.75	0.029
09136	GRAPE JUC, FRZ CONC, SWTND, UNDIL, W/ VIT C	179	0.65	44.37	0.103
14282	GRAPE JUICE DRINK, CANNED	50	0.1	12.9	0
11975	GRAPE LEAVES, CND	69	4.27	11.7	0.312
11974	GRAPE LEAVES, RAW	93	5.6	17.3	0.336
09124	GRAPEFRUIT JUC, CND, SWTND	46	0.58	11.13	0.012
09123	GRAPEFRUIT JUC, CND, UNSWTND	38	0.52	8.96	0.013
09126	GRAPEFRUIT JUC, FRZ CONC, UNSWTND, DIL W/3 VOLUME H2O	41	0.55	9.73	0.019
09125	GRAPEFRUIT JUC, FRZ CONC, UNSWTND, UNDIL	146	1.97	34.56	0.064
09128	GRAPEFRUIT JUC, WHITE, RAW	39	0.5	9.2	0.014
09404	GRAPEFRUIT JUICE, PINK, RAW	39	0.5	9.2	0.014
09111	GRAPEFRUIT, RAW, PINK&RED&WHITE, ALL AREAS	32	0.63	8.08	0.014
09112	GRAPEFRUIT, RAW, PINK&RED, ALL AREAS	30	0.55	7.68	0.014
09113	GRAPEFRUIT, RAW, PINK&RED, CALIFORNIA&ARIZONA	37	0.5	9.69	0.014
09114	GRAPEFRUIT, RAW, PINK&RED, FLORIDA	30	0.55	7.5	0.014
09116	GRAPEFRUIT, RAW, WHITE, ALL AREAS	33	0.69	8.41	0.014
09117	GRAPEFRUIT, RAW, WHITE, CALIFORNIA	37	0.88	9.09	0.014
09118	GRAPEFRUIT, RAW, WHITE, FLORIDA	32	0.63	8.19	0.014
09119	GRAPEFRUIT, SECTIONS, CND, H2O PK, SOL&LIQUIDS	36	0.58	9.15	0.014
09120	GRAPEFRUIT, SECTIONS, CND, JUC PK, SOL&LIQUIDS	37	0.7	9.21	0.012
09121	GRAPEFRUIT, SECTIONS, CND, LT SYRUP PK, SOL&LIQUIDS	60	0.56	15.44	0.014
09131	GRAPES, AMERICAN TYPE (SLIP SKN), RAW	67	0.63	17.15	0.114
09133	GRAPES, CND, THOMPSON SEEDLESS, H2O PK, SOL&LIQUIDS	40	0.5	10.3	0.035
09134	GRAPES, CND, THOMPSON SEEDLESS, HVY SYRUP PK, SOL&LIQUID	73	0.48	19.65	0.033
09132	GRAPES, RED OR GRN(EURO TYPE VAR, SUCH AS, THOMPSON SDLE	71	0.66	17.77	0.189
06114	GRAVY, AU JUS, CANNED	16	1.2	2.5	0.1
06115	GRAVY, AU JUS, DRY	313	9.2	47.49	2.026
06116	GRAVY, BEEF, CANNED	53	3.75	4.81	1.153
06118	GRAVY, BROWN, DRY	367	10.74	59.38	3.319
06119	GRAVY, CHICKEN, CANNED	79	1.93	5.42	1.41
06120	GRAVY, CHICKEN, DRY	381	11.27	62.09	2.92
06565	GRAVY, CUSTOM FOODS, RED LABEL AU JUS BASE, DRY	191	15.68	22.98	2.268
06564	GRAVY, CUSTOM FOODS, SUPERB COUNTRY GRAVY MIX, DRY	481	8.1	53.58	10.427
06567	GRAVY, CUSTOM FOODS, SUPERB INST AU JUS MIX, DRY	296	21.15	39.44	2.766
06570	GRAVY, CUSTOM FOODS, SUPERB INST BF GRAVY MIX, DRY	369	9.8	61.1	4.88

NDB #	Food Description (100 gram portions = 3½ ounces = 20 tsp = ½ cup approx.	Calories	Protein	Carbs	Sat Fat
06562	GRAVY, CUSTOM FOODS, SUPERB INST BROWN GRAVY MIX, DRY	380	8.53	59.78	5.866
06573	GRAVY, CUSTOM FOODS, SUPERB INST CHICK GRAVY MIX, DRY	395	10.2	56.54	4.511
06569	GRAVY, CUSTOM FOODS, SUPERB INST PORK GRAVY MIX, DRY	363	8.33	64.72	3.919
06576	GRAVY, CUSTOM FOODS, SUPERB INST TURKEY GRAVY MIX, DRY	409	11.72	57.56	4.931
06571	GRAVY, CUSTOM FOODS, SUPERB OLD-FASH BISCUIT MIX, DRY	495	6.56	54.23	8.377
06568	GRAVY, CUSTOM FOODS, SUPERB PEPPERED OLD-FASH BISCUIT MI	500	6.57	51.87	8.689
06579	GRAVY, HEINZ, HEINZ HOME STYLE SAVORY BROWN GRAVY, CND	41	1.5	5.69	0.54
06121	GRAVY, MUSHROOM, CANNED	50	1.26	5.47	0.4
06122	GRAVY, MUSHROOM, DEHYD, DRY	328	10	64.66	2.36
06800	GRAVY, NESTLE, CHEF-MATE COUNTRY SAUSAGE GRAVY, RTS	155	4.6	6.28	3.22
06566	GRAVY, NESTLE, TRIO AU JUS GRAVY MIX, DRY	280	0.91	57.83	1.78
06561	GRAVY, NESTLE, TRIO BROWN GRAVY MIX, DRY	406	10.42	57.86	4.29
06574	GRAVY, NESTLE, TRIO CHICK GRAVY MIX, DRY	405	11.4	63.22	4.07
06572	GRAVY, NESTLE, TRIO COUNTRY GRAVY MIX, DRY	433	9.08	64.87	3.99
06563	GRAVY, NESTLE, TRIO SOUTHERN GRAVY MIX, DRY	481	2.46	60.51	5.61
06577	GRAVY, NESTLE, TRIO TURKEY GRAVY MIX, DRY	362	8.57	72.05	0.99
06123	GRAVY, ONION, DEHYD, DRY	322	9	67.64	1.86
06746	GRAVY, PEPPERIDGE FARM HEARTY BF GRAVY, GLASS JAR	43	3	6.2	0.238
06124	GRAVY, PORK, DRY	367	8.78	63.57	4.29
06125	GRAVY, TURKEY, CANNED	51	2.6	5.1	0.62
06126	GRAVY, TURKEY, DRY	367	10.42	65.12	1.975
06127	GRAVY, UNSPEC TYPE, DRY	344	13	58	2.86
22600	GREEN GIANT, BROCCOLI IN CHS FLAV SAU, FRZ	67	2.3	8.9	0.48
22125	GREEN GIANT, HARVEST BURGER, ORIG FLAV, ALL VEG PROT PATTY	153	20	7.8	1.13
09138	GROUNDCHERRIES, (CAPE-GOOSEBERRIES OR POHA), RAW	53	1.9	11.2	
15031	GROUPER, MIXED SPECIES, RAW	92	19.38	0	0.233
15032	GROUPER, MXD SP, CKD, DRY HEAT	118	24.84	0	0.299
09143	GUAVA SAUCE, COOKED	36	0.32	9.48	0.04
09139	GUAVAS, COMMON, RAW	51	0.82	11.88	0.172
09140	GUAVAS, STRAWBERRY, RAW	69	0.58	17.36	0.172
05152	GUINEA HEN, MEAT ONLY, RAW	110	20.64	0	0.64
05151	GUINEA HEN, MEAT&SKN, RAW	158	23.4	0	1.77
15034	HADDOCK, COOKED, DRY HEAT	112	24.24	0	0.167
15033	HADDOCK, RAW	87	18.91	0	0.13
15035	HADDOCK, SMOKED	116	25.23	0	0.173

NDB #	Food Description (100 gram portions = 3½ ounces = 20 tsp = ½ cup approx.	Calories	Protein	Carbs	Sat Fat
15037	HALIBUT, ATLANTIC&PACIFIC, CKD, DRY HEAT	140	26.69	0	0.417
15036	HALIBUT, ATLANTIC&PACIFIC, RAW	110	20.81	0	0.325
15196	HALIBUT, GREENLAND, CKD, DRY HEAT	239	18.42	0	3.102
15038	HALIBUT, GREENLAND, RAW	186	14.37	0	2.419
07938	HAM HONEY SMOKED CKD	122	17.93	7.27	0.795
07033	HAM AND CHEESE SPREAD	245	16.18	2.28	8.62
07031	HAM SALAD SPREAD	216	8.68	10.65	5.06
07032	HAM&CHS LOAF OR ROLL	259	16.62	1.43	7.51
07026	HAM, CHOPPED, CANNED	239	16.06	0.28	6.28
07027	HAM, CHOPPED, NOT CANNED	229	17.12	0	5.73
07030	HAM, MINCED	263	16.28	1.85	7.18
07028	HAM, SLICED, EX LN, (APPROX 5% FAT)	131	19.35	0.97	1.62
07029	HAM, SLICED, REG (APPROX 11% FAT)	182	17.56	3.11	3.39
22601	HANOVER, STIR FRY 2, WHITE RICE&VEG W/ORIENTAL SOY SAU, FRZ	95	3.3	19.7	
12120	HAZELNUTS OR FILBERTS	628	14.95	16.7	4.464
12121	HAZELNUTS OR FILBERTS, BLANCHED	629	13.7	17	4.669
12122	HAZELNUTS OR FILBERTS, DRY RSTD, WO/SALT	646	15.03	17.6	4.511
07034	HEADCHEESE, PORK	212	16	0.3	4.94
22402	HEALTHY CHOIC BF MACARONI, FRZ ENTREE	88	5.89	13.94	0.28
22606	HEALTHY CHOIC CACCIATORE CHICK, PSTA&VEG&CACC SAU, FRZ E	75	6.21	10.13	0.28
22619	HEALTHY CHOIC CNTRY RST TURKY, MSHRM&BRN GRVY, RICE PILA	93	7.91	11.6	0.52
22707	HEALTHY CHOIC MESQ BF, BARBQ SAU, MSH POT, SWTND CORN, F	103	6.88	12.31	0.94
22708	HEALTHY CHOIC SALSBRY STK, MSHRM GRVY, MSH POT, SWT CORN	100	5.53	14.73	0.92
22401	HEALTHY CHOIC SPAGHETTI BOLOGNESE, FRZ ENTREE	90	5.05	15.24	0.35
22709	HEALTHY CHOIC TRADL MT LF, TOM SAU, PARS POT, VEG, DSRT, FR	93	4.51	15.4	0.74
22604	HEALTHY CHOIC, CHEDDAR BROCCOLI POTATOES W/CHS SAU, FRZ	110	4.36	17.8	1
22588	HEALTHY CHOICE CHICK ENCHLDA SUPR, RICE, CORN, AP/RASP CO	93	4.06	14.37	0.97
22587	HEALTHY CHOICE CHICK TERIYAKI, RICE, MXD VEG, AP/CHER COMP,	86	5.47	11.89	0.96
22713	HEALTHY CHOICE MESQ CHICK BBQ, WH RI, MXD VEG, AP/RAISN CO	104	6.06	16.15	0.67
11961	HEARTS OF PALM, CANNED	28	2.52	4.62	0.13
18640	HEINZ, WEIGHT WATCHERS CHOC ECLAIRS, FRZ	238	4	39.8	1.26
15040	HERRING, ATLANTIC, CKD, DRY HEAT	203	23.03	0	2.615
15042	HERRING, ATLANTIC, KIPPERED	217	24.58	0	2.791
15041	HERRING, ATLANTIC, PICKLED	262	14.19	9.64	2.381
15039	HERRING, ATLANTIC, RAW	158	17.96	0	2.04

NDB #	Food Description (100 gram portions = 3½ ounces = 20 tsp = ½ cup approx.	Calories	Protein	Carbs	Sat Fat
15197	HERRING, PACIFIC, CKD, DRY HEAT	250	21.01	0	4.174
15043	HERRING, PACIFIC, RAW	195	16.39	0	3.257
12130	HICKORYNUTS, DRIED	657	12.72	18.25	7.038
18636	HIDDEN VALLEY RANCH, SALAD CRISPINS ITAL STYLE, PARMES CRO	434	11.9	67.8	1.433
22701	HODGSON MILL, WHL WHEAT MACARONI&CHS DINNER, DRY MIX	376	14.1	69.2	1.37
20030	HOMINY, CANNED, WHITE	72	1.48	14.26	0.123
20330	HOMINY, CANNED, YELLOW	72	1.48	14.26	0.123
07035	HONEY LOAF PORK BF	125	15.77	5.33	1.43
07088	HONEY ROLL SAUSAGE, BEEF	182	18.58	2.18	4.08
19296	HONEY, STR OR EXTRACTED	304	0.3	82.4	0
10856	HORMEL ALWAYS TENDER, BNLESS PORK LOIN, FRSH PORK	145	19.02	0.76	2.84
10855	HORMEL ALWAYS TENDER, CNTR CUT CHOPS, FRSH PORK	167	18.74	0.84	3.6
10854	HORMEL ALWAYS TENDER, PORK LOIN FILETS, LEMON GARLIC-FLA	118	17.83	1.79	1.41
10853	HORMEL ALWAYS TENDER, PORK TENDERLOIN, PEPPERCORN-FLA	110	17.21	1.82	1.16
10852	HORMEL ALWAYS TENDER, PORK TENDERLOIN, TERIYAKI-FLAVORE	119	18.2	4.63	1.05
10857	HORMEL CANADIAN STYLE BACON	122	16.88	1.87	1.83
22719	HORMEL CHILI W/BNS, CND ENTREE	97	6.71	13.63	0.74
22705	HORMEL CHILI, NO BNS, CND ENTREE	82	7.2	7.59	0.93
22698	HORMEL CORNED BF HASH, CND ENTREE	164	8.73	9.27	4.32
07278	HORMEL PILLOW PAK SLICED TURKEY PEPPERONI	243	30.99	3.78	3.7
22721	HORMEL RST BF HASH, CND ENTREE	163	9.03	9.71	4.2
07276	HORMEL SPAM LUNCHEON MEAT PORK W/ HAM MINCED CND	310	13.24	3.03	9.88
07277	HORMEL SPAM, LT LUNCH MT, PORK & CHICK, MINCED, CND, VIT C A	191	15.23	1.35	4.49
22706	HORMEL TURKEY CHILI W/BNS, CND ENTREE	82	7.58	10.35	0.27
22720	HORMEL VEGETARIAN CHILI W/BNS, CND ENTREE	83	4.83	15.39	0.05
07279	HORMEL WRANGLER BEEF FRANKS	290	12.58	2.11	10.62
10851	HORMEL, CURE 81 HAM	106	18.43	0.21	1.17
22694	HORMEL, DINTY MOORE BF STEW, CND ENTREE	94	4.79	6.81	2.39
02055	HORSERADISH, PREPARED	48	1.18	11.29	0.09
11222	HORSERADISH-TREE LEAFY TIPS, RAW	64	9.4	8.28	
11786	HORSERADISH-TREE, LEAFY TIPS, CKD, BLD, DRND, W/SALT	60	5.27	11.15	
11223	HORSERADISH-TREE, LEAFY TIPS, CKD, BLD, DRND, WO/SALT	60	5.27	11.15	0.152
11787	HORSERADISH-TREE, PODS, CKD, BLD, DRND, W/SALT	36	2.09	8.18	
11621	HORSERADISH-TREE, PODS, CKD, BLD, DRND, WO/SALT	36	2.09	8.18	0.031
11620	HORSERADISH-TREE, PODS, RAW	37	2.1	8.53	0.033

NDB #	Food Description (100 gram portions = 3½ ounces = 20 tsp = ½ cup approx.	Calories	Protein	Carbs	Sat Fat
22537	HOT POCKETS HAM 'N CHS STUFFED SNDWCH, FRZ	266	11.6	30	4.52
22536	HOT POCKETS PEPPERONI PIZZA STUFFED SNDWCH, FRZ	287	10.6	30.2	5.18
22534	HOT POCKETS, BF&CHEDDAR STUFFED SNDWCH, FRZ	284	11.5	27.6	6.2
22535	HOT POCKETS, CROISSANT POCKTS CHIK, BROC&CHDR STUFD SND	235	8.9	30.4	2.62
18607	HOWARD JOHNSON'S TOASTEES, BLUEBERRY TOASTER MUFFNS, F	331	7.1	45.1	2.16
16158	HUMMUS, COMMERCIAL	166	7.9	14.29	1.437
16137	HUMMUS, HOME-PREPARED	171	4.9	20.17	1.265
18270	HUSH PUPPIES, PREP FROM RECIPE	337	7.7	46	2.108
16368	HYACINTH BNS, MATURE SEEDS, CKD, BLD, W/SALT	117	8.14	20.7	0.099
16068	HYACINTH BNS, MATURE SEEDS, CKD, BLD, WO/SALT	117	8.14	20.7	0.099
16067	HYACINTH BNS, MATURE SEEDS, RAW	344	23.9	60.76	0.288
11788	HYACINTH-BEANS, IMMAT SEEDS, CKD, BLD, DRND, W/SALT	50	2.95	9.2	0.119
11225	HYACINTH-BEANS, IMMAT SEEDS, CKD, BLD, DRND, WO/SALT	50	2.95	9.2	0.119
11224	HYACINTH-BEANS, IMMAT SEEDS, RAW	46	2.1	9.19	0.088
19270	ICE CREAMS, CHOC	216	3.8	28.2	6.8
19114	ICE CREAMS, CHOC, LT	157	4.39	31	1.4
43541	ICE CREAMS, CHOC, RICH	236	2.8	21.6	9.891
19090	ICE CREAMS, FRENCH VANILLA, SOFT-SERVE	215	4.1	22.2	7.48
19259	ICE CREAMS, HEALTHY CHOIC PRALINE & CARAMEL	181	3.79	35.21	0.7
19271	ICE CREAMS, STRAWBERRY	192	3.2	27.6	5.19
19095	ICE CREAMS, VANILLA	201	3.5	23.6	6.79
19088	ICE CREAMS, VANILLA, LT	139	3.8	22.7	2.63
19260	ICE CREAMS, VANILLA, LT, NO SUGAR ADDED	152	4.5	18.9	3.68
19096	ICE CREAMS, VANILLA, LT, SOFT-SERVE	126	4.9	21.8	1.63
19089	ICE CREAMS, VANILLA, RICH	242	3.5	22.62	9.97
18271	ICE CRM CONES, CAKE OR WAFER-TYPE	417	8.1	79	1.222
18272	ICE CRM CONES, SUGAR, ROLLED-TYPE	402	7.9	84.1	0.573
19262	ICE CRM NOVELTIES, KLONDIKE BAR VNLA ICE CRM, W/ CHOC COAT	330	4.2	24.1	13.1
42074	ICE CRM NOVELTIES, VANILLA, LT, NO SUGAR ADDED, CHOCOLATE-	214	6.4	25.8	5.528
19264	ICE CRM NOVLTS, ESKIMO PIE BAR, VNLA ICE CRM, W/ DK CHOC COA	331	4.1	24.5	14.5
19281	ICE NOVELTIES, ITALIAN, REST-PREP	53	0.03	13.5	0
19280	ICE NOVELTIES, LIME	128	0.4	32.6	0
19387	ICE NOVELTIES, PINEAPPLE-COCONUT	113	0	23.9	2.304
19283	ICE NOVELTIES, POP	72	0	18.9	0
19717	ICE NOVELTIES, POP, W/ ADDED VIT C	72	0	18.9	0

NDB #	Food Description (100 gram portions = 3½ ounces = 20 tsp = ½ cup approx.	Calories	Protein	Carbs	Sat Fat
03926	INF FORMULA, CARNATION, ALSOY, W/ IRON, LIQ CONC, NOT RECON	132	4	13.2	1.03
03928	INF FORMULA, CARNATION, ALSOY, W/ IRON, PDR, NOT RECON	520	15.5	51.2	4.05
03925	INF FORMULA, CARNATION, ALSOY, W/ IRON, RTF	67	2	6.6	0.51
03865	INFANT FORM, MEAD JOHNSON, GERBER SOY, W/IRON, LIQ CNC, NO	131	3.94	13.13	2.967
03871	INFANT FORM, MEAD JOHNSON, LACTOFREE, W/IRON, LIQ CONC, N	131	2.89	13.65	3.098
03816	INFANT FORM, MEAD JOHNSON, NUTRAMIGEN, W/IRON, LIQ CNC, NO	131	3.68	14.44	2.809
03901	INFANT FORMULA, CARNATION FOLLOW-UP, W/IRON, LIQ CONC, NOT	131	3.4	17.3	2.28
03913	INFANT FORMULA, CARNATION FOLLOW-UP, W/IRON, PDR, NOT REC	471	12.2	62.2	8.54
03900	INFANT FORMULA, CARNATION FOLLOW-UP, W/IRON, RTF	65	1.7	8.6	1.18
03801	INFANT FORMULA, CARNATION GOOD START, W/IRON, LIQ CONC, N	127	3.1	14.1	2.82
03802	INFANT FORMULA, CARNATION GOOD START, W/IRON, PDR, NOT RE	512	12.5	56	11.66
03800	INFANT FORMULA, CARNATION GOOD START, W/IRON, RTF	66	1.6	7.3	1.47
03807	INFANT FORMULA, MEAD JOHNSON, ENFAMIL, LO IRON, LIQ CNC, NO	131	2.76	14.31	2.967
03809	INFANT FORMULA, MEAD JOHNSON, ENFAMIL, LO IRON, PDR, NOT R	530	11.1	56	11.97
03806	INFANT FORMULA, MEAD JOHNSON, ENFAMIL, LO IRON, RTF	66	1.38	7.15	1.483
03804	INFANT FORMULA, MEAD JOHNSON, ENFAMIL, W/IRON, LIQ CONC, N	131	2.76	14.31	2.967
03805	INFANT FORMULA, MEAD JOHNSON, ENFAMIL, W/IRON, PDR, NOT RE	530	11.1	56	11.97
03803	INFANT FORMULA, MEAD JOHNSON, ENFAMIL, W/IRON, RTF	66	1.38	7.15	1.483
03863	INFANT FORMULA, MEAD JOHNSON, GERBER SOY, W/IRON, PDR, NO	515	15.5	52	11.45
03862	INFANT FORMULA, MEAD JOHNSON, GERBER SOY, W/IRON, RTF	66	1.97	6.56	1.483
03834	INFANT FORMULA, MEAD JOHNSON, GERBER, LO IRON, LIQ CONC, N	131	2.76	14.31	2.967
03835	INFANT FORMULA, MEAD JOHNSON, GERBER, LO IRON, PDR, NOT R	520	10.9	57	11.97
03833	INFANT FORMULA, MEAD JOHNSON, GERBER, LO IRON, RTF	66	1.38	7.15	1.483
03829	INFANT FORMULA, MEAD JOHNSON, GERBER, W/IRON, LIQ CONC, N	131	2.76	14.31	2.967
03831	INFANT FORMULA, MEAD JOHNSON, GERBER, W/IRON, PDR, NOT RE	520	10.9	57	11.97
03828	INFANT FORMULA, MEAD JOHNSON, GERBER, W/IRON, RTF	66	1.38	7.15	1.483
03869	INFANT FORMULA, MEAD JOHNSON, LACTOFREE, W/IRON, PDR, NOT	530	11.6	55	12.38
03868	INFANT FORMULA, MEAD JOHNSON, LACTOFREE, W/IRON, RTF	66	1.44	6.85	1.549
03810	INFANT FORMULA, MEAD JOHNSON, LOFENALAC, W/IRON, PDR, NOT	462	15	60	2.36
03811	INFANT FORMULA, MEAD JOHNSON, LOFENALAC, W/IRON, PREP FR	65	2.14	8.45	0.332
03814	INFANT FORMULA, MEAD JOHNSON, NUTRAMIGEN, W/IRON, PDR, NO	500	13.9	54	10.64
03813	INFANT FORMULA, MEAD JOHNSON, NUTRAMIGEN, W/IRON, RTF	66	1.84	7.22	1.405
03819	INFANT FORMULA, MEAD JOHNSON, PORTAGEN, W/IRON, PDR, NOT	470	16.5	54	20.21
03820	INFANT FORMULA, MEAD JOHNSON, PORTAGEN, W/IRON, PREP FRO	64	2.25	7.4	2.73
03821	INFANT FORMULA, MEAD JOHNSON, PREGESTIMIL, W/IRON, PDR, NO	500	14.1	51	17.08

NDB #	Food Description (100 gram portions = 3½ ounces = 20 tsp = ½ cup approx.	Calories	Protein	Carbs	Sat Fat
03822	INFANT FORMULA, MEAD JOHNSON, PREGESTIMIL, W/IRON, PREP FR	65	1.82	6.7	2.184
03824	INFANT FORMULA, MEAD JOHNSON, PROSOBEE, W/IRON, LIQ CNC,	131	3.94	13.13	2.967
03826	INFANT FORMULA, MEAD JOHNSON, PROSOBEE, W/IRON, PDR, NOT	515	15.5	52	11.45
03823	INFANT FORMULA, MEAD JOHNSON, PROSOBEE, W/IRON, RTF	66	1.97	6.56	1.483
03846	INFANT FORMULA, ROSS, ALIMENTUM, RTF	65	1.8	6.68	1.838
03848	INFANT FORMULA, ROSS, ISOMIL SF, W/IRON, LIQ CONC, NOT RECON	127	3.39	12.86	2.881
03847	INFANT FORMULA, ROSS, ISOMIL SF, W/IRON, RTF	66	1.8	6.6	1.26
03842	INFANT FORMULA, ROSS, ISOMIL, W/IRON, LIQ CONC, NOT RECON	127	3.12	13.12	2.262
03843	INFANT FORMULA, ROSS, ISOMIL, W/IRON, PDR, NOT RECON	516	12.64	53.15	9.167
03841	INFANT FORMULA, ROSS, ISOMIL, W/IRON, RTF	66	1.61	6.76	1.166
03839	INFANT FORMULA, ROSS, SIMILAC NAT CARE, LO IRON, RTF	78	2.1	8.22	2.544
03837	INFANT FORMULA, ROSS, SIMILAC PM 60/40, LO IRON, PDR, NOT REC	536	11.91	54.72	12.214
03836	INFANT FORMULA, ROSS, SIMILAC PM 60/40, LO IRON, RTF	66	1.5	6.7	1.61
03840	INFANT FORMULA, ROSS, SIMILAC SPL CARE 24, W/IRON, RTF	78	2.1	8.22	2.533
03876	INFANT FORMULA, ROSS, SIMILAC TODDLERS BEST, RTF	65	2.28	7.18	1.026
03856	INFANT FORMULA, ROSS, SIMILAC, LO IRON, LIQ CONC, NOT RECON	127	2.64	13.76	2.401
03858	INFANT FORMULA, ROSS, SIMILAC, LO IRON, PDR, NOT RECON	524	10.84	55.32	9.873
03855	INFANT FORMULA, ROSS, SIMILAC, LO IRON, RTF	66	1.36	7.09	1.237
03851	INFANT FORMULA, ROSS, SIMILAC, W/IRON, LIQ CONC, NOT RECON	127	2.64	13.76	2.401
03853	INFANT FORMULA, ROSS, SIMILAC, W/IRON, PDR, NOT RECON	524	10.84	55.32	9.873
03850	INFANT FORMULA, ROSS, SIMILAC, W/IRON, RTF	66	1.36	7.09	1.237
18606	INTERST BRNDS CRP, HOSTESS DING DONGS CHOC SNACK CKE, C	460	3.9	56.7	13.795
18641	INTERSTATE BRANDS CORP, WONDER HAMBURGER ROLLS	273	8.07	50.84	1.013
09420	JACKFRUIT, CND, SYRUP PK	92	0.36	23.94	
09144	JACKFRUIT, RAW	94	1.47	24.01	0.063
22543	JACK'S GREAT COMBINATIONS SAUSAGE&PEPPERONI PIZZA, FRZ	254	12.7	22	4.82
22544	JACK'S ORIGINAL PEPPERONI PIZZA, FRZ	265	12.3	24.2	5.1
19297	JAMS AND PRESERVES	278	0.37	68.86	0.01
19719	JAMS&PRESERVES, APRICOT	242	0.7	64.4	0.01
09145	JAVA-PLUM, (JAMBOLAN), RAW	60	0.72	15.56	
19300	JELLIES	283	0.2	70.47	0.018
22545	JENO'S CRISP 'N TASTY COMBINATION PIZZA, SAUSGE&PEPPERONI,	248	8.5	26.1	2.88
22546	JENO'S CRISP 'N TASTY PEPPERONI PIZZA, FRZ	269	9.7	23.9	3.37
11226	JERUSALEM-ARTICHOKES, RAW	76	2	17.44	0
11230	JEW'S EAR, (PEPEAO), DRIED	298	4.82	81.04	

NDB #	Food Description (100 gram portions = 3½ ounces = 20 tsp = ½ cup approx.	Calories	Protein	Carbs	Sat Fat
11228	JEW'S EAR, (PEPEAO), RAW	25	0.48	6.75	
22364	JIMMY DEAN, SAUSAGE BISCUITS, BRKFST SNDWCH, FRZ	401	9.9	24.1	8.97
09147	JUJUBE, DRIED	287	3.7	73.6	
09146	JUJUBE, RAW	79	1.2	20.23	
11789	JUTE, POTHERB, CKD, BLD, DRND, W/SALT	37	3.68	7.3	0.03
11232	JUTE, POTHERB, CKD, BLD, DRND, WO/SALT	37	3.68	7.3	0.03
11231	JUTE, POTHERB, RAW	34	4.65	5.8	0.038
11790	KALE, CKD, BLD, DRND, W/SALT	28	1.9	5.63	0.052
11234	KALE, CKD, BLD, DRND, WO/SALT	28	1.9	5.63	0.052
11235	KALE, FROZEN, UNPREPARED	28	2.66	4.9	0.059
11791	KALE, FRZ, CKD, BLD, DRND, W/SALT	30	2.84	5.24	0.063
11236	KALE, FRZ, CKD, BLD, DRND, WO/SALT	30	2.84	5.24	0.063
11233	KALE, RAW	50	3.3	10.01	0.091
11792	KALE, SCOTCH, CKD, BLD, DRND, W/SALT	28	1.9	5.63	0.053
11623	KALE, SCOTCH, CKD, BLD, DRND, WO/SALT	28	1.9	5.63	0.053
11622	KALE, SCOTCH, RAW	42	2.8	8.32	0.078
11237	KANPYO, (DRIED GOURD STRIPS)	258	8.58	65.04	0.045
18608	KEEBLER, KEEBLER CHOC GRAHAM SELECTS	465	7.1	71.8	3.09
18609	KEEBLER, KEEBLER GOLDEN VANILLA WAFERS, ARTIFICIALLY FLAV	475	5.2	69.7	3.58
18500	KELLOGG, KELLOGG'S EGGO, BANANA BREAD WAFFLES	272	6.8	41.6	1.71
18499	KELLOGG, KELLOGG'S EGGO, BTTRMLK PANCAKE	233	6	38.1	1.44
18492	KELLOGG, KELLOGG'S LOFAT POP TARTS, BLUEBERRY	369	4.5	76.5	1.2
18493	KELLOGG, KELLOGG'S LOFAT POP TARTS, CHERRY	369	4.5	76.5	1.2
18491	KELLOGG, KELLOGG'S LOFAT POP TARTS, FRSTD APPL CINN	368	4.2	76.9	1.1
18494	KELLOGG, KELLOGG'S LOFAT POP TARTS, FRSTD BROWN SUGAR CI	376	4.7	78.3	1.2
18495	KELLOGG, KELLOGG'S LOFAT POP TARTS, FRSTD CHOC FUDGE	366	5.1	76	1
18497	KELLOGG, KELLOGG'S LOFAT POP TARTS, FRSTD STRAWBERRY	367	4.1	77.5	1.1
18496	KELLOGG, KELLOGG'S LOFAT POP TARTS, STRAWBERRY	369	4.5	76.6	1.2
18501	KELLOGG, KELLOGG'S NUTRI-GRAIN CRL BARS, MXD BERRY	370	4.3	72.8	1.5
18498	KELLOGG, KELLOGG'S POP TARTS, FRSTD WILD WATERMELON	388	4.3	72.9	2.6
18512	KELLOGG'S EGGO GOLDEN OAT WAFFLES	198	6.83	37.52	0.6
18507	KELLOGG'S EGGO LOWFAT BLUEBERRY NUTRI - GRAIN WAFFLES	208	5.95	42.71	0.41
18505	KELLOGG'S EGGO LOWFAT HOMESTYLE WAFFLES	236	7.06	44.15	0.9
18506	KELLOGG'S EGGO LOWFAT NUTRI - GRAIN WAFFLES	203	6.28	40.27	0.47
18508	KELLOGG'S POP-TARTS PASTRY SWIRLS, APPL CINN DANISH	413	4.8	59.7	4.8

NDB #	Food Description (100 gram portions = 3½ ounces = 20 tsp = ½ cup approx.	Calories	Protein	Carbs	Sat Fat
18510	KELLOGG'S POP-TARTS PASTRY SWIRLS, CHS DANISH	407	4.8	59.1	4.8
18509	KELLOGG'S POP-TARTS PASTRY SWIRLS, STRAWBERRY DANISH	410	4.8	60	4.8
22690	KID CUISINE COSMIC CHICK NUGTS, MAC&CHS, CORN, CHOC PUDD,	204	6.9	20.6	2.57
07037	KIELBASA, KOLBASSY, PORK, BF, NONFAT DRY MILK	310	13.26	2.14	9.91
07934	KIELBASA, POLISH, TURKEY & BF, SMOKED	226	13.1	3.9	6.23
09148	KIWI FRUIT, (CHINESE GOOSEBERRIES), FRSH, RAW	61	0.99	14.88	0.029
09405	KIWIFRUIT, (CHINESE GOOSEBERRIES), HELD IN STORAGE, RAW	61	0.99	14.88	
07038	KNACKWURST KNOCKWURST PORK BF	307	11.1	3.2	10.21
11793	KOHLRABI, CKD, BLD, DRND, W/SALT	29	1.8	6.69	0.014
11242	KOHLRABI, CKD, BLD, DRND, WO/SALT	29	1.8	6.69	0.014
11241	KOHLRABI, RAW	27	1.7	6.2	0.013
01194	KRAFT BREAKSTONE'S FREE FAT FREE SOUR CRM	91	4.7	15.1	0.8
01193	KRAFT BREAKSTONE'S RED FAT SOUR CRM	152	4.5	6.5	7.6
01195	KRAFT BREYERS LOWFAT STRAWBERRY YOGURT (1% MILKFAT)	96	3.8	18.2	0.5
01196	KRAFT BREYERS LT N' LVLY LOWFAT STR'BERY YOGURT (1% MILKF	108	3.2	21.9	0.5
01198	KRAFT BREYERS LT NONFAT STR'BERY YOGURT (W/ASPRT&FRUCT	55	3.4	9.9	0.1
01197	KRAFT BREYERS SMOTH&CRMY LOWFAT STR'BERY YOGURT (1% MI	102	3.8	19.9	0.5
01189	KRAFT CHEEZ WHIZ LT PAST PROCESS CHS PRODUCT	215	16.3	16.2	6.4
01188	KRAFT CHEEZ WHIZ PAST PROCESS CHS SAU	276	12	9.2	13.1
18637	KRAFT FOODS, SHAKE 'N' BAKE ORIG RECIPE, COATING FOR PORK,	377	6.1	79.8	
01190	KRAFT FREE SINGLES AMERICAN NONFAT PAST PROCESS CHS PRO	148	22.7	11.7	0.7
22005	KRAFT MACARONI & CHEESE DINNER ORIGINAL FLAVOR, UNPREP	370	16.2	67.9	1.8
01192	KRAFT VELVEETA LT RED FAT PAST PROCESS CHS PRODUCT	222	19.6	11.8	7.1
01191	KRAFT VELVEETA PAST PROCESS CHS SPRD	303	16.3	9.8	14.4
14272	KRAFT, CAPRI SUN ALL NAT JUC DRK FRUIT PUNCH, RTD	47	0	12.5	0
14273	KRAFT, CRYSTAL LT SG FR LO CAL SOFT DRK MIX LEMONAD, W/SWN	228	3.3	7.6	0
14377	KRAFT, CRYSTAL LT SUGAR FREE LO CAL ICED TEA MIX, W/ASPRT, P	283	6.3	42.9	0
14232	KRAFT, GENERAL FOODS INT COFFEE SGR&FAT FR LO CAL FRN VN I	363	3.1	76	0.8
14205	KRAFT, GENERAL FOODS INTRN COFF SGR&FT FR MOCHA FLV INST,	337	5.4	72.8	1.4
14230	KRAFT, GENERAL FOODS INTRN COFFEE CAFE FRANCAIS FLV INST,	480	4.2	55.3	6.4
14231	KRAFT, GENERAL FOODS INTRN COFFEE FRENCH VAN FLV INST, PD	463	2.5	71.1	4.6
14225	KRAFT, GENERAL FOODS INTRN COFFEE SUISSE MOCHA FLV INST, P	440	3.5	72.1	4.3
19286	KRAFT, JELLO FAT FR CK&SRV RD CAL PUDD&PIE FLNG CHC, RG, P	360	1.7	91	0.6
19287	KRAFT, JELLO FAT FR CK&SRV RD CL PUDD&PIE FLNG VAN, RG, PDR	374	0.1	94.3	0.1
19275	KRAFT, JELLO FAT& SUGR FR INST RED CAL PUD&PIE FLNG CHOC,	310	4.9	74.6	1

NDB #	Food Description (100 gram portions = 3½ ounces = 20 tsp = ½ cup approx.	Calories	Protein	Carbs	Sat Fat
19276	KRAFT, JELLO FAT&SGR FR INST RED CAL PUD&PIE FLNG VAN, W/ A,	331	0.8	77.9	0.1
19277	KRAFT, JELLO SGR FR CK&SRV RED CAL PUD&PIE FLNG CHOC, W/ A	310	6.1	74.5	1.6
19278	KRAFT, JELLO SGR FR CK&SRV RED CAL PUDD&PIE FLNG VAN, W/A,	349	1	82.3	0.1
19291	KRAFT, JELLO SGR FR LO CAL GELATIN SNACKS STRAWBERRY, W/ A	8	1.4	0	0
19290	KRAFT, JELLO SGR FR LO CAL GELATIN STRWBRY, W/ A, PDR	333	56.8	4.9	0
14276	KRAFT, KOOL-AID BURSTS SOFT DRK TROPICAL PUNCH, RTD	43	0	11.6	0
14178	KRAFT, KOOL-AID SPLASH SOFT DRINK GRAPE BERRY PUNCH, RTD	46	0	12.2	0
14275	KRAFT, KOOL-AID SUGAR SWTND SOFT DRK MIX TROPICAL PUNCH,	375	0	95.6	0
14274	KRAFT, KOOL-AID UNSWTND SOFT DRK MIX TROPICAL PUNCH, PDR	198	0	9.6	0
18567	KRAFT, STOVE TOP STUFFING MIX CHICKEN FLAVOR	381	12.6	73.1	0.8
14129	KRAFT, SUGAR FREE COUNTRY TIME PINK LEMONADE MIX, W/VIT C	270	2.7	88.7	
14127	KRAFT, SUGAR FREE KOOL-AID MIX, W/ASPRT&VIT C, CHERRY FLAV	290	6.1	84.9	
14128	KRAFT. COUNTRY TIME LEMONADE MIX, W/VIT C	354	0.1	98.1	
18610	KRUSTEAZ ALMND POPPYSD MUFF MIX, ARTIFIC FLAV, DRY	418	6	76.1	2.84
18611	KRUSTEAZ BTTRMLK MINI PANCAKES, FRZ, READY TO MICROWAVE	215	6.7	40.2	0.434
09149	KUMQUATS, RAW	63	0.9	16.43	0.014
17281	LAMB, AUS, IMP, FRSH, COMP OF RTL CUTS, LN&FAT, 1/8"FAT, CKD	256	24.52	0	7.94
17280	LAMB, AUS, IMP, FRSH, COMP OF RTL CUTS, LN&FAT, 1/8"FAT, RAW	229	17.84	0	8.189
17283	LAMB, AUS, IMP, FRSH, COMP OF RTL CUTS, LN, 1/8"FAT, CKD	201	26.71	0	4.048
17282	LAMB, AUS, IMP, FRSH, COMP OF RTL CUTS, LN, 1/8"FAT, RAW	142	20.25	0	2.54
17285	LAMB, AUS, IMP, FRSH, FAT, CKD	639	9.42	0	34.751
17284	LAMB, AUS, IMP, FRSH, FAT, RAW	648	6.27	0	35.353
17287	LAMB, AUS, IMP, FRSH, FORESHANK, LN&FAT, 1/8"FAT, CKD, BRSD	236	24.78	0	6.794
17286	LAMB, AUS, IMP, FRSH, FORESHANK, LN&FAT, 1/8"FAT, RAW	195	18.85	0	5.981
17289	LAMB, AUS, IMP, FRSH, FORESHANK, LN, 1/8"FAT, CKD, BRSD	165	27.5	0	1.884
17288	LAMB, AUS, IMP, FRSH, FORESHANK, LN, 1/8"FAT, RAW	123	20.83	0	1.344
17307	LAMB, AUS, IMP, FRSH, LEG, CNTR SLCE, BNE-IN, LN&FT, 1/8"FT, CKD,	215	25.54	0	5.32
17306	LAMB, AUS, IMP, FRSH, LEG, CNTR SLICE, BONE-IN, LN&FAT, 1/8"FAT,	195	19.17	0	5.813
17309	LAMB, AUS, IMP, FRSH, LEG, CNTR SLICE, BONE-IN, LN, 1/8"FAT, CKD,	183	26.75	0	3.111
17308	LAMB, AUS, IMP, FRSH, LEG, CNTR SLICE, BONE-IN, LN, 1/8"FAT, RAW	143	20.65	0	2.413
17295	LAMB, AUS, IMP, FRSH, LEG, SHANK HALF, LN&FAT, 1/8"FAT, CKD, RS	231	25.25	0	6.341
17294	LAMB, AUS, IMP, FRSH, LEG, SHANK HALF, LN&FAT, 1/8"FAT, RAW	201	18.59	0	6.389
17297	LAMB, AUS, IMP, FRSH, LEG, SHANK HALF, LN, 1/8"FAT, CKD, RSTD	182	27.18	0	2.918
17296	LAMB, AUS, IMP, FRSH, LEG, SHANK HALF, LN, 1/8"FAT, RAW	133	20.45	0	2.008
17302	LAMB, AUS, IMP, FRSH, LEG, SIRL CHOPS, BNLESS, LN&FAT, 1/8"FAT,	208	18.33	0	6.898

NDB #	Food Description (100 gram portions = 3½ ounces = 20 tsp = ½ cup approx.	Calories	Protein	Carbs	Sat Fat
17305	LAMB, AUS, IMP, FRSH, LEG, SIRL CHOPS, BNLESS, LN, 1/8"FAT, CKD,	188	27.63	0	3.159
17303	LAMB, AUS, IMP, FRSH, LEG, SIRL CHPS, BNLESS, LN&FT, 1/8"FT, CKD	235	25.75	0	6.414
17301	LAMB, AUS, IMP, FRSH, LEG, SIRL HALF, BNLESS, LN, 1/8"FAT, CKD, R	215	27.75	0	4.508
17299	LAMB, AUS, IMP, FRSH, LEG, SIRL HLF, BNLESS, LN&FT, 1/8"FAT, CKD,	281	24.88	0	9.245
17304	LAMB, AUS, IMP, FRSH, LEG, SIRLOIN CHOPS, BNLESS, LN, 1/8"FAT, R	132	20.43	0	1.948
17298	LAMB, AUS, IMP, FRSH, LEG, SIRLOIN HALF, BNLESS, LN&FAT, 1/8"FA	254	17.25	0	9.754
17300	LAMB, AUS, IMP, FRSH, LEG, SIRLOIN HALF, BNLESS, LN, 1/8"FAT, RA	138	20.48	0	2.308
17291	LAMB, AUS, IMP, FRSH, LEG, WHL (SHK&SIRL), LN&FAT, 1/8"FAT, CKD,	244	25.16	0	7.091
17290	LAMB, AUS, IMP, FRSH, LEG, WHL (SHK&SIRL), LN&FAT, 1/8"FAT, RAW	215	18.24	0	7.288
17293	LAMB, AUS, IMP, FRSH, LEG, WHL (SHK&SIRL), LN, 1/8"FAT, CKD, RST	190	27.31	0	3.297
17292	LAMB, AUS, IMP, FRSH, LEG, WHL (SHK&SIRL), LN, 1/8"FAT, RAW	135	20.46	0	2.081
17311	LAMB, AUS, IMP, FRSH, LOIN, LN&FAT, 1/8"FAT, CKD, BRLD	219	25.49	0	5.572
17310	LAMB, AUS, IMP, FRSH, LOIN, LN&FAT, 1/8"FAT, RAW	203	19.32	0	6.401
17313	LAMB, AUS, IMP, FRSH, LOIN, LN, 1/8"FAT, CKD, BRLD	192	26.53	0	3.687
17312	LAMB, AUS, IMP, FRSH, LOIN, LN, 1/8"FAT, RAW	146	21	0	2.673
17315	LAMB, AUS, IMP, FRSH, RIB, LN&FAT, 1/8"FAT, CKD, RSTD	277	22.24	0	9.734
17314	LAMB, AUS, IMP, FRSH, RIB, LN&FAT, 1/8"FAT, RAW	289	16.46	0	11.925
17317	LAMB, AUS, IMP, FRSH, RIB, LN, 1/8"FAT, CKD, RSTD	210	24.63	0	5.072
17316	LAMB, AUS, IMP, FRSH, RIB, LN, 1/8"FAT, RAW	160	20.12	0	3.533
17323	LAMB, AUS, IMP, FRSH, SHLDR, ARM, LN&FAT, 1/8"FAT, CKD, BRSD	311	29.7	0	9.696
17322	LAMB, AUS, IMP, FRSH, SHLDR, ARM, LN&FAT, 1/8"FAT, RAW	243	17.06	0	9.125
17325	LAMB, AUS, IMP, FRSH, SHLDR, ARM, LN, 1/8"FAT, CKD, BRSD	238	34.17	0	4.173
17324	LAMB, AUS, IMP, FRSH, SHLDR, ARM, LN, 1/8"FAT, RAW	137	19.88	0	2.335
17327	LAMB, AUS, IMP, FRSH, SHLDR, BLADE, LN&FAT, 1/8"FAT, CKD, BRLD	291	21.71	0	10.51
17326	LAMB, AUS, IMP, FRSH, SHLDR, BLADE, LN&FAT, 1/8"FAT, RAW	262	16.48	0	10.3
17329	LAMB, AUS, IMP, FRSH, SHLDR, BLADE, LN, 1/8"FAT, CKD, BRLD	231	23.83	0	6.334
17328	LAMB, AUS, IMP, FRSH, SHLDR, BLADE, LN, 1/8"FAT, RAW	164	19.1	0	3.883
17319	LAMB, AUS, IMP, FRSH, SHLDR, WHL (ARM&BLD), LN&FAT, 1/8"FAT, C	296	23.58	0	10.324
17318	LAMB, AUS, IMP, FRSH, SHLDR, WHL (ARM&BLD), LN&FAT, 1/8"FAT, R	256	16.68	0	9.907
17321	LAMB, AUS, IMP, FRSH, SHLDR, WHL (ARM&BLD), LN, 1/8"FAT, CKD	233	26.18	0	5.843
17320	LAMB, AUS, IMP, FRSH, SHLDR, WHL (ARM&BLD), LN, 1/8"FAT, RAW	155	19.36	0	3.355
17006	LAMB, DOM, COMP OF RTL CUTS, FAT, 1/4"FAT, CHOIC, CKD	586	12.16	0	27.02
17005	LAMB, DOM, COMP OF RTL CUTS, FAT, 1/4"FAT, CHOIC, RAW	665	6.65	0	32.24
17002	LAMB, DOM, COMP OF RTL CUTS, LN&FAT, 1/4"FAT, CHOIC, CKD	294	24.52	0	8.83
17001	LAMB, DOM, COMP OF RTL CUTS, LN&FAT, 1/4"FAT, CHOIC, RAW	267	16.88	0	9.47

NDB #	Food Description (100 gram portions = 3½ ounces = 20 tsp = ½ cup approx.	Calories	Protein	Carbs	Sat Fat
17227	LAMB, DOM, COMP OF RTL CUTS, LN&FAT, 1/8"FAT, CHOIC, CKD	271	25.51	0	7.45
17226	LAMB, DOM, COMP OF RTL CUTS, LN&FAT, 1/8"FAT, CHOIC, RAW	243	17.54	0	8.07
17004	LAMB, DOM, COMP OF RTL CUTS, LN, 1/4"FAT, CHOIC, CKD	206	28.22	0	3.4
17003	LAMB, DOM, COMP OF RTL CUTS, LN, 1/4"FAT, CHOIC, RAW	134	20.29	0	1.88
17061	LAMB, DOM, CUBED FOR STEW (LEG&SHLDR), LN, 1/4"FAT, CKD, BR	186	28.08	0	2.62
17060	LAMB, DOM, CUBED FOR STEW (LEG&SHLDR), LN, 1/4"FAT, CKD, BR	223	33.69	0	3.15
17059	LAMB, DOM, CUBED FOR STEW OR KABOB (LEG&SHLDR), LN, 1/4"FA	134	20.21	0	1.89
17008	LAMB, DOM, FORESHANK, LN&FAT, 1/4"FAT, CHOIC, CKD, BRSD	243	28.37	0	5.63
17007	LAMB, DOM, FORESHANK, LN&FAT, 1/4"FAT, CHOIC, RAW	201	18.91	0	5.83
17228	LAMB, DOM, FORESHANK, LN&FAT, 1/8"FAT, CHOIC, RAW	201	18.91	0	5.83
17229	LAMB, DOM, FORESHANK, LN&FAT, 1/8"FAT, CKD, BRSD	243	28.37	0	5.63
17010	LAMB, DOM, FORESHANK, LN, 1/4"FAT, CHOIC, CKD, BRSD	187	31.01	0	2.15
17009	LAMB, DOM, FORESHANK, LN, 1/4"FAT, CHOIC, RAW	120	21.08	0	1.18
17016	LAMB, DOM, LEG, SHANK HALF, LN&FAT, 1/4"FAT, CHOIC, CKD, RSTD	225	26.41	0	5.09
17015	LAMB, DOM, LEG, SHANK HALF, LN&FAT, 1/4"FAT, CHOIC, RAW	201	18.58	0	5.8
17233	LAMB, DOM, LEG, SHANK HALF, LN&FAT, 1/8"FAT, CHOIC, CKD, RSTD	217	26.73	0	4.6
17232	LAMB, DOM, LEG, SHANK HALF, LN&FAT, 1/8"FAT, CHOIC, RAW	185	18.99	0	4.88
17018	LAMB, DOM, LEG, SHANK HALF, LN, 1/4"FAT, CHOIC, CKD, RSTD	180	28.17	0	2.38
17017	LAMB, DOM, LEG, SHANK HALF, LN, 1/4"FAT, CHOIC, RAW	125	20.52	0	1.5
17020	LAMB, DOM, LEG, SIRLOIN HALF, LN&FAT, 1/4"FAT, CHOIC, CKD, RST	292	24.63	0	8.74
17019	LAMB, DOM, LEG, SIRLOIN HALF, LN&FAT, 1/4"FAT, CHOIC, RAW	272	16.94	0	9.73
17235	LAMB, DOM, LEG, SIRLOIN HALF, LN&FAT, 1/8"FAT, CHOIC, CKD, RST	284	24.95	0	8.26
17234	LAMB, DOM, LEG, SIRLOIN HALF, LN&FAT, 1/8"FAT, CHOIC, RAW	261	17.21	0	9.12
17022	LAMB, DOM, LEG, SIRLOIN HALF, LN, 1/4"FAT, CHOIC, CKD, RSTD	204	28.35	0	3.28
17021	LAMB, DOM, LEG, SIRLOIN HALF, LN, 1/4"FAT, CHOIC, RAW	134	20.55	0	1.82
17012	LAMB, DOM, LEG, WHL (SHK&SIRL), LN&FAT, 1/4"FAT, CHOIC, CKD, R	258	25.55	0	6.89
17011	LAMB, DOM, LEG, WHL (SHK&SIRL), LN&FAT, 1/4"FAT, CHOIC, RAW	230	17.91	0	7.43
17231	LAMB, DOM, LEG, WHL (SHK&SIRL), LN&FAT, 1/8"FAT, CHOIC, CKD, R	242	26.2	0	5.92
17230	LAMB, DOM, LEG, WHL (SHK&SIRL), LN&FAT, 1/8"FAT, CHOIC, RAW	209	18.47	0	6.21
17014	LAMB, DOM, LEG, WHL (SHK&SIRL), LN, 1/4"FAT, CHOIC, CKD, RSTD	191	28.3	0	2.76
17013	LAMB, DOM, LEG, WHL (SHK&SIRL), LN, 1/4"FAT, CHOIC, RAW	128	20.56	0	1.61
17024	LAMB, DOM, LOIN, LN&FAT, 1/4"FAT, CHOIC, CKD, BRLD	316	25.17	0	9.83
17025	LAMB, DOM, LOIN, LN&FAT, 1/4"FAT, CHOIC, CKD, RSTD	309	22.55	0	10.24
17023	LAMB, DOM, LOIN, LN&FAT, 1/4"FAT, CHOIC, RAW	310	16.32	0	11.76
17237	LAMB, DOM, LOIN, LN&FAT, 1/8"FAT, CHOIC, CKD, BRLD	297	26.06	0	8.65

NDB #	Food Description (100 gram portions = 3½ ounces = 20 tsp = ½ cup approx.	Calories	Protein	Carbs	Sat Fat
17238	LAMB, DOM, LOIN, LN&FAT, 1/8"FAT, CHOIC, CKD, RSTD	290	23.27	0	9.08
17236	LAMB, DOM, LOIN, LN&FAT, 1/8"FAT, CHOIC, RAW	279	17.18	0	9.95
17027	LAMB, DOM, LOIN, LN, 1/4"FAT, CHOIC, CKD, BRLD	216	29.99	0	3.48
17028	LAMB, DOM, LOIN, LN, 1/4"FAT, CHOIC, CKD, RSTD	202	26.59	0	3.72
17026	LAMB, DOM, LOIN, LN, 1/4"FAT, CHOIC, RAW	143	20.88	0	2.13
17030	LAMB, DOM, RIB, LN&FAT, 1/4"FAT, CHOIC, CKD, BRLD	361	22.13	0	12.7
17031	LAMB, DOM, RIB, LN&FAT, 1/4"FAT, CHOIC, CKD, RSTD	359	21.12	0	12.77
17029	LAMB, DOM, RIB, LN&FAT, 1/4"FAT, CHOIC, RAW	372	14.52	0	15.16
17240	LAMB, DOM, RIB, LN&FAT, 1/8"FAT, CHOIC, CKD, BRLD	340	23.06	0	11.36
17241	LAMB, DOM, RIB, LN&FAT, 1/8"FAT, CHOIC, CKD, RSTD	341	21.82	0	11.66
17239	LAMB, DOM, RIB, LN&FAT, 1/8"FAT, CHOIC, RAW	342	15.32	0	13.43
17033	LAMB, DOM, RIB, LN, 1/4"FAT, CHOIC, CKD, BRLD	235	27.74	0	4.65
17034	LAMB, DOM, RIB, LN, 1/4"FAT, CHOIC, CKD, RSTD	232	26.16	0	4.76
17032	LAMB, DOM, RIB, LN, 1/4"FAT, CHOIC, RAW	169	19.98	0	3.3
17045	LAMB, DOM, SHLDR, ARM, LN&FAT, 1/4"FAT, CHOIC, CKD, BRLD	281	24.44	0	8.37
17044	LAMB, DOM, SHLDR, ARM, LN&FAT, 1/4"FAT, CHOIC, CKD, BRSD	346	30.39	0	9.87
17046	LAMB, DOM, SHLDR, ARM, LN&FAT, 1/4"FAT, CHOIC, CKD, RSTD	279	22.53	0	8.74
17043	LAMB, DOM, SHLDR, ARM, LN&FAT, 1/4"FAT, CHOIC, RAW	260	16.79	0	9.15
17247	LAMB, DOM, SHLDR, ARM, LN&FAT, 1/8"FAT, CHOIC, CKD, BRSD	337	31.1	0	9.21
17246	LAMB, DOM, SHLDR, ARM, LN&FAT, 1/8"FAT, CHOIC, RAW	244	17.19	0	8.24
17249	LAMB, DOM, SHLDR, ARM, LN&FAT, 1/8"FAT, CHOIC, RSTD	267	22.93	0	8.04
17248	LAMB, DOM, SHLDR, ARM, LN&FAT, 1/8"FAT, CKD, BRLD	269	24.91	0	7.66
17049	LAMB, DOM, SHLDR, ARM, LN, 1/4"FAT, CHOIC, CKD, BRLD	200	27.71	0	3.42
17048	LAMB, DOM, SHLDR, ARM, LN, 1/4"FAT, CHOIC, CKD, BRSD	279	35.54	0	5.03
17050	LAMB, DOM, SHLDR, ARM, LN, 1/4"FAT, CHOIC, CKD, RSTD	192	25.46	0	3.59
17047	LAMB, DOM, SHLDR, ARM, LN, 1/4"FAT, CHOIC, RAW	132	19.99	0	1.86
17053	LAMB, DOM, SHLDR, BLADE, LN&FAT, 1/4"FAT, CHOIC, CKD, BRLD	278	23.08	0	8.18
17052	LAMB, DOM, SHLDR, BLADE, LN&FAT, 1/4"FAT, CHOIC, CKD, BRSD	345	28.51	0	10.29
17054	LAMB, DOM, SHLDR, BLADE, LN&FAT, 1/4"FAT, CHOIC, CKD, RSTD	281	22.25	0	8.64
17051	LAMB, DOM, SHLDR, BLADE, LN&FAT, 1/4"FAT, CHOIC, RAW	259	16.63	0	8.93
17252	LAMB, DOM, SHLDR, BLADE, LN&FAT, 1/8"FAT, CHOIC, CKD, BRLD	267	23.48	0	7.49
17251	LAMB, DOM, SHLDR, BLADE, LN&FAT, 1/8"FAT, CHOIC, CKD, BRSD	339	28.92	0	9.88
17253	LAMB, DOM, SHLDR, BLADE, LN&FAT, 1/8"FAT, CHOIC, CKD, RSTD	270	22.62	0	7.96
17250	LAMB, DOM, SHLDR, BLADE, LN&FAT, 1/8"FAT, CHOIC, RAW	244	17.01	0	8.04
17057	LAMB, DOM, SHLDR, BLADE, LN, 1/4"FAT, CHOIC, CKD, BRLD	211	25.48	0	4.04

NDB #	Food Description (100 gram portions = 3½ ounces = 20 tsp = ½ cup approx.	Calories	Protein	Carbs	Sat Fat
17056	LAMB, DOM, SHLDR, BLADE, LN, 1/4"FAT, CHOIC, CKD, BRSD	288	32.35	0	6.37
17058	LAMB, DOM, SHLDR, BLADE, LN, 1/4"FAT, CHOIC, CKD, RSTD	209	24.61	0	4.34
17055	LAMB, DOM, SHLDR, BLADE, LN, 1/4"FAT, CHOIC, RAW	151	19.29	0	2.73
17037	LAMB, DOM, SHLDR, WHL (ARM&BLD), LN&FAT, 1/4"FAT, CHOIC, CKD	278	24.42	0	8.04
17036	LAMB, DOM, SHLDR, WHL (ARM&BLD), LN&FAT, 1/4"FAT, CHOIC, CKD	344	28.68	0	10.34
17038	LAMB, DOM, SHLDR, WHL (ARM&BLD), LN&FAT, 1/4"FAT, CHOIC, CKD	276	22.51	0	8.44
17035	LAMB, DOM, SHLDR, WHL (ARM&BLD), LN&FAT, 1/4"FAT, CHOIC, RAW	264	16.58	0	9.28
17244	LAMB, DOM, SHLDR, WHL (ARM&BLD), LN&FAT, 1/8"FAT, CHOIC, CKD	268	23.84	0	7.53
17243	LAMB, DOM, SHLDR, WHL (ARM&BLD), LN&FAT, 1/8"FAT, CHOIC, CKD	338	29.46	0	9.71
17245	LAMB, DOM, SHLDR, WHL (ARM&BLD), LN&FAT, 1/8"FAT, CHOIC, CKD	269	22.7	0	7.98
17242	LAMB, DOM, SHLDR, WHL (ARM&BLD), LN&FAT, 1/8"FAT, CHOIC, RAW	244	17.07	0	8.1
17041	LAMB, DOM, SHLDR, WHL (ARM&BLD), LN, 1/4"FAT, CHOIC, CKD, BRL	210	27.12	0	3.88
17040	LAMB, DOM, SHLDR, WHL (ARM&BLD), LN, 1/4"FAT, CHOIC, CKD, BRS	283	32.81	0	6.17
17042	LAMB, DOM, SHLDR, WHL (ARM&BLD), LN, 1/4"FAT, CHOIC, CKD, RST	204	24.94	0	4.08
17039	LAMB, DOM, SHLDR, WHL (ARM&BLD), LN, 1/4"FAT, CHOIC, RAW	144	19.55	0	2.42
17225	LAMB, GROUND, CKD, BRLD	283	24.75	0	8.12
17224	LAMB, GROUND, RAW	282	16.56	0	10.19
17067	LAMB, NZ, IMP, FRZ, COMP OF RTL CUTS, FAT, CKD	586	9.72	0	31.51
17066	LAMB, NZ, IMP, FRZ, COMP OF RTL CUTS, FAT, RAW	640	6.92	0	35.29
17255	LAMB, NZ, IMP, FRZ, COMP OF RTL CUTS, LN&FAT, 1/8"FAT, CKD	270	25.26	0	8.76
17254	LAMB, NZ, IMP, FRZ, COMP OF RTL CUTS, LN&FAT, 1/8"FAT, RAW	232	17.95	0	8.64
17063	LAMB, NZ, IMP, FRZ, COMP OF RTL CUTS, LN&FAT, CKD	305	24.42	0	11.05
17062	LAMB, NZ, IMP, FRZ, COMP OF RTL CUTS, LN&FAT, RAW	277	16.74	0	11.57
17065	LAMB, NZ, IMP, FRZ, COMP OF RTL CUTS, LN, CKD	206	29.59	0	3.86
17064	LAMB, NZ, IMP, FRZ, COMP OF RTL CUTS, LN, RAW	128	20.75	0	1.88
17257	LAMB, NZ, IMP, FRZ, FORESHANK, LN&FAT, 1/8"FAT, CKD, BRSD	258	26.97	0	7.82
17256	LAMB, NZ, IMP, FRZ, FORESHANK, LN&FAT, 1/8"FAT, RAW	223	18.04	0	8.18
17069	LAMB, NZ, IMP, FRZ, FORESHANK, LN&FAT, CKD, BRSD	258	26.97	0	7.82
17068	LAMB, NZ, IMP, FRZ, FORESHANK, LN&FAT, RAW	223	18.04	0	8.18
17071	LAMB, NZ, IMP, FRZ, FORESHANK, LN, CKD, BRSD	186	30.76	0	2.61
17070	LAMB, NZ, IMP, FRZ, FORESHANK, LN, RAW	118	20.82	0	1.4
17259	LAMB, NZ, IMP, FRZ, LEG, WHL (SHK&SIRL), LN&FAT, 1/8"FAT, CKD, RS	234	25.34	0	6.75
17258	LAMB, NZ, IMP, FRZ, LEG, WHL (SHK&SIRL), LN&FAT, 1/8"FAT, RAW	201	18.76	0	6.67
17073	LAMB, NZ, IMP, FRZ, LEG, WHL (SHK&SIRL), LN&FAT, CKD, RSTD	246	24.81	0	7.61
17072	LAMB, NZ, IMP, FRZ, LEG, WHL (SHK&SIRL), LN&FAT, RAW	216	18.34	0	7.68

NDB #	Food Description (100 gram portions = 3½ ounces = 20 tsp = ½ cup approx.	Calories	Protein	Carbs	Sat Fat
17075	LAMB, NZ, IMP, FRZ, LEG, WHL (SHK&SIRL), LN, CKD, RSTD	181	27.68	0	3.05
17074	LAMB, NZ, IMP, FRZ, LEG, WHL (SHK&SIRL), LN, RAW	123	20.85	0	1.62
17261	LAMB, NZ, IMP, FRZ, LOIN, LN&FAT, 1/8"FAT, CKD, BRLD	296	24.41	0	10.56
17260	LAMB, NZ, IMP, FRZ, LOIN, LN&FAT, 1/8"FAT, RAW	273	17.18	0	11.23
17077	LAMB, NZ, IMP, FRZ, LOIN, LN&FAT, CKD, BRLD	315	23.43	0	11.96
17076	LAMB, NZ, IMP, FRZ, LOIN, LN&FAT, RAW	303	16.33	0	13.24
17079	LAMB, NZ, IMP, FRZ, LOIN, LN, CKD, BRLD	199	29.31	0	3.58
17078	LAMB, NZ, IMP, FRZ, LOIN, LN, RAW	130	21.17	0	1.87
17263	LAMB, NZ, IMP, FRZ, RIB, LN&FAT, 1/8"FAT, CKD, RSTD	317	19.86	0	12.82
17262	LAMB, NZ, IMP, FRZ, RIB, LN&FAT, 1/8"FAT, RAW	311	15.87	0	13.7
17081	LAMB, NZ, IMP, FRZ, RIB, LN&FAT, CKD, RSTD	340	18.98	0	14.45
17080	LAMB, NZ, IMP, FRZ, RIB, LN&FAT, RAW	346	14.92	0	15.99
17083	LAMB, NZ, IMP, FRZ, RIB, LN, CKD, RSTD	196	24.42	0	4.43
17082	LAMB, NZ, IMP, FRZ, RIB, LN, RAW	142	20.49	0	2.58
17265	LAMB, NZ, IMP, FRZ, SHLDR, WHL (ARM&BLD), LN&FAT, 1/8"FAT, CKD,	342	29.43	0	11.5
17264	LAMB, NZ, IMP, FRZ, SHLDR, WHL (ARM&BLD), LN&FAT, 1/8"FAT, RAW	251	17.19	0	9.9
17085	LAMB, NZ, IMP, FRZ, SHLDR, WHL (ARM&BLD), LN&FAT, CKD, BRSD	357	28.21	0	12.74
17084	LAMB, NZ, IMP, FRZ, SHLDR, WHL (ARM&BLD), LN&FAT, RAW	272	16.65	0	11.22
17087	LAMB, NZ, IMP, FRZ, SHLDR, WHL (ARM&BLD), LN, CKD, BRSD	285	34.06	0	6.81
17086	LAMB, NZ, IMP, FRZ, SHLDR, WHL (ARM&BLD), LN, RAW	135	20.25	0	2.31
17186	LAMB, VAR MEATS&BY-PRODUCTS, BRAIN, CKD, BRSD	145	12.55	0	2.6
17187	LAMB, VAR MEATS&BY-PRODUCTS, BRAIN, CKD, PAN-FRIED	273	16.97	0	5.67
17185	LAMB, VAR MEATS&BY-PRODUCTS, BRAIN, RAW	122	10.4	0	2.19
17192	LAMB, VAR MEATS&BY-PRODUCTS, HEART, CKD, BRSD	185	24.97	1.93	3.14
17191	LAMB, VAR MEATS&BY-PRODUCTS, HEART, RAW	122	16.47	0.21	2.25
17196	LAMB, VAR MEATS&BY-PRODUCTS, KIDNEYS, CKD, BRSD	137	23.65	0.99	1.23
17195	LAMB, VAR MEATS&BY-PRODUCTS, KIDNEYS, RAW	97	15.74	0.82	1
17200	LAMB, VAR MEATS&BY-PRODUCTS, LIVER, CKD, BRSD	220	30.57	2.53	3.41
17201	LAMB, VAR MEATS&BY-PRODUCTS, LIVER, CKD, PAN-FRIED	238	25.53	3.78	4.9
17199	LAMB, VAR MEATS&BY-PRODUCTS, LIVER, RAW	139	20.38	1.78	1.94
17206	LAMB, VAR MEATS&BY-PRODUCTS, LUNGS, CKD, BRSD	113	19.88	0	1.06
17205	LAMB, VAR MEATS&BY-PRODUCTS, LUNGS, RAW	95	16.7	0	0.89
17209	LAMB, VAR MEATS&BY-PRODUCTS, MECHANICALLY SEPARATED, RA	276	14.97	0	11.79
17211	LAMB, VAR MEATS&BY-PRODUCTS, PANCREAS, CKD, BRSD	234	22.83	0	6.84
17210	LAMB, VAR MEATS&BY-PRODUCTS, PANCREAS, RAW	152	14.84	0	4.44

NDB #	Food Description (100 gram portions = 3½ ounces = 20 tsp = ½ cup approx.	Calories	Protein	Carbs	Sat Fat
17215	LAMB, VAR MEATS&BY-PRODUCTS, SPLEEN, CKD, BRSD	156	26.46	0	1.58
17214	LAMB, VAR MEATS&BY-PRODUCTS, SPLEEN, RAW	101	17.2	0	1.03
17221	LAMB, VAR MEATS&BY-PRODUCTS, TONGUE, CKD, BRSD	275	21.57	0	7.83
17220	LAMB, VAR MEATS&BY-PRODUCTS, TONGUE, RAW	222	15.7	0	6.63
11794	LAMBS QUARTERS, CKD, BLD, DRND, W/SALT	32	3.2	5	0.052
11245	LAMBSQUARTERS, CKD, BLD, DRND, WO/SALT	32	3.2	5	0.052
11244	LAMBSQUARTERS, RAW	43	4.2	7.3	0.059
04002	LARD	902	0	0	39.2
22613	LAS CAMPANAS BF&BEAN BURRITO, FRZ	260	7.6	33.5	3.67
22538	LEAN POCKETS GLAZED CHICK SUPREME STUFFED SANDWICHES, F	182	7.7	26.7	1.5
18369	LEAVENING AGENTS, BAKING PDR, DOUBLE-ACTING, NA AL SULFAT	53	0	27.7	0
18370	LEAVENING AGENTS, BAKING PDR, DOUBLE-ACTING, STRAIGHT PO4	51	0.1	24.1	0
18371	LEAVENING AGENTS, BAKING PDR, LOW-SODIUM	97	0.1	46.9	0.073
18372	LEAVENING AGENTS, BAKING SODA	0	0	0	0
18373	LEAVENING AGENTS, CRM OF TARTAR	258	0	61.5	0
18375	LEAVENING AGENTS, YEAST, BAKER'S, ACTIVE DRY	295	38.3	38.2	0.595
18374	LEAVENING AGENTS, YEAST, BAKER'S, COMPRESSED	105	8.4	18.1	0.243
07039	LEBANON BOLOGNA BF	196	19.17	0.19	5.84
11795	LEEKS, (BULB&LOWER LEAF-PORTION), CKD, BLD, DRND, W/SALT	31	0.81	7.62	0.027
11247	LEEKS, (BULB&LOWER LEAF-PORTION), CKD, BLD, DRND, WO/SALT	31	0.81	7.62	0.027
11246	LEEKS, (BULB&LOWER LEAF-PORTION), RAW	61	1.5	14.15	0.04
11624	LEEKS, (BULB&LOWER-LEAF PORTION), FREEZE-DRIED	321	15.2	74.65	0.279
11972	LEMON GRASS (CITRONELLA), RAW	99	1.82	25.29	0.119
09153	LEMON JUC, CND OR BTLD	21	0.4	6.48	0.038
09154	LEMON JUC, FRZ, UNSWTND, SINGLE STRENGTH	22	0.46	6.5	0.043
09152	LEMON JUICE, RAW	25	0.38	8.63	0
09156	LEMON PEEL, RAW	47	1.5	16	0.039
14542	LEMONADE, FRZ CONC, PINK	181	0.3	47.1	0.026
14543	LEMONADE, FRZ CONC, PINK, PREP W/H2O	40	0.1	10.5	0.006
14292	LEMONADE, FRZ CONC, WHITE	181	0.3	47.1	0.026
14293	LEMONADE, FRZ CONC, WHITE, PREP W/H2O	40	0.1	10.5	0.006
14289	LEMONADE, LO CAL, W/ASPRT, PDR	332	3.6	83.7	0.039
14290	LEMONADE, LO CAL, W/ASPRT, PDR, PREP W/H2O	2	0	0.5	0
14288	LEMONADE, PDR, PREP W/H2O	39	0	10.2	0
14287	LEMONADE, POWDER	376	0	98.8	0.003

NDB #	Food Description (100 gram portions = 3½ ounces = 20 tsp = ½ cup approx.	Calories	Protein	Carbs	Sat Fat
14296	LEMONADE-FLAVOR DRK, PDR	387	0.1	98.8	0.157
14297	LEMONADE-FLAVOR DRK, PDR, PREP W/H2O	42	0	10.8	0.017
09151	LEMONS, RAW, WITH PEEL	20	1.2	10.7	0.039
09150	LEMONS, RAW, WITHOUT PEEL	29	1.1	9.32	0.039
18504	LENDER'S BAGEL SHOP BLUEBERRY BAGELS	259	10.5	52.33	0.3
18502	LENDER'S BIG'N CRUSTY BLUEBERRY BAGEL	252	9.26	53.96	0.2
18503	LENDER'S PREMIUM REFR BLUEBERRY BAGELS	258	10.43	52.51	0.33
16370	LENTILS, MATURE SEEDS, CKD, BLD, W/SALT	116	9.02	20.14	0.053
16070	LENTILS, MATURE SEEDS, CKD, BLD, WO/SALT	116	9.02	20.14	0.053
16069	LENTILS, MATURE SEEDS, RAW	338	28.06	57.09	0.135
16144	LENTILS, PINK, RAW	346	24.95	59.15	0.379
11926	LENTILS, SPROUTED, CKD, STIR-FRIED, W/SALT	101	8.8	21.25	0.053
11249	LENTILS, SPROUTED, CKD, STIR-FRIED, WO/SALT	101	8.8	21.25	0.053
11248	LENTILS, SPROUTED, RAW	106	8.96	22.14	0.057
11250	LETTUCE, BUTTERHEAD (INCL BOSTON&BIBB TYPES), RAW	13	1.29	2.32	0.029
11251	LETTUCE, COS OR ROMAINE, RAW	14	1.62	2.37	0.026
11252	LETTUCE, ICEBERG (INCL CRISPHEAD TYPES), RAW	12	1.01	2.09	0.025
11253	LETTUCE, LOOSELEAF, RAW	18	1.3	3.5	0.039
22697	LIBBY'S SPREADABLES RTS SNDWCH SALAD, CHICKEN, SHELF STA	145	4.9	10.1	1.95
11714	LIMA BNS, IMMAT SEEDS, CKD, BLD, DRND, W/SALT	123	6.81	23.64	0.073
11032	LIMA BNS, IMMAT SEEDS, CKD, BLD, DRND, WO/SALT	123	6.81	23.64	0.073
11715	LIMA BNS, IMMAT SEEDS, CND, NO SALT, SOL&LIQUIDS	71	4.07	13.33	0.066
11716	LIMA BNS, IMMAT SEEDS, FRZ, BABY, CKD, BLD, DRND, W/SALT	105	6.65	19.45	0.068
11040	LIMA BNS, IMMAT SEEDS, FRZ, BABY, CKD, BLD, DRND, WO/SALT	105	6.65	19.45	0.068
11039	LIMA BNS, IMMAT SEEDS, FRZ, BABY, UNPREP	132	7.59	25.13	0.102
11717	LIMA BNS, IMMAT SEEDS, FRZ, FORDHOOK, CKD, BLD, DRND, W/SAL	100	6.07	18.8	0.077
11038	LIMA BNS, IMMAT SEEDS, FRZ, FORDHOOK, CKD, BLD, DRND, WO/SA	100	6.07	18.8	0.077
11037	LIMA BNS, IMMAT SEEDS, FRZ, FORDHOOK, UNPREP	106	6.4	19.83	0.081
11031	LIMA BNS, IMMAT SEEDS, RAW	113	6.84	20.16	0.198
16372	LIMA BNS, LRG, MATURE SEEDS, CKD, BLD, W/SALT	115	7.8	20.89	0.089
16072	LIMA BNS, LRG, MATURE SEEDS, CKD, BLD, WO/SALT	115	7.8	20.89	0.089
16073	LIMA BNS, LRG, MATURE SEEDS, CND	79	4.93	14.91	0.039
16071	LIMA BNS, LRG, MATURE SEEDS, RAW	338	21.46	63.38	0.161
16375	LIMA BNS, THIN SEEDED (BABY), MATURE SEEDS, CKD, BLD, W/SALT	126	8.04	23.31	0.088
16075	LIMA BNS, THIN SEEDED (BABY), MATURE SEEDS, CKD, BLD, WO/SA	126	8.04	23.31	0.088

NDB #	Food Description (100 gram portions = 3½ ounces = 20 tsp = ½ cup approx.	Calories	Protein	Carbs	Sat Fat
16074	LIMA BNS, THIN SEEDED (BABY), MATURE SEEDS, RAW	335	20.62	62.83	0.219
09161	LIME JUC, CND OR BTLD, UNSWTND	21	0.25	6.69	0.026
09160	LIME JUICE, RAW	27	0.44	9.01	0.011
14302	LIMEADE, FRZ CONC	187	0.2	49.5	0.011
14303	LIMEADE, FRZ CONC, PREP W/H2O	41	0	11	0.002
09159	LIMES, RAW	30	0.7	10.54	0.022
15198	LING, COOKED, DRY HEAT	111	24.35	0	
15044	LING, RAW	87	18.99	0	0.12
15199	LINGCOD, COOKED, DRY HEAT	109	22.64	0	0.255
15045	LINGCOD, RAW	85	17.66	0	0.197
22702	LIPTON, ALFREDO EGG NOODLES IN A CREAMY SAU, DRY MIX	418	15.5	62.4	4.57
09165	LITCHIS, DRIED	277	3.8	70.7	0.27
09164	LITCHIS, RAW	66	0.83	16.53	0.099
07040	LIVER CHEESE, PORK	304	15.2	2.1	8.96
07041	LIVER SAUSAGE, LIVERWURST, PORK	326	14.1	2.2	10.6
07911	LIVERWURST SPRD	302	12.38	5.89	9
15148	LOBSTER, NORTHERN, CKD, MOIST HEAT	98	20.5	1.28	0.107
15147	LOBSTER, NORTHERN, RAW	90	18.8	0.5	0.18
09167	LOGANBERRIES, FROZEN	55	1.52	13.02	0.011
09173	LONGANS, DRIED	286	4.9	74	
09172	LONGANS, RAW	60	1.31	15.14	
09174	LOQUATS, RAW	47	0.43	12.14	0.04
11796	LOTUS ROOT, CKD, BLD, DRND, W/SALT	66	1.58	16.03	0.021
11255	LOTUS ROOT, CKD, BLD, DRND, WO/SALT	66	1.58	16.03	0.021
11254	LOTUS ROOT, RAW	74	2.6	17.24	0.03
12013	LOTUS SEEDS, DRIED	332	15.41	64.47	0.33
12205	LOTUS SEEDS, RAW	89	4.13	17.28	0.088
07254	LOUIS RICH TURKEY BACON	250	15.1	1.7	5.27
07251	LOUIS RICH, CHICK (WHITE, OVEN RSTD)	128	17	2.3	1.452
07250	LOUIS RICH, CHICK BREAST (OVEN RSTD DELUXE)	101	18.3	2.5	0.541
07249	LOUIS RICH, CHICK BREAST CLASSIC BKD /GRILL (CARVING BOARD)	98	19.7	3.7	0.162
07252	LOUIS RICH, FRANKS (TURKEY & CHICK CHEESE)	201	12.7	5.1	5.19
07253	LOUIS RICH, FRANKS (TURKEY & CHICKEN)	188	11.2	5.3	3.839
07258	LOUIS RICH, TURKEY (HONEY RSTD, FAT FREE)	102	19.3	4.5	0.234
07255	LOUIS RICH, TURKEY BOLOGNA	183	11.3	4.85	3.79

NDB #	Food Description (100 gram portions = 3½ ounces = 20 tsp = ½ cup approx.	Calories	Protein	Carbs	Sat Fat
07256	LOUIS RICH, TURKEY BREAST & WHITE TURKEY (OVEN ROASTED)	99	17.1	3.2	0.468
07259	LOUIS RICH, TURKEY BREAST (OVEN RSTD, FAT FREE)	84	15	4.5	0.205
07260	LOUIS RICH, TURKEY BREAST (OVEN RSTD, PORTION FAT FREE)	90	19.1	1.9	0.207
07261	LOUIS RICH, TURKEY BREAST (SMOKED, CARVING BOARD)	94	19.7	1.6	0.3
07262	LOUIS RICH, TURKEY BREAST (SMOKED, PORTION FAT FREE)	93	19.3	2.2	0.234
07257	LOUIS RICH, TURKEY BREAST&WHITE TURKEY (SMOKED SLICED)	100	17.6	2.4	0.63
07264	LOUIS RICH, TURKEY HAM (10% H2O)	113	18.2	0.9	1.06
07265	LOUIS RICH, TURKEY NUGGETS/STICKS (BREADED)	276	14.3	15.4	3.39
07266	LOUIS RICH, TURKEY SALAMI	147	15.3	0.4	2.783
07267	LOUIS RICH, TURKEY SALAMI COTTO	149	15	0.9	2.9
07268	LOUIS RICH, TURKEY SMOKED SAUSAGE	161	14.8	3.2	2.67
07042	LUNCHEON MEAT, BEEF, LOAVED	308	14.4	2.9	11.18
07043	LUNCHEON MEAT, BF, THIN SLICED	177	28.11	5.71	1.65
07047	LUNCHEON MEAT, PORK, BEEF	353	12.59	2.33	11.59
07045	LUNCHEON MEAT, PORK, CANNED	334	12.5	2.1	10.79
07090	LUNCHEON SAUSAGE, PORK&BF	260	15.38	1.58	7.62
16377	LUPINS, MATURE SEEDS, CKD, BLD, W/SALT	119	15.57	9.88	0.346
16077	LUPINS, MATURE SEEDS, CKD, BLD, WO/SALT	119	15.57	9.88	0.346
16076	LUPINS, MATURE SEEDS, RAW	371	36.17	40.38	1.156
07060	LUXURY LOAF, PORK	141	18.4	4.9	1.58
12632	MACADAMIA NUTS, DRY RSTD, W/SALT	716	7.79	12.83	11.947
12132	MACADAMIA NUTS, DRY RSTD, WO/SALT	718	7.79	13.38	11.947
12131	MACADAMIA NUTS, RAW	718	7.91	13.82	12.061
07940	MACARONI & CHS LOAF CHICK PORK & BF	230	11.76	11.94	5.614
22247	MACARONI&CHS, CND	79	3	11.5	1.2
20400	MACARONI, CKD, UNENR	141	4.77	28.34	0.095
20100	MACARONI, COOKED, ENRICHED	141	4.77	28.34	0.095
20099	MACARONI, DRY, ENR	371	12.78	74.69	0.225
20499	MACARONI, DRY, UNENRICHED	371	12.78	74.69	0.225
20102	MACARONI, PROTEIN-FORTIFIED, CKD, ENR, (N X 5.70)	164	8.08	31.66	0.032
20302	MACARONI, PROTEIN-FORTIFIED, CKD, ENR, (N X 6.25)	164	8.86	30.88	0.032
20101	MACARONI, PROTEIN-FORTIFIED, DRY, ENR, (N X 5.70)	375	19.86	67.56	0.328
20301	MACARONI, PROTEIN-FORTIFIED, DRY, ENR, (N X 6.25)	374	21.78	65.65	0.328
20106	MACARONI, VEG, CKD, ENR	128	4.53	26.61	0.016
20105	MACARONI, VEG, DRY, ENR	367	13.14	74.88	0.15

NDB #	Food Description (100 gram portions = 3½ ounces = 20 tsp = ½ cup approx.	Calories	Protein	Carbs	Sat Fat
20108	MACARONI, WHOLE-WHEAT, CKD	124	5.33	26.54	0.099
20107	MACARONI, WHOLE-WHEAT, DRY	348	14.63	75.03	0.258
02022	MACE, GROUND	475	6.71	50.5	9.51
15047	MACKEREL, ATLANTIC, CKD, DRY HEAT	262	23.85	0	4.176
15046	MACKEREL, ATLANTIC, RAW	205	18.6	0	3.257
15048	MACKEREL, JACK, CND, DRND SOL	156	23.19	0	1.857
15200	MACKEREL, KING, CKD, DRY HEAT	134	26	0	0.465
15049	MACKEREL, KING, RAW	105	20.28	0	0.363
15201	MACKEREL, PACIFIC&JACK, MXD SP, CKD, DRY HEAT	201	25.73	0	2.881
15050	MACKEREL, PACIFIC&JACK, MXD SP, RAW	158	20.07	0	2.247
15052	MACKEREL, SPANISH, CKD, DRY HEAT	158	23.59	0	1.801
15051	MACKEREL, SPANISH, RAW	139	19.29	0	1.828
11986	MALABAR SPINACH, COOKED	23	2.98	2.71	
14305	MALT BEVERAGE	60	0.29	13.44	0.024
14317	MALTED DRK MIX, CHOC, PDR	375	5.1	87.8	2.159
14318	MALTED DRK MIX, CHOC, PDR, PREP W/ WHL MILK	89	3.44	11.32	2.013
14315	MALTED DRK MIX, CHOC, W/ ADDED NUTR, PDR	358	4.9	84.4	1.964
14316	MALTED DRK MIX, CHOC, W/ ADDED NUTR, PDR, PREP W/ WHL MILK	88	3.42	11.05	1.998
14311	MALTED DRK MIX, NAT, PDR	414	11.2	75.8	4.199
14312	MALTED DRK MIX, NAT, PDR, PREP W/ WHL MILK	90	3.92	10.36	2.169
14309	MALTED DRK MIX, NAT, W/ ADDED NUTR, PDR	383	8.8	81.2	1.483
14310	MALTED DRK MIX, NAT, W/ ADDED NUTR, PDR, PREP W/ WHL MILK	88	3.73	10.8	1.96
09175	MAMMY-APPLE, (MAMEY), RAW	51	0.5	12.5	0.136
09176	MANGOS, RAW	65	0.51	17	0.066
09177	MANGOSTEEN, CND, SYRUP PK	73	0.41	17.91	
04630	MARGARINE SPRD, APPROX 48% FAT, TUB	424	0.2	0.86	8.792
04632	MARGARINE SPRD, FAT-FREE, BOTTLE	46	0	5.58	0.374
04631	MARGARINE SPRD, FAT-FREE, TUB	44	0.1	4.34	2.128
04629	MARGARINE, 70% VEG OIL SPRD, SOYBN & SOYBEAN(HYDROGENAT	619	0.21	1.13	12.623
04628	MARGARINE, 80% FAT, STK, INCL REG & HYDR CORN & SOYBN OILS	705	0.18	1.94	14.787
04522	MARGARINE, REG, HARD, COCNT (HYDR&REG)&SAFFLOWER&PALM	719	0.9	0.9	56.9
04065	MARGARINE, REG, HARD, CORN (HYDR&REG)	719	0.9	0.9	14
04071	MARGARINE, REG, HARD, CORN (HYDR)	719	0.9	0.9	13.2
04067	MARGARINE, REG, HARD, CORN&SOYBN (HYDR)&CTTNSD (HYDR),	719	0.9	0.9	15
04068	MARGARINE, REG, HARD, CORN&SOYBN (HYDR)&CTTNSD (HYDR),	714	0.5	0.5	15

NDB #	Food Description (100 gram portions = 3½ ounces = 20 tsp = ½ cup approx.	Calories	Protein	Carbs	Sat Fat
04091	MARGARINE, REG, HARD, LARD (HYDR)	733	0.9	0.9	31.6
04089	MARGARINE, REG, HARD, SAFFLOWER&SOYBN (HYDR&REG)&CTTN	719	0.9	0.9	14.4
04078	MARGARINE, REG, HARD, SAFFLOWER&SOYBN (HYDR)	719	0.9	0.9	13.8
04079	MARGARINE, REG, HARD, SAFFLOWER&SOYBN (HYDR)&CTTNSD (H	719	0.9	0.9	13.3
04080	MARGARINE, REG, HARD, SOYBN (HYDR&REG)	719	0.9	0.9	13.1
04073	MARGARINE, REG, HARD, SOYBN (HYDR)	719	0.9	0.9	16.7
04074	MARGARINE, REG, HARD, SOYBN (HYDR)&CORN&CTTNSD (HYDR)	719	0.9	0.9	19.8
04075	MARGARINE, REG, HARD, SOYBN (HYDR)&CTTNSD	719	0.9	0.9	16.3
04076	MARGARINE, REG, HARD, SOYBN (HYDR)&CTTNSD (HYDR)	719	0.9	0.9	15.1
04082	MARGARINE, REG, HARD, SOYBN (HYDR)&PALM (HYDR&REG)	719	0.9	0.9	17.5
04077	MARGARINE, REG, HARD, SOYBN (HYDR)&PALM (HYDR)	719	0.9	0.9	15.1
04083	MARGARINE, REG, HARD, SOYBN (HYDR), CTTNSD (HYDR), &SOYBN	719	0.9	0.9	15.6
04081	MARGARINE, REG, HARD, SOYBN, SOYBN (HYDR), &CTTNSD (HYDR)	719	0.9	0.9	15.6
04521	MARGARINE, REG, HARD, SUNFLOWER&SOYBN (HYDR)&CTTNSD (H	719	0.9	0.9	11.9
04105	MARGARINE, REG, LIQ, SOYBN (HYDR&REG)&CTTNSD	721	1.9	0	13.2
04132	MARGARINE, REG, UNSPEC OILS, W/SALT	719	0.9	0.9	15.8
04131	MARGARINE, REG, UNSPEC OILS, WO/ SALT	714	0.5	0.5	15
04092	MARGARINE, SOFT, CORN (HYDR&REG)	716	0.8	0.5	14.1
04102	MARGARINE, SOFT, SAFFLOWER (HYDR&REG)	716	0.8	0.5	9.2
04101	MARGARINE, SOFT, SAFFLOWER&CTTNSD (HYDR)&PNUT (HYDR)	716	0.8	0.5	13.4
04094	MARGARINE, SOFT, SOYBN (HYDR&REG), W/SALT	716	0.8	0.5	13.5
04095	MARGARINE, SOFT, SOYBN (HYDR)&CTTNSD	716	0.8	0.5	16.5
04097	MARGARINE, SOFT, SOYBN (HYDR)&CTTNSD (HYDR), W/SALT	716	0.8	0.5	14.2
04096	MARGARINE, SOFT, SOYBN (HYDR)&CTTNSD (HYDR), WO/SALT	716	0.8	0.9	14.1
04523	MARGARINE, SOFT, SOYBN (HYDR)&PALM (HYDR&REG)	716	0.8	0.5	17.1
04524	MARGARINE, SOFT, SOYBN (HYDR)&SAFFLOWER	716	0.8	0.5	10.4
04099	MARGARINE, SOFT, SOYBN (HYDR), CTTNSD (HYDR), &SOYBN	716	0.8	0.5	15.3
04093	MARGARINE, SOFT, SOYBN (HYDROGENATE&REG), WO/SALT	716	0.8	0.9	13.5
04103	MARGARINE, SOFT, SOYBN, SOYBN (HYDR), &CTTNSD (HYDR)	716	0.8	0.5	16.1
04525	MARGARINE, SOFT, SUNFLOWER&CTTNSD (HYDR)&PNUT (HYDR)	716	0.8	0.5	12.8
04130	MARGARINE, SOFT, UNSPEC OILS, W/SALT	716	0.8	0.5	13.8
04129	MARGARINE, SOFT, UNSPEC OILS, WO/ SALT	716	0.8	0.9	13.8
04585	MARGARINE-BUTTER BLEND, 60% CORN OIL MARGARINE&40% BUTT	718	0.88	0.65	28.442
04107	MARGARINE-LIKE SPRD, (APPROX 40% FAT), CORN (HYDR&REG)	345	0.5	0.4	6.4
04110	MARGARINE-LIKE SPRD, (APPROX 40% FAT), SOY(HYDR)&CTTNSD(H	345	0.5	0.4	7.2

NDB #	Food Description (100 gram portions = 3½ ounces = 20 tsp = ½ cup approx.	Calories	Protein	Carbs	Sat Fat
04108	MARGARINE-LIKE SPRD, (APPROX 40% FAT), SOY(HYDR)&PLM(HYDR	345	0.5	0.4	10.1
04109	MARGARINE-LIKE SPRD, (APPROX 40% FAT), SOYBN (HYDR)	345	0.5	0.4	6.5
04112	MARGARINE-LIKE SPRD, (APPROX 40% FAT), SOYBN (HYDR)&CTTNS	345	0.5	0.4	8.3
04128	MARGARINE-LIKE SPRD, (APPROX 40% FAT), UNSPEC OILS	345	0.5	0.4	7.7
04526	MARGARINE-LIKE SPRD, APPROX 60% FAT, STK, SOYBN HYDR&PALM	540	0.6	0	14.1
04561	MARGARINE-LIKE SPRD, APPROX 60% FAT, TUB, UNSPEC OILS	540	0.6	0	12.8
04106	MARGARINE-LIKE SPRD, APPRX 60% FAT, TUB, SOYBN HYDR&CTTNS	540	0.6	0	12
04527	MARGARINE-LIKE SPRD, APPRX 60%FAT, TUB, SOYBN HYDR&PALM	540	0.6	0	13.5
22677	MARIE CALLENDER'S BF STROGANOFF&NOODLES W/CARROTS&PE	163	8.26	15.95	3.01
22526	MARIE CALLENDER'S CHICK POT PIE, FRZ ENTREE	214	5.28	18.87	5.4
22685	MARIE CALLENDER'S ESCALLOPED NOODLES&CHICK, FRZ ENTREE	171	5.6	16.53	3.13
22599	MARIE CALLENDER'S TURKEY W/GRAVY&DRSNG W/BROCCOLI, FRZ	127	7.82	13.06	2.29
02023	MARJORAM, DRIED	271	12.66	60.56	0.529
19303	MARMALADE, ORANGE	246	0.3	66.3	0
22676	MARQUEZ PRIMERA SHRED BF, GRN CHILI&MONT JACK CHS BURRIT	228	10.5	28.1	2.65
18613	MARTHA WHITE FOODS, MARTHA WHITE'S ART BLUEBERRY MUFFIN	404	5.1	76.1	2.141
18615	MARTHA WHITE FOODS, MARTHA WHITE'S BTTRMLK BISCUIT MIX, D	418	7.4	64.5	2.723
18614	MARTHA WHITE'S CHEWY FUDGE BRWNIE MIX, DRY	408	4.7	83	1.58
18612	MCKEE BAKING, LITTL DEBBI NUT BAR, WAFER W/PNUT BUTE, CHOC	548	8	55.2	6.29
16106	MEAT EXTENDER	313	38.11	38.32	0.424
09185	MELON BALLS, FROZEN	33	0.84	7.94	0.064
09181	MELONS, CANTALOUPE, RAW	35	0.88	8.36	0.071
09183	MELONS, CASABA, RAW	26	0.9	6.2	0.025
09184	MELONS, HONEYDEW, RAW	35	0.46	9.18	0.025
22608	MICHELINA'S SPAGHETTI, MEATBALL&POMODORO SAU, LOFAT FRZ	110	4.8	17.1	0.779
01110	MILK SHAKES, THICK CHOC	119	3.05	21.15	1.681
01111	MILK SHAKES, THICK VANILLA	112	3.86	17.75	1.886
01075	MILK SUBSTITUTES, FLUID W/HYDR VEG OILS	61	1.75	6.16	0.767
01076	MILK SUBSTITUTES, FLUID, W/LAURIC ACID OIL	61	1.75	6.16	3.037
01088	MILK, BTTRMLK, FLUID, CULTURED, LOWFAT	40	3.31	4.79	0.548
01094	MILK, BUTTERMILK, DRIED	387	34.3	49	3.598
01105	MILK, CHOC BEV, HOT COCOA, HOMEMADE	77	3.91	11.79	1.438
01102	MILK, CHOC, FLUID, COMM,	83	3.17	10.34	2.104
01104	MILK, CHOC, FLUID, COMM, LOWFAT	63	3.24	10.44	0.616
01103	MILK, CHOC, FLUID, COMM, RED FAT	72	3.21	10.4	1.239

NDB #	Food Description (100 gram portions = 3½ ounces = 20 tsp = ½ cup approx.	Calories	Protein	Carbs	Sat Fat
01095	MILK, CND, COND, SWTND	321	7.91	54.4	5.486
01097	MILK, CND, EVAP, NONFAT	78	7.55	11.35	0.121
01153	MILK, CND, EVAP, W/ VIT A	134	6.81	10.04	4.591
01096	MILK, CND, EVAP, WO/ VIT A	134	6.81	10.04	4.591
01093	MILK, DRY, NONFAT, CA RED	354	35.5	51.8	0.124
01092	MILK, DRY, NONFAT, INST, W/ VIT A	358	35.1	52.19	0.467
01155	MILK, DRY, NONFAT, INST, WO/ VIT A	358	35.1	52.19	0.47
01154	MILK, DRY, NONFAT, REG, W/ VIT A	362	36.16	51.98	0.499
01091	MILK, DRY, NONFAT, REG, WO/ VIT A	362	36.16	51.98	0.499
01090	MILK, DRY, WHOLE	496	26.32	38.42	16.742
01059	MILK, FILLED, FLUID, W/BLEND OF HYDR VEG OILS	63	3.33	4.74	0.768
01060	MILK, FILLED, FLUID, W/LAURIC ACID OIL	63	3.33	4.74	3.101
01077	MILK, FLUID, 3.25% MILKFAT	61	3.29	4.66	2.079
01106	MILK, GOAT, FLUID	69	3.56	4.45	2.667
01107	MILK, HUMAN, MATURE, FLUID	70	1.03	6.89	2.009
01108	MILK, INDIAN BUFFALO, FLUID	97	3.75	5.18	4.597
01089	MILK, LOW SODIUM, FLUID	61	3.1	4.46	2.154
01084	MILK, LOWFAT, FLUID, 1% MILKFAT, PROT FORT, W/ VIT A	48	3.93	5.52	0.728
01083	MILK, LOWFAT, FLUID, 1% MILKFAT, W/ NONFAT MILK SOL&VIT A	43	3.48	4.97	0.604
01082	MILK, LOWFAT, FLUID, 1% MILKFAT, W/ VIT A	42	3.29	4.78	0.66
01087	MILK, NONFAT, FLUID, PROT FORT, W/ VIT A (FAT FREE/SKIM)	41	3.96	5.56	0.162
01086	MILK, NONFAT, FLUID, W/ NONFAT MILK SOL&VIT A (FAT FREE/SKIM)	37	3.57	5.02	0.162
01085	MILK, NONFAT, FLUID, W/ VIT A (FAT FREE OR SKIM)	35	3.41	4.85	0.117
01151	MILK, NONFAT, FLUID, WO/ VIT A (FAT FREE OR SKIM)	35	3.41	4.85	0.117
01078	MILK, PRODUCER, FLUID, 3.7% MILKFAT	64	3.28	4.65	2.278
01081	MILK, RED FAT, FLUID, 2% MILKFAT, PROT FORT, W/ VIT A	56	3.95	5.49	1.232
01080	MILK, RED FAT, FLUID, 2% MILKFAT, W/ NONFAT MILK SOL&VIT A	51	3.48	4.97	1.195
01152	MILK, RED FAT, FLUID, 2% MILKFAT, W/ NONFAT MILK SOL, WO/ VIT A	56	3.95	5.49	1.232
01079	MILK, RED FAT, FLUID, 2% MILKFAT, W/ VIT A	50	3.33	4.8	1.195
01109	MILK, SHEEP, FLUID	108	5.98	5.36	4.603
15202	MILKFISH, COOKED, DRY HEAT	190	26.32	0	
15053	MILKFISH, RAW	148	20.53	0	1.66
20032	MILLET, COOKED	119	3.51	23.67	0.172
20031	MILLET, RAW	378	11.02	72.85	0.723
16112	MISO	206	11.81	27.96	0.878

NDB #	Food Description (100 gram portions = 3½ ounces = 20 tsp = ½ cup approx.	Calories	Protein	Carbs	Sat Fat
18616	MISSION FOODS, MISSION FLR TORTILLAS, SOFT TACO, 8 INCH	287	8.7	49.6	0.695
12635	MIXED NUTS, DRY RSTD, W/PNUTS, W/SALT	594	17.3	25.35	6.899
12135	MIXED NUTS, DRY RSTD, W/PNUTS, WO/SALT	594	17.3	25.35	6.899
12637	MIXED NUTS, OIL RSTD, W/PNUTS, W/SALT	617	16.76	21.41	8.725
12137	MIXED NUTS, OIL RSTD, W/PNUTS, WO/SALT	617	16.76	21.41	8.725
12138	MIXED NUTS, OIL RSTD, WO/PNUTS, WO/SALT	615	15.52	22.27	9.087
12638	MIXED NUTS, WO/PNUTS, OIL RSTD, W/SALT	615	15.52	22.27	9.087
19304	MOLASSES	266	0	68.8	0.018
19305	MOLASSES, BLACKSTRAP	235	0	60.8	0
15203	MONKFISH, COOKED, DRY HEAT	97	18.56	0	
15054	MONKFISH, RAW	76	14.48	0	0.34
16163	MORI-NU, TOFU, SILKEN, EX FIRM	55	7.4	2	0.3
16162	MORI-NU, TOFU, SILKEN, FIRM	62	6.9	2.4	0.406
16165	MORI-NU, TOFU, SILKEN, LITE EX FIRM	38	7	1	0.116
16161	MORI-NU, TOFU, SILKEN, SOFT	55	4.8	2.9	0.357
16164	MOR-NU, TOFU, SILKEN, LITE FIRM	37	6.3	1.1	0.133
07050	MORTADELLA, BEEF, PORK	311	16.37	3.05	9.51
16379	MOTHBEANS, MATURE SEEDS, CKD, BLD, W/SALT	117	7.81	20.96	0.124
16079	MOTHBEANS, MATURE SEEDS, CKD, BLD, WO/SALT	117	7.81	20.96	0.124
16078	MOTHBEANS, MATURE SEEDS, RAW	343	22.94	61.52	0.364
07061	MOTHER'S LOAF, PORK	282	12.07	7.53	7.95
11927	MOUNTAIN YAM, HAWAII, CKD, STMD, W/SALT	82	1.73	20	0.018
11259	MOUNTAIN YAM, HAWAII, CKD, STMD, WO/SALT	82	1.73	20	0.018
11258	MOUNTAIN YAM, HAWAII, RAW	67	1.34	16.31	0.022
22539	MRS PATERSON'S AUSSIE PIE, HAND HELD CHICK PIE, FRZ	278	9.4	25.5	4.6
18274	MUFFINS, BLUEBERRY, COMMLY PREP	277	5.5	48	1.397
18275	MUFFINS, BLUEBERRY, DRY MIX	366	4.9	63.2	2.489
18278	MUFFINS, BLUEBERRY, PREP FROM RECIPE, MADE W/LOFAT (2%) MI	285	6.5	40.7	2.03
18277	MUFFINS, BLUEBERRY, TOASTER-TYPE	313	4.6	53.3	1.398
18386	MUFFINS, BLUEBERRY, TOASTER-TYPE, TSTD	333	4.9	56.7	1.551
18279	MUFFINS, CORN, COMMLY PREP	305	5.9	50.9	1.354
18280	MUFFINS, CORN, DRY MIX, PREP	321	7.4	49.1	2.797
18282	MUFFINS, CORN, PREP FROM RECIPE, MADE W/LOFAT (2%) MILK	316	7.1	44.2	2.311
18281	MUFFINS, CORN, TOASTER-TYPE	346	5.3	57.9	1.681
18283	MUFFINS, OAT BRAN	270	7	48.3	1.087

NDB #	Food Description (100 gram portions = 3½ ounces = 20 tsp = ½ cup approx.	Calories	Protein	Carbs	Sat Fat
18273	MUFFINS, PLN, PREP FROM RECIPE, MADE W/LOFAT (2%) MILK	296	6.9	41.4	2.156
18284	MUFFINS, WHEAT BRAN, DRY MIX	396	7.1	73	2.939
18286	MUFFINS, WHEAT BRAN, TOASTER-TYPE W/RAISINS	295	5.2	52.2	1.357
18388	MUFFINS, WHEAT BRAN, TOASTER-TYPE W/RAISINS, TSTD	313	5.5	55.5	1.5
09190	MULBERRIES, RAW	43	1.44	9.8	0.027
15056	MULLET, STRIPED, CKD, DRY HEAT	150	24.81	0	1.431
15055	MULLET, STRIPED, RAW	117	19.35	0	1.116
16381	MUNG BNS, MATURE SEEDS, CKD, BLD, W/SALT	105	7.02	19.14	0.116
16081	MUNG BNS, MATURE SEEDS, CKD, BLD, WO/SALT	105	7.02	19.14	0.116
16080	MUNG BNS, MATURE SEEDS, RAW	347	23.86	62.62	0.348
11718	MUNG BNS, MATURE SEEDS, SPROUTED, CKD, BLD, DRND, W/SALT	21	2.03	4.19	0.025
11044	MUNG BNS, MATURE SEEDS, SPROUTED, CKD, BLD, DRND, WO/SAL	21	2.03	4.19	0.025
11045	MUNG BNS, MATURE SEEDS, SPROUTED, CKD, STIR-FRIED	50	4.3	10.59	0.039
11043	MUNG BNS, MATURE SEEDS, SPROUTED, RAW	30	3.04	5.93	0.046
16384	MUNGO BNS, MATURE SEEDS, CKD, BLD, W/SALT	105	7.54	18.34	0.038
16084	MUNGO BNS, MATURE SEEDS, CKD, BLD, WO/SALT	105	7.54	18.34	0.038
16083	MUNGO BNS, MATURE SEEDS, RAW	341	25.21	58.99	0.114
11987	MUSHROOM, OYSTER, RAW	37	4.14	6.22	
11266	MUSHROOMS, BROWN, ITALIAN, OR CRIMINI, RAW	22	2.5	4.12	0.014
11797	MUSHROOMS, CKD, BLD, DRND, W/SALT	27	2.17	5.14	0.061
11261	MUSHROOMS, CKD, BLD, DRND, WO/SALT	27	2.17	5.14	0.061
11264	MUSHROOMS, CND, DRND SOL	24	1.87	4.96	0.038
11950	MUSHROOMS, ENOKI, RAW	34	2.37	7.02	0.043
11265	MUSHROOMS, PORTABELLA, RAW	26	2.5	5.07	0.026
11260	MUSHROOMS, RAW	25	2.9	4.08	0.046
11798	MUSHROOMS, SHIITAKE, CKD, W/SALT	55	1.56	14.28	0.055
11269	MUSHROOMS, SHIITAKE, CKD, WO/SALT	55	1.56	14.28	0.055
11268	MUSHROOMS, SHIITAKE, DRIED	296	9.58	75.37	0.247
11989	MUSHROOMS, STRAW, CND, DRND SOL	32	3.83	4.65	0.089
15165	MUSSEL, BLUE, CKD, MOIST HEAT	172	23.8	7.39	0.85
15164	MUSSEL, BLUE, RAW	86	11.9	3.69	0.425
11270	MUSTARD GREENS, RAW	26	2.7	4.9	0.01
11799	MUSTARD GRNS, CKD, BLD, DRND, W/SALT	15	2.26	2.1	0.012
11271	MUSTARD GRNS, CKD, BLD, DRND, WO/SALT	15	2.26	2.1	0.012
11800	MUSTARD GRNS, FRZ, CKD, BLD, DRND, W/SALT	19	2.27	3.12	0.013

NDB #	Food Description (100 gram portions = 3½ ounces = 20 tsp = ½ cup approx.	Calories	Protein	Carbs	Sat Fat
11273	MUSTARD GRNS, FRZ, CKD, BLD, DRND, WO/SALT	19	2.27	3.12	0.013
11272	MUSTARD GRNS, FRZ, UNPREP	20	2.49	3.41	0.014
02024	MUSTARD SEED, YELLOW	469	24.94	34.94	1.46
11801	MUSTARD SPINACH, (TENDERGREEN), CKD, BLD, DRND, W/SALT	16	1.7	2.8	
11275	MUSTARD SPINACH, (TENDERGREEN), CKD, BLD, DRND, WO/SALT	16	1.7	2.8	
11274	MUSTARD SPINACH, (TENDERGREEN), RAW	22	2.2	3.9	0.015
02046	MUSTARD, PREPARED, YELLOW	66	3.95	7.78	0.158
14119	MXD VEG&FRUIT JUC DRK	110	0.22	28	0.006
14118	NABISCO, KNOX DRINKING GELATIN, ORANGE FLVR, W/ASPRT, LO C	375	67.2	24.91	0.45
18617	NABISCO, NABISCO GRAHAMS CRACKERS	424	6.99	76.2	1.56
18618	NABISCO, NABISCO NILLA PIE CRUST, READY TO USE	513	3.5	63.1	5.15
18619	NABISCO, NABISCO OREO CRUNCHIES, COOKIE CRUMB TOPPING	476	4.78	70.23	4.14
18620	NABISCO, NABISCO ORIGINAL PREMIUM SALTINE CRACKERS	420	10.9	71.1	1.85
18621	NABISCO, NABISCO RITZ CRACKERS	492	7.2	64.2	3.92
18650	NABISCO, NABISCO SNACKWELL'S CARAMEL DELIGHTS COOKIES	383	4.5	69.85	2.734
18645	NABISCO, NABISCO SNACKWELL'S CRACKED PEPPER CRACKER	439	9.26	74.69	1.959
18651	NABISCO, NABISCO SNACKWELL'S FAT FREE DEVIL'S FD COOKIE CA	305	5	74.25	0.427
18648	NABISCO, NABISCO SNACKWELL'S FRENCH ONION SNACK CRACKE	428	7.14	77	1.802
18647	NABISCO, NABISCO SNACKWELL'S ITALIAN RANCH SNACK CRACKER	428	7.07	77.77	2
18649	NABISCO, NABISCO SNACKWELL'S MINT CREME COOKIES	432	3.8	75.95	3.48
18646	NABISCO, NABISCO SNACKWELL'S SALSA SNACK CRACKERS	427	7	77.84	1.811
18652	NABISCO, NABISCO SNACKWELL'S WHEAT CRACKER	415	7.94	77	
18622	NABISCO, NABISCO SNACKWELL'S ZESTY CHS CRACKERS	431	7.45	77	2.239
18624	NABISCO, NABISCO WHEAT THINS CRACKERS, BKD	470	8.3	69.1	3.19
22513	NALLEY CHILI CON CARNE W/BNS, CND ENTREE	109	15.6	4.6	1.08
16113	NATTO	212	17.72	14.35	1.591
09191	NECTARINES, RAW	49	0.94	11.78	0.051
22215	NESTLE, CHEF-MATE CHILI W/BNS, CND	163	7.01	11.48	4.32
22216	NESTLE, CHEF-MATE CHILI WO/BNS, CND	172	7.42	7.04	5.75
22217	NESTLE, CHEF-MATE CORNED BF HASH, CND	192	9.58	11.49	5.3
14137	NESTLE, NESTEA ICE TEA, LEMON FLAVOR, RTD	37	0	8.5	0.024
07091	NEW ENGLAND BRAND SAUSAGE, PORK, BF	161	17.27	4.83	2.56
11802	NEW ZEALAND SPINACH, CKD, BLD, DRND, W/SALT	12	1.3	2.2	0.027
11277	NEW ZEALAND SPINACH, CKD, BLD, DRND, WO/SALT	12	1.3	2.2	0.027
11276	NEW ZEALAND SPINACH, RAW	14	1.5	2.5	0.032

NDB #	Food Description (100 gram portions = 3½ ounces = 20 tsp = ½ cup approx.	Calories	Protein	Carbs	Sat Fat
16082	NOODLES, CHINESE, CELLOPHANE OR LONG RICE (MUNG BNS), DE	351	0.16	86.1	0.017
20113	NOODLES, CHINESE, CHOW MEIN	527	8.38	57.54	4.384
20110	NOODLES, EGG, CKD, ENR	133	4.75	24.84	0.31
20310	NOODLES, EGG, CKD, ENR, W/ SALT	133	4.75	24.84	0.31
20510	NOODLES, EGG, CKD, UNENR, W/ SALT	133	4.75	24.84	0.31
20410	NOODLES, EGG, CKD, UNENR, WO/ SALT	133	4.75	24.84	0.31
20109	NOODLES, EGG, DRY, ENRICHED	381	14.02	71.13	0.889
20409	NOODLES, EGG, DRY, UNENR	381	14.02	71.13	0.889
20112	NOODLES, EGG, SPINACH, CKD, ENR	132	5.04	24.25	0.361
20111	NOODLES, EGG, SPINACH, DRY, ENR	382	14.61	70.32	1.047
20115	NOODLES, JAPANESE, SOBA, CKD	99	5.06	21.44	0.019
20114	NOODLES, JAPANESE, SOBA, DRY	336	14.38	74.62	0.136
20117	NOODLES, JAPANESE, SOMEN, CKD	131	4	27.54	0.025
20116	NOODLES, JAPANESE, SOMEN, DRY	356	11.35	74.1	0.115
11964	NOPALES, CKD, WO/SALT	15	1.35	3.27	0.006
11963	NOPALES, RAW	16	1.28	3.39	0.016
02025	NUTMEG, GROUND	525	5.84	49.29	25.94
12087	NUTS, CASHEW NUTS, RAW	566	18.22	27.13	8.328
20034	OAT BRAN, COOKED	40	3.21	11.44	0.163
20033	OAT BRAN, RAW	246	17.3	66.22	1.328
20038	OATS	389	16.89	66.27	1.217
15058	OCEAN PERCH, ATLANTIC, CKD, DRY HEAT	121	23.88	0	0.313
15057	OCEAN PERCH, ATLANTIC, RAW	94	18.62	0	0.244
15230	OCTOPUS, COMMON, CKD, MOIST HEAT	164	29.82	4.4	0.453
15166	OCTOPUS, COMMON, RAW	82	14.91	2.2	0.227
09192	OHELOBERRIES, RAW	28	0.38	6.84	
04053	OIL, OLIVE, SALAD OR COOKING	884	0	0	13.5
04042	OIL, PNUT, SALAD OR COOKING	884	0	0	16.9
04058	OIL, SESAME, SALAD OR COOKING	884	0	0	14.2
04044	OIL, SOYBN, SALAD OR COOKING	884	0	0	14.4
04034	OIL, SOYBN, SALAD OR COOKING, (HYDR)	884	0	0	14.9
04543	OIL, SOYBN, SALAD OR COOKING, (HYDR)&CTTNSD	884	0	0	18
04518	OIL, VEG CORN, SALAD OR COOKING	884	0	0	12.7
04510	OIL, VEG SAFFLOWER, SALAD OR COOKING, LINOLEIC, (OVER 70%)	884	0	0	6.203
04511	OIL, VEG SAFFLOWER, SALAD OR COOKING, OLEIC, OVER 70%	884	0	0	6.203

NDB #	Food Description (100 gram portions = 3½ ounces = 20 tsp = ½ cup approx.	Calories	Protein	Carbs	Sat Fat
04530	OIL, VEG, APRICOT KERNEL	884	0	0	6.3
04501	OIL, VEG, COCOA BUTTER	884	0	0	59.7
04502	OIL, VEG, CTTNSD, SALAD OR COOKING	884	0	0	25.9
04572	OIL, VEG, NUTMEG BUTTER	884	0	0	90
04060	OIL, VEG, SUNFLOWER, LINOLEIC (LESS THAN 60%)	884	0	0	10.1
04506	OIL, VEG, SUNFLOWER, LINOLEIC, (60%&OVER)	884	0	0	10.3
04545	OIL, VEG, SUNFLOWER, LINOLEIC, (HYDR)	884	0	0	13
04573	OIL, VEG, UCUHUBA BUTTER	884	0	0	85.2
04529	OIL, VEGETABLE, ALMOND	884	0	0	8.2
04534	OIL, VEGETABLE, BABASSU	884	0	0	81.2
04541	OIL, VEGETABLE, CUPU ASSU	884	0	0	53.2
04517	OIL, VEGETABLE, GRAPESEED	884	0	0	9.6
04532	OIL, VEGETABLE, HAZELNUT	884	0	0	7.4
04055	OIL, VEGETABLE, PALM	884	0	0	49.3
04514	OIL, VEGETABLE, POPPYSEED	884	0	0	13.5
04037	OIL, VEGETABLE, RICE BRAN	884	0	0	19.7
04536	OIL, VEGETABLE, SHEANUT	884	0	0	46.6
04516	OIL, VEGETABLE, TEASEED	884	0	0	21.1
04515	OIL, VEGETABLE, TOMATOSEED	884	0	0	19.7
04528	OIL, VEGETABLE, WALNUT	884	0	0	9.1
04038	OIL, WHEAT GERM	884	0	0	18.8
11803	OKRA, CKD, BLD, DRND, W/SALT	32	1.87	7.21	0.045
11279	OKRA, CKD, BLD, DRND, WO/SALT	32	1.87	7.21	0.045
11280	OKRA, FROZEN, UNPREPARED	30	1.69	6.64	0.065
11804	OKRA, FRZ, CKD, BLD, DRND, W/SALT	28	2.08	5.75	0.079
11281	OKRA, FRZ, CKD, BLD, DRND, WO/SALT	28	2.08	5.75	0.079
11278	OKRA, RAW	33	2	7.63	0.026
22514	OLD EL PASO CHILI W/BNS, CND ENTREE	109	7.7	9.5	0.904
07051	OLIVE LOAF, PORK	235	11.8	9.2	5.85
09194	OLIVES, RIPE, CND (JUMBO-SUPER COLOSSAL)	81	0.97	5.61	0.909
09193	OLIVES, RIPE, CND (SMALL-EXTRA LRG)	115	0.84	6.26	1.415
02026	ONION POWDER	347	10.12	80.67	0.183
11296	ONION RINGS, BREADED, PAR FR, FRZ, PREP, HTD IN OVEN	407	5.34	38.16	8.585
11295	ONION RINGS, BREADED, PAR FR, FRZ, UNPREP	258	3.15	30.53	4.534
11805	ONIONS, CKD, BLD, DRND, W/SALT	44	1.36	10.15	0.031

NDB #	Food Description (100 gram portions = 3½ ounces = 20 tsp = ½ cup approx.	Calories	Protein	Carbs	Sat Fat
11283	ONIONS, CKD, BLD, DRND, WO/SALT	44	1.36	10.15	0.031
11285	ONIONS, CND, SOL&LIQUIDS	19	0.85	4.01	0.016
11284	ONIONS, DEHYDRATED FLAKES	349	8.95	83.28	0.078
11806	ONIONS, FRZ, CHOPD, CKD, BLD, DRND, W/SALT	28	0.77	6.6	0.016
11288	ONIONS, FRZ, CHOPD, CKD, BLD, DRND, WO/SALT	28	0.77	6.6	0.016
11287	ONIONS, FRZ, CHOPD, UNPREP	29	0.79	6.81	0.017
11807	ONIONS, FRZ, WHL, CKD, BLD, DRND, W/SALT	28	0.71	6.7	0.009
11290	ONIONS, FRZ, WHL, CKD, BLD, DRND, WO/SALT	28	0.71	6.7	0.009
11289	ONIONS, FRZ, WHL, UNPREP	35	0.89	8.44	0.011
11282	ONIONS, RAW	38	1.16	8.63	0.026
11291	ONIONS, SPRING OR SCALLIONS (INCL TOPS&BULB), RAW	32	1.83	7.34	0.032
11293	ONIONS, WELSH, RAW	34	1.9	6.5	0.067
14323	ORANGE DRINK, CANNED	51	0	12.9	0.002
14426	ORANGE DRK, BRKFST TYPE, W/JUC&PULP, FRZ CONC	153	0.4	39	0.002
14427	ORANGE DRK, BRKFST TYPE, W/JUC&PULP, FRZ CONC, PREP W/H2O	45	0.1	11.3	0.001
09406	ORANGE JUC, CALIFORNIA, CHILLED, INCL FROM CONC	44	0.8	10.06	0.029
09209	ORANGE JUC, CHILLED, INCL FROM CONC	44	0.8	10.06	0.029
09207	ORANGE JUC, CND, UNSWTND	42	0.59	9.85	0.018
09215	ORANGE JUC, FRZ CONC, UNSWTND, DIL W/3 VOLUME H2O	45	0.68	10.78	0.007
09214	ORANGE JUC, FRZ CONC, UNSWTND, UNDIL	159	2.39	38.17	0.024
09206	ORANGE JUICE, RAW	45	0.7	10.4	0.024
09216	ORANGE PEEL, RAW	97	1.5	25	0.024
14327	ORANGE&APRICOT JUC DRK, CND	51	0.3	12.7	0.01
14409	ORANGE-FLAVOR DRK, BRKFST TYPE, LO CAL, PDR	217	3.6	85.9	0
14407	ORANGE-FLAVOR DRK, BRKFST TYPE, PDR	366	0	91.5	0
14408	ORANGE-FLAVOR DRK, BRKFST TYPE, PDR, PREP W/ H2O	47	0	11.7	0
14424	ORANGE-FLAVOR DRK, BRKFST TYPE, W/PULP, FRZ CONC	172	0.1	42.9	0.078
14425	ORANGE-FLAVOR DRK, BRKFST TYPE, W/PULP, FRZ CONC, PREP W/	49	0	12.2	0.022
14403	ORANGE-FLAVOR DRK, KRAFT, TANG DRK MIX	366	0	98.4	0
14404	ORANGE-FLAVOR DRK, KRAFT, TANG SUGAR FREE LO CAL DRK MIX	217	3.6	85.9	0
09217	ORANGE-GRAPEFRUIT JUC, CND, UNSWTND	43	0.6	10.28	0.011
09200	ORANGES, RAW, ALL COMM VAR	47	0.94	11.75	0.015
09202	ORANGES, RAW, CALIFORNIA, NAVELS	46	1.03	11.63	0.011
09201	ORANGES, RAW, CALIFORNIA, VALENCIAS	49	1.04	11.89	0.035
09203	ORANGES, RAW, FLORIDA	46	0.7	11.54	0.025

NDB #	Food Description (100 gram portions = 3½ ounces = 20 tsp = ½ cup approx.	Calories	Protein	Carbs	Sat Fat
09205	ORANGES, RAW, WITH PEEL	63	1.3	15.5	0.035
02027	OREGANO, GROUND	306	11	64.43	2.66
19031	ORIENTAL MIX, RICE-BASED	549	17.31	51.62	3.785
07205	OSCAR MAYER BOLOGNA LIGHT (PORK CHICK BEEF)	201	11.5	5.65	5.62
07209	OSCAR MAYER CHICKEN BREAST (HONEY GLAZED)	109	19.85	3.95	0.394
07211	OSCAR MAYER HAM & CHEESE LOAF	234	13.85	3.75	6.561
07213	OSCAR MAYER HAM (WATER ADDED BKD CKD 96% FAT FREE)	104	16.3	1.83	0.851
07233	OSCAR MAYER SMOKIES (BEEF)	296	12.25	1.9	11.25
07242	OSCAR MAYER WIENERS (BEEF FRANKS BUN LENGTH)	327	11.1	2.8	12.53
07202	OSCAR MAYER, BOLOGNA (BEEF LIGHT)	200	11.75	5.55	5.82
07201	OSCAR MAYER, BOLOGNA (BEEF)	316	11.05	2.45	12.85
07200	OSCAR MAYER, BOLOGNA (CHICK, PORK, BF)	318	10.9	2.4	10.49
07203	OSCAR MAYER, BOLOGNA (FAT FREE)	79	12.6	6	0.235
07208	OSCAR MAYER, BRAUNSCHWEIGER LIVER SAUSAGE (SAREN TUBE)	341	14.2	2.3	10.89
07207	OSCAR MAYER, BRAUNSCHWEIGER LIVER SAUSAGE (SLICED)	331	14.25	2.55	10.94
07210	OSCAR MAYER, CHICK BREAST (OVEN RSTD, FAT FREE)	85	18.3	1.7	0.17
07217	OSCAR MAYER, HAM (40%HAM/WATER PRODUCT, SMOKED, FAT FRE	72	14.6	1.9	0.221
07212	OSCAR MAYER, HAM (CHOPPED W/ NAT JUICE)	180	16.3	3.65	4.056
07214	OSCAR MAYER, HAM (H2O , BLD)	104	16.6	1.2	1.247
07215	OSCAR MAYER, HAM (H2O , HONEY)	111	16.7	3.1	1.167
07216	OSCAR MAYER, HAM (H2O , SMOKED, CKD)	99	16.6	0.1	1.222
07218	OSCAR MAYER, HEAD CHEESE	185	15.7	0	4.299
07220	OSCAR MAYER, LIVER CHS (PORK FAT WRAPPED)	299	15.45	2.05	9.3
07221	OSCAR MAYER, LUNCHEON LOAF (SPICED)	234	13.5	7	5.367
07222	OSCAR MAYER, OLD FASHIONED LOAF	231	13.1	8	5.6
07223	OSCAR MAYER, OLIVE LOAF (CHICK, PORK, TURKEY)	263	9.9	6.9	7.02
07224	OSCAR MAYER, PICKLE PIMIENTO LOAF (W/CHICK)	269	9.6	9.1	6.99
07225	OSCAR MAYER, PORK SAUSAGE LINKS (CKD)	343	16.3	1	10.69
07228	OSCAR MAYER, SALAMI (FOR BEER)	225	13.5	1.9	6.388
07229	OSCAR MAYER, SALAMI (GENOA)	388	20.7	1.2	12.04
07230	OSCAR MAYER, SALAMI (HARD)	368	25.9	1.6	11.085
07226	OSCAR MAYER, SALAMI BF COTTO	206	14.2	1.9	6.74
07227	OSCAR MAYER, SALAMI COTTO (BF, PORK, CHICK)	245	13.4	2.2	8.47
07237	OSCAR MAYER, SMMR SAUSAGE BF THURINGER CERVELAT	309	14.6	1.9	11.8
07238	OSCAR MAYER, SMMR SAUSAGE THURINGER CERVALAT	304	14.9	0.9	10.727

NDB #	Food Description (100 gram portions = 3½ ounces = 20 tsp = ½ cup approx.	Calories	Protein	Carbs	Sat Fat
07232	OSCAR MAYER, SMOKIE LINKS SAUSAGE	302	12.4	1.7	9.38
07234	OSCAR MAYER, SMOKIES (CHS)	303	12.9	1.8	10.16
07235	OSCAR MAYER, SMOKIES SAUSAGE LITTLE (PORK, TURKEY)	301	12.4	1.8	9.444
07236	OSCAR MAYER, SMOKIES SAUSAGE LITTLE CHS (PORK, TURKEY)	315	13.5	1.7	11.16
07231	OSCAR MAYER, SNDWCH SPRD (PORK, CHICK, BF)	237	6.5	15.4	5.754
07239	OSCAR MAYER, TURKEY BREAST (SMOKED, FAT FREE)	80	14.9	3.6	0.18
07241	OSCAR MAYER, WIENERS (BEEF FRANKS)	327	11.35	2.35	12.46
07243	OSCAR MAYER, WIENERS (BEEF FRANKS, FAT FREE)	78	13.2	5.1	0.225
07244	OSCAR MAYER, WIENERS (BEEF FRANKS, LIGHT)	193	10.7	4.1	6.32
07245	OSCAR MAYER, WIENERS (CHEESE HOT DOGS W/ TURKEY)	318	12	2.8	10.025
07246	OSCAR MAYER, WIENERS (FAT FREE HOT DOGS)	73	12.6	4.3	0.2
07247	OSCAR MAYER, WIENERS (LIGHT PORK, TURKEY, BEEF)	194	12.1	2.8	5.199
07240	OSCAR MAYER, WIENERS (PORK, TURKEY)	324	10.95	2.65	9.467
07248	OSCAR MAYER, WIENERS LITTLE (PORK, TURKEY)	311	10.9	2.3	11.15
07206	OSCAR MAYER. BOLOGNA (WISCONSIN MADE RING)	313	11.8	2.6	11.14
05643	OSTRICH, FAN, RAW	117	21.81	0	0.95
05642	OSTRICH, GROUND, CKD, PAN-BROILED	175	26.15	0	1.793
05641	OSTRICH, GROUND, RAW	165	20.22	0	2.177
05645	OSTRICH, INSIDE LEG, CKD	141	29.01	0	0.7
05644	OSTRICH, INSIDE LEG, RAW	111	22.39	0	0.6
05647	OSTRICH, INSIDE STRIP, CKD	164	29.37	0	1.71
05646	OSTRICH, INSIDE STRIP, RAW	127	23.69	0	0.923
05648	OSTRICH, OUTSIDE LEG, RAW	115	22.86	0	0.61
05650	OSTRICH, OUTSIDE STRIP, CKD	156	28.55	0	1.43
05649	OSTRICH, OUTSIDE STRIP, RAW	120	23.36	0	0.771
05652	OSTRICH, OYSTER, CKD	159	28.81	0	1.69
05651	OSTRICH, OYSTER, RAW	125	21.55	0	
05653	OSTRICH, RND, RAW	116	21.99	0	0.81
05654	OSTRICH, TENDERLOIN, RAW	123	22.07	0	1.17
05656	OSTRICH, TIP CKD	145	28.49	0	1
05655	OSTRICH, TIP RAW	114	21.85	0	0.86
05658	OSTRICH, TOP LOIN, CKD	155	28.12	0	1.32
05657	OSTRICH, TOP LOIN, RAW	119	21.67	0	1.2
07935	OVEN-ROASTED CHICK BREAST ROLL	134	14.59	1.79	2.48
15170	OYSTER, EASTERN, CANNED	69	7.06	3.91	0.631

NDB #	Food Description (100 gram portions = 3½ ounces = 20 tsp = ½ cup approx.	Calories	Protein	Carbs	Sat Fat
15168	OYSTER, EASTERN, CKD, BREADED&FRIED	197	8.77	11.62	3.197
15246	OYSTER, EASTERN, FARMED, CKD, DRY HEAT	79	7	7.28	0.683
15245	OYSTER, EASTERN, FARMED, RAW	59	5.22	5.53	0.443
15244	OYSTER, EASTERN, WILD, CKD, DRY HEAT	72	8.25	4.8	0.55
15169	OYSTER, EASTERN, WILD, CKD, MOIST HEAT	137	14.1	7.82	1.544
15167	OYSTER, EASTERN, WILD, RAW	68	7.05	3.91	0.772
15231	OYSTER, PACIFIC, CKD, MOIST HEAT	163	18.9	9.9	1.02
15171	OYSTER, PACIFIC, RAW	81	9.45	4.95	0.51
18288	PANCAKES PLN, FRZ, RTH (INCL BTTRMLK)	229	5.2	43.6	0.767
18294	PANCAKES, BLUEBERRY, PREP FROM RECIPE	222	6.1	29	1.986
18390	PANCAKES, BTTRMLK, PREP FROM RECIPE	227	6.8	28.7	1.832
18295	PANCAKES, BUCKWHEAT, DRY MIX, INCOMPLETE	340	10.9	71.3	0.439
18289	PANCAKES, PLN, DRY MIX, COMPLETE (INCL BTTRMLK)	376	10.1	71.3	0.984
18290	PANCAKES, PLN, DRY MIX, COMPLETE, PREP	194	5.2	36.7	0.507
18291	PANCAKES, PLN, DRY MIX, INCOMPLETE (INCL BTTRMLK)	355	10	73.6	0.25
18292	PANCAKES, PLN, DRY MIX, INCOMPLETE, PREP	218	7.8	28.9	2.045
18293	PANCAKES, PLN, PREP FROM RECIPE	227	6.4	28.3	2.122
18297	PANCAKES, SPL DIETARY, DRY MIX	349	8.9	73.9	0.202
18299	PANCAKES, WHOLE-WHEAT, DRY MIX, INCOMPLETE	344	12.8	71	0.244
18300	PANCAKES, WHOLE-WHEAT, DRY MIX, INCOMPLETE, PREP	208	8.5	29.4	1.749
09229	PAPAYA NECTAR, CANNED	57	0.17	14.51	0.047
09226	PAPAYAS, RAW	39	0.61	9.81	0.043
22548	PAPPALO'S FOR ONE, DEEP DISH PEPPERONI PIZZA, FRZ	264	11.4	32.5	3.69
02028	PAPRIKA	289	14.76	55.74	2.1
02029	PARSLEY, DRIED	276	22.42	51.66	0.115
11625	PARSLEY, FREEZE-DRIED	271	31.3	42.38	
11297	PARSLEY, RAW	36	2.97	6.33	0.132
11808	PARSNIPS, CKD, BLD, DRND, W/SALT	81	1.32	19.53	0.05
11299	PARSNIPS, CKD, BLD, DRND, WO/SALT	81	1.32	19.53	0.05
11298	PARSNIPS, RAW	75	1.2	17.99	0.05
09232	PASSION-FRUIT JUC, PURPLE, RAW	51	0.39	13.6	0.004
09233	PASSION-FRUIT JUC, YEL, RAW	60	0.67	14.45	0.015
09231	PASSION-FRUIT, (GRANADILLA), PURPLE, RAW	97	2.2	23.38	0.059
22907	PASTA W/MEATBALLS IN TOMATO SAU, CND ENTREE	103	4.32	12.29	1.59
22522	PASTA W/SLICED FRANKS IN TOMATO SAU, CND ENTREE	104	3.7	11.9	1.47

NDB #	Food Description (100 gram portions = 3½ ounces = 20 tsp = ½ cup approx.	Calories	Protein	Carbs	Sat Fat
20092	PASTA, CORN, COOKED	126	2.63	27.91	0.102
20091	PASTA, CORN, DRY	357	7.46	79.26	0.29
20093	PASTA, FRESH-REFRIGERATED, PLN, AS PURCHASED	288	11.31	54.73	0.328
20094	PASTA, FRESH-REFRIGERATED, PLN, CKD	131	5.15	24.93	0.15
20095	PASTA, FRESH-REFRIGERATED, SPINACH, AS PURCHASED	289	11.26	55.72	0.483
20096	PASTA, FRESH-REFRIGERATED, SPINACH, CKD	130	5.06	25.04	0.217
20097	PASTA, HOMEMADE, MADE W/EGG, CKD	130	5.28	23.54	0.408
20098	PASTA, HOMEMADE, MADE WO/EGG, CKD	124	4.37	25.12	0.14
07925	PASTRAMI BF 98% FAT-FREE	95	19.6	1.54	0
07052	PASTRAMI, TURKEY	141	18.36	1.66	1.81
07942	PATE TRUFFLE FLAVOR	327	11.2	6.3	10.1
05282	PATE DE FOIE GRAS, CND (GOOSE LIVER PATE), SMOKED	462	11.4	4.67	14.45
07053	PATE, CHICKEN LIVER, CANNED	201	13.45	6.55	4
07054	PATE, GOOSE LIVER, SMOKED, CND	462	11.4	4.67	14.45
07055	PATE, LIVER, NOT SPECIFIED, CND	319	14.2	1.5	9.57
22584	PATIO BF&BEAN BURRITO W/GRN CHILI, MILD, FRZ	232	7.09	31.7	2.85
22586	PATIO MEX STY DIN, TAMALE, BF ENCHLDA&CHILI SAU, BNS&RICE, F	135	3.7	18.2	1.8
09407	PEACH NECTAR, CND, W/ VIT C	54	0.27	13.92	0.002
09251	PEACH NECTAR, CND, WO/ VIT C	54	0.27	13.92	0.002
09242	PEACHES, CND, EX HVY SYRUP PK, SOL&LIQUIDS	96	0.47	26.06	0.003
09239	PEACHES, CND, EX LT SYRUP, SOL&LIQUIDS	42	0.4	11.1	0.011
09237	PEACHES, CND, H2O PK, SOL&LIQUIDS	24	0.44	6.11	0.006
09241	PEACHES, CND, HVY SYRUP PK, SOL&LIQUIDS	74	0.45	19.94	0.01
09238	PEACHES, CND, JUC PK, SOL&LIQUIDS	44	0.63	11.57	0.004
09240	PEACHES, CND, LT SYRUP PK, SOL&LIQUIDS	54	0.45	14.55	0.003
09245	PEACHES, DEHYD (LOW-MOISTURE), SULFURED, STWD	133	2.01	34.14	0.045
09244	PEACHES, DEHYD (LOW-MOISTURE), SULFURED, UNCKD	325	4.89	83.18	0.111
09248	PEACHES, DRIED, SULFURED, STWD, W/ SUGAR	103	1.06	26.6	0.024
09247	PEACHES, DRIED, SULFURED, STWD, WO/ SUGAR	77	1.16	19.69	0.026
09246	PEACHES, DRIED, SULFURED, UNCKD	239	3.61	61.33	0.082
09250	PEACHES, FRZ, SLICED, SWTND	94	0.63	23.98	0.014
09236	PEACHES, RAW	43	0.7	11.1	0.01
09243	PEACHES, SPICED, CND, HVY SYRUP PK, SOL&LIQUIDS	75	0.41	20.08	0.011
16097	PEANUT BUTTER, CHUNK STYLE, W/SALT	589	24.05	21.59	9.58
16397	PEANUT BUTTER, CHUNK STYLE, WO/SALT	589	24.05	21.59	9.58

NDB #	Food Description (100 gram portions = 3½ ounces = 20 tsp = ½ cup approx.	Calories	Protein	Carbs	Sat Fat
16098	PEANUT BUTTER, SMOOTH STYLE, W/SALT	593	25.21	19.28	10.344
16398	PEANUT BUTTER, SMOOTH STYLE, WO/SALT	593	25.21	19.28	10.344
16099	PEANUT FLOUR, DEFATTED	327	52.2	34.7	0.063
16100	PEANUT FLOUR, LOW FAT	428	33.8	31.27	3.04
16088	PEANUTS, ALL TYPES, CKD, BLD, W/SALT	318	13.5	21.26	3.055
16090	PEANUTS, ALL TYPES, DRY-ROASTED, W/SALT	585	23.68	21.51	6.893
16390	PEANUTS, ALL TYPES, DRY-ROASTED, WO/SALT	585	23.68	21.51	6.893
16089	PEANUTS, ALL TYPES, OIL-ROASTED, W/SALT	581	26.35	18.93	6.843
16389	PEANUTS, ALL TYPES, OIL-ROASTED, WO/SALT	581	26.35	18.93	6.843
16087	PEANUTS, ALL TYPES, RAW	567	25.8	16.14	6.834
16092	PEANUTS, SPANISH, OIL-ROASTED, W/SALT	579	28.01	17.45	7.555
16392	PEANUTS, SPANISH, OIL-ROASTED, WO/SALT	579	28.01	17.45	7.555
16091	PEANUTS, SPANISH, RAW	570	26.15	15.82	7.642
16094	PEANUTS, VALENCIA, OIL-ROASTED, W/SALT	589	27.04	16.3	7.894
16394	PEANUTS, VALENCIA, OIL-ROASTED, WO/SALT	589	27.04	16.3	7.894
16093	PEANUTS, VALENCIA, RAW	570	25.09	20.91	7.329
16096	PEANUTS, VIRGINIA, OIL-ROASTED, W/SALT	578	25.87	19.86	6.345
16396	PEANUTS, VIRGINIA, OIL-ROASTED, WO/SALT	578	25.87	19.86	6.345
16095	PEANUTS, VIRGINIA, RAW	563	25.19	16.54	6.361
09408	PEAR NECTAR, CND, W/ VIT C	60	0.11	15.76	0.001
09262	PEAR NECTAR, CND, WO/ VIT C	60	0.11	15.76	0.001
09340	PEARS, ASIAN, RAW	42	0.5	10.65	0.012
09258	PEARS, CND, EX HVY SYRUP PK, SOL&LIQUIDS	97	0.19	25.25	0.007
09255	PEARS, CND, EX LT SYRUP PK, SOL&LIQUIDS	47	0.3	12.2	0.006
09253	PEARS, CND, H2O PK, SOL&LIQUIDS	29	0.19	7.81	0.002
09257	PEARS, CND, HVY SYRUP PK, SOL&LIQUIDS	74	0.2	19.17	0.007
09254	PEARS, CND, JUC PK, SOL&LIQUIDS	50	0.34	12.94	0.004
09256	PEARS, CND, LT SYRUP PK, SOL&LIQUIDS	57	0.19	15.17	0.002
09261	PEARS, DRIED, SULFURED, STWD, W/ SUGAR	140	0.86	37.14	0.016
09260	PEARS, DRIED, SULFURED, STWD, WO/ SUGAR	127	0.91	33.81	0.017
09259	PEARS, DRIED, SULFURED, UNCKD	262	1.87	69.7	0.035
09252	PEARS, RAW	59	0.39	15.11	0.022
11816	PEAS&CARROTS, CND, NO SALT, SOL&LIQUIDS	38	2.17	8.48	0.049
11318	PEAS&CARROTS, CND, REG PK, SOL&LIQUIDS	38	2.17	8.48	0.049
11817	PEAS&CARROTS, FRZ, CKD, BLD, DRND, W/SALT	48	3.09	10.12	0.077

NDB #	Food Description (100 gram portions = 3½ ounces = 20 tsp = ½ cup approx.	Calories	Protein	Carbs	Sat Fat
11323	PEAS&CARROTS, FRZ, CKD, BLD, DRND, WO/SALT	48	3.09	10.12	0.077
11322	PEAS&CARROTS, FRZ, UNPREP	53	3.4	11.15	0.084
11324	PEAS&ONIONS, CND, SOL&LIQUIDS	51	3.28	8.57	0.068
11818	PEAS&ONIONS, FRZ, CKD, BLD, DRND, W/SALT	45	2.54	8.63	0.036
11327	PEAS&ONIONS, FRZ, CKD, BLD, DRND, WO/SALT	45	2.54	8.63	0.036
11326	PEAS&ONIONS, FRZ, UNPREP	70	3.98	13.51	0.057
11809	PEAS, EDIBLE-PODDED, CKD, BLD, DRND, W/SALT	42	3.27	7.05	0.044
11301	PEAS, EDIBLE-PODDED, CKD, BLD, DRND, WO/SALT	42	3.27	7.05	0.044
11810	PEAS, EDIBLE-PODDED, FRZ, CKD, BLD, DRND, W/SALT	52	3.5	9.02	0.073
11303	PEAS, EDIBLE-PODDED, FRZ, CKD, BLD, DRND, WO/SALT	52	3.5	9.02	0.073
11302	PEAS, EDIBLE-PODDED, FRZ, UNPREP	42	2.8	7.2	0.058
11300	PEAS, EDIBLE-PODDED, RAW	42	2.8	7.56	0.039
11304	PEAS, GREEN, RAW	81	5.42	14.46	0.071
11811	PEAS, GRN, CKD, BLD, DRND, W/SALT	84	5.36	15.64	0.039
11305	PEAS, GRN, CKD, BLD, DRND, WO/SALT	84	5.36	15.64	0.039
11813	PEAS, GRN, CND, NO SALT, DRND SOL	69	4.42	12.58	0.062
11812	PEAS, GRN, CND, NO SALT, SOL&LIQUIDS	53	3.19	9.75	0.054
11308	PEAS, GRN, CND, REG PK, DRND SOL	69	4.42	12.58	0.062
11306	PEAS, GRN, CND, REG PK, SOL&LIQUIDS	53	3.19	9.75	0.05
11310	PEAS, GRN, CND, SEASONED, SOL&LIQUIDS	50	3.09	9.25	0.048
11814	PEAS, GRN, FRZ, CKD, BLD, DRND, W/SALT	78	5.15	14.26	0.049
11313	PEAS, GRN, FRZ, CKD, BLD, DRND, WO/SALT	78	5.15	14.26	0.049
11312	PEAS, GRN, FRZ, UNPREP	77	5.21	13.7	0.066
11815	PEAS, MATURE SEEDS, SPROUTED, CKD, BLD, DRND, W/SALT	118	7.05	21.86	0.09
11317	PEAS, MATURE SEEDS, SPROUTED, CKD, BLD, DRND, WO/SALT	118	7.05	21.86	0.09
11316	PEAS, MATURE SEEDS, SPROUTED, RAW	128	8.8	28.26	0.124
16386	PEAS, SPLIT, MATURE SEEDS, CKD, BLD, W/SALT	118	8.34	21.11	0.054
16086	PEAS, SPLIT, MATURE SEEDS, CKD, BLD, WO/SALT	118	8.34	21.11	0.054
16085	PEAS, SPLIT, MATURE SEEDS, RAW	341	24.55	60.38	0.161
12142	PECANS	691	9.17	13.86	6.18
12643	PECANS, DRY RSTD, W/SALT	710	9.5	13.55	6.283
12143	PECANS, DRY RSTD, WO/SALT	710	9.5	13.55	6.283
12644	PECANS, OIL RSTD, W/SALT	715	9.2	13.01	7.238
12144	PECANS, OIL RSTD, WO/SALT	715	9.2	13.01	7.238
42063	PECTIN, LIQUID	11	0	2.8	0

NDB #	Food Description (100 gram portions = 3½ ounces = 20 tsp = ½ cup approx.	Calories	Protein	Carbs	Sat Fat
19310	PECTIN, UNSWTND, DRY MIX	325	0.3	90.4	0.05
11978	PEPPER, ANCHO, DRIED	281	11.86	51.41	0.82
11976	PEPPER, BANANA, RAW	27	1.66	5.35	0.048
02030	PEPPER, BLACK	255	10.95	64.81	0.98
02031	PEPPER, RED OR CAYENNE	318	12.01	56.63	3.26
11977	PEPPER, SERRANO, RAW	32	1.74	6.7	0.059
02032	PEPPER, WHITE	296	10.4	68.61	0.626
07056	PEPPERED LOAF PORK BF	145	17.27	4.59	2.28
18628	PEPPERIDGE FARM APPL TURNOVERS, FRZ, READY TO BAKE	319	4.2	35.1	4.53
18626	PEPPERIDGE FARM CLASSIC STYLE CROUTONS, SEASONED	465	13.6	61.1	3.72
18627	PEPPERIDGE FARM CRUSTY ITALIAN BREAD, GARLIC	372	8.3	41.6	4.822
02064	PEPPERMINT, FRESH	70	3.75	14.89	0.246
22903	PEPPERONI PIZZA, FROZEN	274	11.09	24.8	4.84
07057	PEPPERONI, PORK, BEEF	497	20.97	2.84	16.13
11980	PEPPERS, CHILI, GRN, CND	21	0.72	4.6	0.028
11962	PEPPERS, HOT CHILE, SUN-DRIED	324	10.58	69.86	0.813
11329	PEPPERS, HOT CHILI, GRN, CND, PODS, EXCLUDING SEEDS, SOL&LI	21	0.9	5.1	0.01
11670	PEPPERS, HOT CHILI, GRN, RAW	40	2	9.46	0.021
11820	PEPPERS, HOT CHILI, RED, CND, EXCLUDING SEEDS, SOL&LIQUIDS	21	0.9	5.1	0.01
11819	PEPPERS, HOT CHILI, RED, RAW	40	2	9.46	0.021
11981	PEPPERS, HUNGARIAN, RAW	29	0.8	6.68	0.046
11632	PEPPERS, JALAPENO, CND, SOL&LIQUIDS	27	0.92	4.72	0.097
11979	PEPPERS, JALAPENO, RAW	30	1.35	5.91	0.062
11982	PEPPERS, PASILLA, DRIED	345	12.35	51.13	
11333	PEPPERS, SWEET, GREEN, RAW	27	0.89	6.43	0.028
11821	PEPPERS, SWEET, RED, RAW	27	0.89	6.43	0.028
11951	PEPPERS, SWEET, YELLOW, RAW	27	1	6.32	0.031
11822	PEPPERS, SWT, GRN, CKD, BLD, DRND, W/SALT	28	0.92	6.7	0.029
11334	PEPPERS, SWT, GRN, CKD, BLD, DRND, WO/SALT	28	0.92	6.7	0.029
11335	PEPPERS, SWT, GRN, CND, SOL&LIQUIDS	18	0.8	3.9	0.045
11634	PEPPERS, SWT, GRN, FREEZE-DRIED	314	17.9	68.7	0.447
11338	PEPPERS, SWT, GRN, FRZ, CHOPD, BLD, DRND, WO/SALT	18	0.95	3.9	0.027
11825	PEPPERS, SWT, GRN, FRZ, CHOPD, CKD, BLD, DRND, W/SALT	18	0.95	3.9	0.027
11337	PEPPERS, SWT, GRN, FRZ, CHOPD, UNPREP	20	1.08	4.45	0.031
11824	PEPPERS, SWT, RED, CKD, BLD, DRND, W/SALT	28	0.92	6.7	0.029

NDB #	Food Description (100 gram portions = 3½ ounces = 20 tsp = ½ cup approx.	Calories	Protein	Carbs	Sat Fat
11823	PEPPERS, SWT, RED, CKD, BLD, DRND, WO/SALT	28	0.92	6.7	0.029
11916	PEPPERS, SWT, RED, CND, SOL&LIQUIDS	18	0.8	3.9	0.045
11931	PEPPERS, SWT, RED, FREEZE-DRIED	314	17.9	68.7	0.447
11919	PEPPERS, SWT, RED, FRZ, CHOPD, CKD, BLD, DRND, W/SALT	18	0.95	3.9	0.027
11918	PEPPERS, SWT, RED, FRZ, CHOPD, CKD, BLD, DRND, WO/SALT	18	0.95	3.9	0.027
11917	PEPPERS, SWT, RED, FRZ, CHOPD, UNPREP	20	1.08	4.45	0.031
15060	PERCH, MIXED SPECIES, RAW	91	19.39	0	0.185
15061	PERCH, MXD SP, CKD, DRY HEAT	117	24.86	0	0.237
09264	PERSIMMONS, JAPANESE, DRIED	274	1.38	73.43	
09263	PERSIMMONS, JAPANESE, RAW	70	0.58	18.59	0.02
09265	PERSIMMONS, NATIVE, RAW	127	0.8	33.5	
05155	PHEASANT, BREAST, MEAT ONLY, RAW	133	24.37	0	1.1
05156	PHEASANT, LEG, MEAT ONLY, RAW	134	22.2	0	1.46
05154	PHEASANT, RAW, MEAT ONLY	133	23.57	0	1.24
05153	PHEASANT, RAW, MEAT&SKN	181	22.7	0	2.7
18338	PHYLLO DOUGH	299	7.1	52.6	1.47
11958	PICKLE RELISH, HAMBURGER	129	0.63	34.48	0.052
11944	PICKLE RELISH, HOT DOG	91	1.5	23.35	0.044
11945	PICKLE RELISH, SWEET	130	0.37	35.05	0.055
07058	PICKLE&PIMIENTO LOAF, PORK	262	11.5	5.9	7.84
11941	PICKLE, CUCUMBER, SOUR	11	0.33	2.25	0.052
11946	PICKLE, CUCUMBER, SOUR, LO NA	11	0.33	2.25	0.052
11940	PICKLE, CUCUMBER, SWEET	117	0.37	31.81	0.067
11948	PICKLE, CUCUMBER, SWT, LO NA	117	0.37	31.81	0.067
11937	PICKLES, CUCUMBER, DILL	18	0.62	4.13	0.048
11947	PICKLES, CUCUMBER, DILL, LO NA	18	0.62	4.13	0.048
07062	PICNIC LOAF, PORK, BEEF	232	14.92	4.76	6.07
18399	PIE CRUST, COOKIE-TYPE, PREP FR RECIPE, GRAHAM CRACKER, CHI	484	4.1	63.9	5.092
18398	PIE CRUST, COOKIE-TYPE, PREP FROM RECIPE, CHOC WAFER, CHILL	506	5.1	54.4	6.732
18330	PIE CRUST, COOKIE-TYPE, PREP FROM RECIPE, GRAHAM CRACKER,	494	4.2	65.2	5.196
18401	PIE CRUST, COOKIE-TYPE, PREP FROM RECIPE, VANILLA WAFER, CHI	531	3.7	50.2	7.434
18332	PIE CRUST, STANDARD-TYPE, DRY MIX	518	6.9	52.1	7.974
18333	PIE CRUST, STANDARD-TYPE, DRY MIX, PREP, BKD	501	6.7	50.4	7.711
18335	PIE CRUST, STANDARD-TYPE, FRZ, RTB, BKD	514	4.4	49.6	10.583
18334	PIE CRUST, STANDARD-TYPE, FRZ, RTB, ENR	457	3.9	44.1	4.357

NDB #	Food Description (100 gram portions = 3½ ounces = 20 tsp = ½ cup approx.	Calories	Protein	Carbs	Sat Fat
18446	PIE CRUST, STANDARD-TYPE, FRZ, RTB, UNENR	457	3.9	44.1	4.357
18336	PIE CRUST, STANDARD-TYPE, PREP FROM RECIPE, BKD	527	6.4	47.5	8.622
18402	PIE CRUST, STANDARD-TYPE, PREP FROM RECIPE, UNBAKED	469	5.7	42.3	7.674
19312	PIE FILLINGS, CANNED, APPLE	101	0.1	26.2	0.02
19314	PIE FILLINGS, CND, CHERRY	115	0.37	28	0.018
18301	PIE, APPL, COMMLY PREP, ENR FLR	237	1.9	34	3.797
18443	PIE, APPL, COMMLY PREP, UNENR FLR	237	1.9	34	3.797
18302	PIE, APPL, PREP FROM RECIPE	265	2.4	37.1	3.05
18303	PIE, BANANA CRM, PREP FROM MIX, NO-BAKE TYPE	251	3.4	31.6	6.904
18304	PIE, BANANA CRM, PREP FROM RECIPE	269	4.4	32.9	3.758
18305	PIE, BLUEBERRY, COMMLY PREP	232	1.8	34.9	1.679
18306	PIE, BLUEBERRY, PREP FROM RECIPE	245	2.7	33.5	2.911
18308	PIE, CHERRY, COMMLY PREP	260	2	39.8	2.562
18309	PIE, CHERRY, PREP FROM RECIPE	270	2.8	38.5	2.985
18310	PIE, CHOC CREME, COMMLY PREP	304	2.6	33.6	4.968
18312	PIE, CHOC MOUSSE, PREP FROM MIX, NO-BAKE TYPE	260	3.5	29.6	8.195
18313	PIE, COCNT CREME, COMMLY PREP	298	2.1	37.2	6.976
18314	PIE, COCNT CRM, PREP FROM MIX, NO-BAKE TYPE	276	2.8	28.5	8.934
18316	PIE, COCNT CUSTARD, COMMLY PREP	260	5.9	30.2	5.854
18317	PIE, EGG CUSTARD, COMMLY PREP	210	5.5	20.8	2.349
18444	PIE, FRIED PIES, CHERRY	316	3	42.6	2.457
18319	PIE, FRIED PIES, FRUIT	316	3	42.6	2.457
18445	PIE, FRIED PIES, LEMON	316	3	42.6	2.457
18320	PIE, LEMON MERINGUE, COMMLY PREP	268	1.5	47.2	1.766
18321	PIE, LEMON MERINGUE, PREP FROM RECIPE	285	3.8	39.1	3.185
18322	PIE, MINCE, PREP FROM RECIPE	289	2.6	48	2.682
18323	PIE, PEACH	223	1.9	32.9	1.508
18324	PIE, PECAN, COMMLY PREP	400	4	57.2	3.545
18325	PIE, PECAN, PREP FROM RECIPE	412	4.9	52.2	3.989
18326	PIE, PUMPKIN, COMMLY PREP	210	3.9	27.3	1.785
18327	PIE, PUMPKIN, PREP FROM RECIPE	204	4.5	26.4	3.171
18328	PIE, VANILLA CRM, PREP FROM RECIPE	278	4.8	32.6	4.03
16402	PIGEON PEAS (RED GM), MATURE SEEDS, CKD, BLD, W/SALT	121	6.76	23.25	0.083
16102	PIGEON PEAS (RED GM), MATURE SEEDS, CKD, BLD, WO/SALT	121	6.76	23.25	0.083
16101	PIGEON PEAS (RED GM), MATURE SEEDS, RAW	343	21.7	62.78	0.33

NDB #	Food Description (100 gram portions = 3½ ounces = 20 tsp = ½ cup approx.	Calories	Protein	Carbs	Sat Fat
11826	PIGEONPEAS, IMMAT SEEDS, CKD, BLD, DRND, W/SALT	111	5.96	19.49	0.365
11345	PIGEONPEAS, IMMAT SEEDS, CKD, BLD, DRND, WO/SALT	111	5.96	19.49	0.365
11344	PIGEONPEAS, IMMAT SEEDS, RAW	136	7.2	23.88	0.354
15063	PIKE, NORTHERN, CKD, DRY HEAT	113	24.69	0	0.151
15062	PIKE, NORTHERN, RAW	88	19.26	0	0.118
15204	PIKE, WALLEYE, CKD, DRY HEAT	119	24.54	0	0.319
15064	PIKE, WALLEYE, RAW	93	19.14	0	0.249
12145	PILINUTS-CANARYTREE, DRIED	719	10.8	3.98	31.184
18629	PILLSBURY BTTRMLK BISCUITS, ART FLAVOR, REFR DOUGH	241	7.8	47.5	0.445
18635	PILLSBURY CINN ROLLS W/ICING, REFR DOUGH	341	5.4	54.3	2.84
18633	PILLSBURY GRANDS BTTRMLK BISCUITS, REFR DOUGH	319	6.8	41.1	3.86
18634	PILLSBURY HUNGRY JACK BTTRMLK BISCUITS, ART FLAVOR, REFR	319	7	42.5	2.705
18630	PILLSBURY, CHOC CHIP COOKIES, REFR DOUGH	455	4.3	63.9	6.494
18631	PILLSBURY, CRUSTY FRENCH LOAF, REFR DOUGH	249	9.3	46.6	0.831
18632	PILLSBURY, TRADITIONAL FUDGE BROWNIE MIX, DRY	441	4.8	78.3	2.59
11943	PIMENTO, CANNED	23	1.1	5.1	0.045
12147	PINE NUTS, PIGNOLIA, DRIED	566	24	14.22	7.797
12149	PINE NUTS, PINYON, DRIED	629	11.57	19.3	9.377
09273	PINEAPPLE JUC, CND, UNSWTND, WO/ VIT C	56	0.32	13.78	0.005
09409	PINEAPPLE JUC, CND, W/ VIT C, UNSWTND	56	0.32	13.78	0.005
09275	PINEAPPLE JUC, FRZ CONC, UNSWTND, DIL W/3 VOLUME H2O	52	0.4	12.77	0.002
09274	PINEAPPLE JUC, FRZ CONC, UNSWTND, UNDIL	179	1.3	44.3	0.007
14334	PINEAPPLE&GRAPEFRUIT JUC DRK, CND	47	0.2	11.6	0.006
14341	PINEAPPLE&ORANGE JUC DRK, CND	50	1.3	11.8	0
09271	PINEAPPLE, CND, EX HVY SYRUP PK, SOL&LIQUIDS	83	0.34	21.5	0.009
09267	PINEAPPLE, CND, H2O PK, SOL&LIQUIDS	32	0.43	8.3	0.006
09270	PINEAPPLE, CND, HVY SYRUP PK, SOL&LIQUIDS	78	0.35	20.2	0.009
09268	PINEAPPLE, CND, JUC PK, SOL&LIQUIDS	60	0.42	15.7	0.006
09269	PINEAPPLE, CND, LT SYRUP PK, SOL&LIQUIDS	52	0.36	13.45	0.009
09272	PINEAPPLE, FRZ, CHUNKS, SWTND	85	0.4	22.2	0.007
09266	PINEAPPLE, RAW	49	0.39	12.39	0.032
12652	PISTACHIO NUTS, DRY RSTD, W/SALT	568	21.35	26.78	5.555
12152	PISTACHIO NUTS, DRY RSTD, WO/SALT	571	21.35	27.65	5.555
12151	PISTACHIO NUTS, RAW	557	20.61	27.97	5.44
09276	PITANGA, (SURINAM-CHERRY), RAW	33	0.8	7.49	

NDB #	Food Description (100 gram portions = 3½ ounces = 20 tsp = ½ cup approx.	Calories	Protein	Carbs	Sat Fat
09278	PLANTAINS, COOKED	116	0.79	31.15	0.069
09277	PLANTAINS, RAW	122	1.3	31.89	0.143
09285	PLUMS, CND, PURPLE, EX HVY SYRUP PK, SOL&LIQUIDS	101	0.36	26.31	0.008
09281	PLUMS, CND, PURPLE, H2O PK, SOL&LIQUIDS	41	0.39	11.03	0.001
09284	PLUMS, CND, PURPLE, HVY SYRUP PK, SOL&LIQUIDS	89	0.36	23.24	0.008
09282	PLUMS, CND, PURPLE, JUC PK, SOL&LIQUIDS	58	0.51	15.15	0.002
09283	PLUMS, CND, PURPLE, LT SYRUP PK, SOL&LIQUIDS	63	0.37	16.28	0.008
09279	PLUMS, RAW	55	0.79	13.01	0.049
11349	POI	112	0.38	27.23	0.029
11827	POKEBERRY SHOOTS, (POKE), CKD, BLD, DRND, W/SALT	20	2.3	3.1	
11351	POKEBERRY SHOOTS, (POKE), CKD, BLD, DRND, WO/SALT	20	2.3	3.1	0.092
11350	POKEBERRY SHOOTS, (POKE), RAW	23	2.6	3.7	
19257	POLANER ALL-FRUIT STRAWBERRY SPRD	231	0.7	57	
07059	POLISH SAUSAGE, PORK	326	14.1	1.63	10.33
15205	POLLOCK, ATLANTIC, CKD, DRY HEAT	118	24.92	0	0.17
15065	POLLOCK, ATLANTIC, RAW	92	19.44	0	0.135
15067	POLLOCK, WALLEYE, CKD, DRY HEAT	113	23.51	0	0.231
15066	POLLOCK, WALLEYE, RAW	81	17.18	0	0.164
09286	POMEGRANATES, RAW	68	0.95	17.17	0.038
15069	POMPANO, FLORIDA, CKD, DRY HEAT	211	23.69	0	4.499
15068	POMPANO, FLORIDA, RAW	164	18.48	0	3.509
19034	POPCORN, AIR-POPPED	382	12	77.9	0.57
19806	POPCORN, AIR-POPPED, WHITE POPCORN	382	12	77.9	0.57
19036	POPCORN, CAKES	384	9.7	80.1	0.48
19038	POPCORN, CARAMEL-COATED, W/PNUTS	400	6.4	80.7	1.04
19039	POPCORN, CARAMEL-COATED, WO/PNUTS	431	3.8	79.1	3.61
19040	POPCORN, CHEESE-FLAVOR	526	9.3	51.6	6.41
19035	POPCORN, OIL-POPPED	500	9	57.2	4.89
19807	POPCORN, OIL-POPPED, WHITE POPCORN	500	9	57.2	4.89
18339	POPOVERS, DRY MIX, ENRICHED	371	10.4	71	0.983
18447	POPOVERS, DRY MIX, UNENR	371	10.4	71	0.983
02033	POPPY SEED	533	18.04	23.69	4.87
07064	PORK SAUSAGE, FRESH, COOKED	369	19.65	1.03	10.81
07063	PORK SAUSAGE, FRESH, RAW	417	11.69	1.02	14.47
19408	PORK SKINS, BARBECUE-FLAVOR	538	57.9	1.6	11.56

NDB #	Food Description (100 gram portions = 3½ ounces = 20 tsp = ½ cup approx.	Calories	Protein	Carbs	Sat Fat
19041	PORK SKINS, PLAIN	545	61.3	0	11.37
07065	PORK&BF SAUSAGE, FRSH, CKD	396	13.8	2.7	12.96
10124	PORK, CURED, BACON, CKD, BRLD, PAN-FRIED OR RSTD	576	30.45	0.59	17.42
10123	PORK, CURED, BACON, RAW	556	8.66	0.09	21.26
10129	PORK, CURED, BRKFST STRIPS, CKD	459	28.95	1.05	12.77
10128	PORK, CURED, BRKFST STRIPS, RAW OR UNHTD	388	11.74	0.7	12.91
10131	PORK, CURED, CANADIAN-STYLE BACON, GRILLED	185	24.24	1.35	2.84
10130	PORK, CURED, CANADIAN-STYLE BACON, UNHTD	157	20.64	1.68	2.22
10167	PORK, CURED, FAT (FROM HAM&ARM PICNIC), RSTD	591	7.64	0	22.69
10166	PORK, CURED, FAT (FROM HAM&ARM PICNIC), UNHTD	579	5.68	0.09	22.52
10132	PORK, CURED, FEET, PICKLED	203	13.52	0.02	5.57
10134	PORK, CURED, HAM, BNLESS, EX LN (APPROX 5% FAT), RSTD	145	20.93	1.5	1.81
10183	PORK, CURED, HAM, BNLESS, EX LN&REG, RSTD	165	21.97	0.5	2.61
10182	PORK, CURED, HAM, BNLESS, EX LN&REG, UNHTD	162	18.26	2.28	2.7
10136	PORK, CURED, HAM, BNLESS, REG (APPROX 11% FAT), RSTD	178	22.62	0	3.12
10141	PORK, CURED, HAM, CNTR SLICE, COUNTRY-STYLE, LN, RAW	195	27.8	0.3	2.78
10142	PORK, CURED, HAM, CNTR SLICE, LN&FAT, UNHTD	203	20.17	0.05	4.572
10138	PORK, CURED, HAM, EX LN (APPROX 4% FAT), CND, RSTD	136	21.16	0.52	1.6
10137	PORK, CURED, HAM, EX LN (APPROX 4% FAT), CND, UNHTD	120	18.49	0	1.51
10185	PORK, CURED, HAM, EX LN&REG, CND, RSTD	167	20.94	0.49	2.81
10184	PORK, CURED, HAM, EX LN&REG, CND, UNHTD	144	17.97	0	2.45
10147	PORK, CURED, HAM, PATTIES, GRILLED	342	13.3	1.7	11.09
10146	PORK, CURED, HAM, PATTIES, UNHTD	315	12.78	1.69	10.13
10140	PORK, CURED, HAM, REG (APPROX 13% FAT), CND, RSTD	226	20.53	0.42	5.04
10139	PORK, CURED, HAM, REG (APPROX 13% FAT), CND, UNHTD	190	16.97	0.02	4.25
10149	PORK, CURED, HAM, STEAK, BNLESS, EX LN, UNHTD	122	19.56	0	1.44
10151	PORK, CURED, HAM, WHL, LN&FAT, RSTD	243	21.57	0	5.98
10150	PORK, CURED, HAM, WHL, LN&FAT, UNHTD	246	18.49	0.06	6.62
10153	PORK, CURED, HAM, WHL, LN, RSTD	157	25.05	0	1.84
10152	PORK, CURED, HAM, WHL, LN, UNHTD	147	22.32	0.05	1.92
10165	PORK, CURED, SALT PORK, RAW	748	5.05	0	29.38
10168	PORK, CURED, SHLDR, ARM PICNIC, LN&FAT, RSTD	280	20.43	0	7.67
10169	PORK, CURED, SHLDR, ARM PICNIC, LN, RSTD	170	24.94	0	2.36
10171	PORK, CURED, SHLDR, BLADE ROLL, LN&FAT, RSTD	287	17.28	0.37	8.38
10170	PORK, CURED, SHLDR, BLADE ROLL, LN&FAT, UNHTD	269	16.47	0	7.939

NDB #	Food Description (100 gram portions = 3½ ounces = 20 tsp = ½ cup approx.	Calories	Protein	Carbs	Sat Fat
10004	PORK, FRESH, BACKFAT, RAW	812	2.92	0	32.21
10220	PORK, FRESH, GROUND, COOKED	297	25.69	0	7.72
10219	PORK, FRESH, GROUND, RAW	263	16.88	0	7.87
10193	PORK, FRSH, BACKRIBS, LN&FAT, CKD, RSTD	370	24.26	0	10.99
10192	PORK, FRSH, BACKRIBS, LN&FAT, RAW	282	16.12	0	8.73
10005	PORK, FRSH, BELLY, RAW	518	9.34	0	19.33
10001	PORK, FRSH, CARCASS, LN&FAT, RAW	376	13.91	0	12.44
10188	PORK, FRSH, COMP (LEG, LOIN, SHLDR, &SPARERIBS), LN&FAT, CKD	273	27.57	0	6.22
10187	PORK, FRSH, COMP (LEG, LOIN, SHLDR, &SPARERIBS), LN&FAT, RAW	216	18.95	0	5.28
10003	PORK, FRSH, COMP OF LEG, LOIN, SHLDR, &SPARERIBS, LN&FAT, RA	227	18.25	0	5.77
10093	PORK, FRSH, COMP OF RTL CUTS (LEG, LOIN, &SHLDR), LN, CKD	212	29.27	0	3.41
10002	PORK, FRSH, COMP OF RTL CUTS (LEG, LOIN, SHLDR), LN, RAW	143	21.07	0	2.03
10227	PORK, FRSH, COMP OF RTL CUTS (LOIN&SHLDR BLADE), LN&FAT, C	252	27.78	0	5.3
10226	PORK, FRSH, COMP OF RTL CUTS (LOIN&SHLDR BLADE), LN&FAT, R	200	19.53	0	4.47
10229	PORK, FRSH, COMP OF RTL CUTS (LOIN&SHLDR BLADE), LN, CKD	211	29.47	0	3.34
10228	PORK, FRSH, COMP OF RTL CUTS (LOIN&SHLDR BLADE), LN, RAW	144	21.23	0	2.03
10007	PORK, FRSH, FAT, CKD	629	12.2	0	24.49
10006	PORK, FRSH, FAT, RAW	638	6.34	0	23.52
10013	PORK, FRSH, LEG (HAM), RUMP HALF, LN&FAT, CKD, RSTD	252	28.88	0	5.25
10012	PORK, FRSH, LEG (HAM), RUMP HALF, LN&FAT, RAW	222	18.74	0	5.44
10015	PORK, FRSH, LEG (HAM), RUMP HALF, LN, CKD, RSTD	206	30.94	0	2.87
10014	PORK, FRSH, LEG (HAM), RUMP HALF, LN, RAW	137	21.24	0	1.79
10017	PORK, FRSH, LEG (HAM), SHANK HALF, LN&FAT, CKD, RSTD	289	25.34	0	7.36
10016	PORK, FRSH, LEG (HAM), SHANK HALF, LN&FAT, RAW	263	17.08	0	7.29
10019	PORK, FRSH, LEG (HAM), SHANK HALF, LN, CKD, RSTD	215	28.21	0	3.63
10018	PORK, FRSH, LEG (HAM), SHANK HALF, LN, RAW	139	20.62	0	1.94
10009	PORK, FRSH, LEG (HAM), WHL, LN&FAT, CKD, RSTD	273	26.83	0	6.47
10008	PORK, FRSH, LEG (HAM), WHL, LN&FAT, RAW	245	17.43	0	6.54
10011	PORK, FRSH, LEG (HAM), WHL, LN, CKD, RSTD	211	29.41	0	3.3
10010	PORK, FRSH, LEG (HAM), WHL, LN, RAW	136	20.48	0	1.87
10028	PORK, FRSH, LOIN, BLADE (CHOPS OR ROASTS), BONE-IN, LN&FAT,	285	15.82	0	8.37
10032	PORK, FRSH, LOIN, BLADE (CHOPS OR ROASTS), BONE-IN, LN, RAW	157	19.27	0	2.85
10030	PORK, FRSH, LOIN, BLADE (CHOPS), BONE-IN, LN&FAT, CKD, BRLD	320	22.47	0	9.31
10029	PORK, FRSH, LOIN, BLADE (CHOPS), BONE-IN, LN&FAT, CKD, BRSD	323	21.91	0	9.54
10178	PORK, FRSH, LOIN, BLADE (CHOPS), BONE-IN, LN&FAT, CKD, PAN-FRI	342	21.49	0	10.17

NDB #	Food Description (100 gram portions = 3½ ounces = 20 tsp = ½ cup approx.	Calories	Protein	Carbs	Sat Fat
10034	PORK, FRSH, LOIN, BLADE (CHOPS), BONE-IN, LN, CKD, BRLD	234	25.36	0	5.06
10033	PORK, FRSH, LOIN, BLADE (CHOPS), BONE-IN, LN, CKD, BRSD	225	25.03	0	4.74
10120	PORK, FRSH, LOIN, BLADE (CHOPS), BONE-IN, LN, CKD, PAN-FRIED	241	24.74	0	5.16
10031	PORK, FRSH, LOIN, BLADE (ROASTS), BONE-IN, LN&FAT, CKD, RSTD	323	23.72	0	9.15
10035	PORK, FRSH, LOIN, BLADE (ROASTS), BONE-IN, LN, CKD, RSTD	247	26.6	0	5.31
10040	PORK, FRSH, LOIN, CNTR LOIN (CHOPS OR ROASTS), BONE-IN, LN, R	140	22.04	0	1.74
10038	PORK, FRSH, LOIN, CNTR LOIN (CHOPS), BONE-IN, LN&FAT, CKD, BRL	240	28.71	0	4.8
10037	PORK, FRSH, LOIN, CNTR LOIN (CHOPS), BONE-IN, LN&FAT, CKD, BR	247	27.94	0	5.32
10042	PORK, FRSH, LOIN, CNTR LOIN (CHOPS), BONE-IN, LN, CKD, BRLD	202	30.19	0	2.95
10041	PORK, FRSH, LOIN, CNTR LOIN (CHOPS), BONE-IN, LN, CKD, BRSD	202	29.78	0	3.07
10176	PORK, FRSH, LOIN, CNTR LOIN (CHOPS), BONE-IN, LN, CKD, PAN-FRI	232	32.18	0	3.64
10039	PORK, FRSH, LOIN, CNTR LOIN (ROASTS), BONE-IN, LN&FAT, CKD, RS	234	26.31	0	5.06
10043	PORK, FRSH, LOIN, CNTR LOIN (ROASTS), BONE-IN, LN, CKD, RSTD	199	27.55	0	3.34
10036	PORK, FRSH, LOIN, CNTR LOIN CHOPS OR ROASTS, BONE-IN, LN&FA	200	20.12	0	4.4
10179	PORK, FRSH, LOIN, CNTR LOIN CHOPS, BONE-IN, LN&FAT, CKD, PAN-	277	29.91	0	6.01
10194	PORK, FRSH, LOIN, CNTR RIB (CHOPS OR ROASTS), BNLESS, LN&FA	211	19.9	0	4.86
10199	PORK, FRSH, LOIN, CNTR RIB (CHOPS OR ROASTS), BNLESS, LN, RA	152	21.8	0	2.24
10044	PORK, FRSH, LOIN, CNTR RIB (CHOPS OR ROASTS), BONE-IN, LN&FA	209	20.17	0	4.71
10048	PORK, FRSH, LOIN, CNTR RIB (CHOPS OR ROASTS), BONE-IN, LN, RA	149	22.11	0	2.07
10196	PORK, FRSH, LOIN, CNTR RIB (CHOPS), BNLESS, LN&FAT, CKD, BRLD	260	27.63	0	5.79
10195	PORK, FRSH, LOIN, CNTR RIB (CHOPS), BNLESS, LN&FAT, CKD, BRSD	255	26.29	0	6.12
10197	PORK, FRSH, LOIN, CNTR RIB (CHOPS), BNLESS, LN&FAT, CKD, PAN-	224	27.68	0	4.3
10201	PORK, FRSH, LOIN, CNTR RIB (CHOPS), BNLESS, LN, CKD, BRLD	216	29.46	0	3.57
10200	PORK, FRSH, LOIN, CNTR RIB (CHOPS), BNLESS, LN, CKD, BRSD	211	27.95	0	3.96
10202	PORK, FRSH, LOIN, CNTR RIB (CHOPS), BNLESS, LN, CKD, PAN-FRIED	224	27.68	0	4.3
10046	PORK, FRSH, LOIN, CNTR RIB (CHOPS), BONE-IN, LN&FAT, CKD, BRL	263	28.79	0	5.69
10045	PORK, FRSH, LOIN, CNTR RIB (CHOPS), BONE-IN, LN&FAT, CKD, BRS	250	26.67	0	5.84
10180	PORK, FRSH, LOIN, CNTR RIB (CHOPS), BONE-IN, LN&FAT, CKD, PAN-	265	26.28	0	6.34
10050	PORK, FRSH, LOIN, CNTR RIB (CHOPS), BONE-IN, LN, CKD, BRLD	219	30.76	0	3.46
10049	PORK, FRSH, LOIN, CNTR RIB (CHOPS), BONE-IN, LN, CKD, BRSD	206	28.35	0	3.67
10177	PORK, FRSH, LOIN, CNTR RIB (CHOPS), BONE-IN, LN, CKD, PAN-FRIE	218	28.11	0	3.98
10198	PORK, FRSH, LOIN, CNTR RIB (ROASTS), BNLESS, LN&FAT, CKD, RST	252	26.99	0	5.35
10203	PORK, FRSH, LOIN, CNTR RIB (ROASTS), BNLESS, LN, CKD, RSTD	214	28.81	0	3.54
10047	PORK, FRSH, LOIN, CNTR RIB (ROASTS), BONE-IN, LN&FAT, CKD, RST	255	27.43	0	5.92
10051	PORK, FRSH, LOIN, CNTR RIB (ROASTS), BONE-IN, LN, CKD, RSTD	223	28.72	0	4.35

NDB #	Food Description (100 gram portions = 3½ ounces = 20 tsp = ½ cup approx.	Calories	Protein	Carbs	Sat Fat
10205	PORK, FRSH, LOIN, COUNTRY-STYLE RIBS, LN&FAT, CKD, BRSD	296	23.87	0	8.01
10206	PORK, FRSH, LOIN, COUNTRY-STYLE RIBS, LN&FAT, CKD, RSTD	328	23.4	0	9.21
10204	PORK, FRSH, LOIN, COUNTRY-STYLE RIBS, LN&FAT, RAW	241	16.99	0	6.49
10208	PORK, FRSH, LOIN, COUNTRY-STYLE RIBS, LN, CKD, BRSD	234	26.04	0	4.94
10209	PORK, FRSH, LOIN, COUNTRY-STYLE RIBS, LN, CKD, RSTD	247	26.6	0	5.31
10207	PORK, FRSH, LOIN, COUNTRY-STYLE RIBS, LN, RAW	157	19.27	0	2.85
10210	PORK, FRSH, LOIN, SIRLOIN (CHOPS OR ROASTS), BNLESS, LN&FAT,	145	20.57	0	2.18
10214	PORK, FRSH, LOIN, SIRLOIN (CHOPS OR ROASTS), BNLESS, LN, RAW	128	21.06	0	1.46
10052	PORK, FRSH, LOIN, SIRLOIN (CHOPS OR ROASTS), BONE-IN, LN&FAT,	205	19.19	0	4.72
10056	PORK, FRSH, LOIN, SIRLOIN (CHOPS OR ROASTS), BONE-IN, LN, RAW	142	21.06	0	1.99
10212	PORK, FRSH, LOIN, SIRLOIN (CHOPS), BNLESS, LN&FAT, CKD, BRLD	208	30.52	0	2.88
10211	PORK, FRSH, LOIN, SIRLOIN (CHOPS), BNLESS, LN&FAT, CKD, BRSD	189	26.54	0	3.03
10216	PORK, FRSH, LOIN, SIRLOIN (CHOPS), BNLESS, LN, CKD, BRLD	193	31.13	0	2.22
10215	PORK, FRSH, LOIN, SIRLOIN (CHOPS), BNLESS, LN, CKD, BRSD	175	27	0	2.34
10054	PORK, FRSH, LOIN, SIRLOIN (CHOPS), BONE-IN, LN&FAT, CKD, BRLD	259	26.65	0	5.93
10053	PORK, FRSH, LOIN, SIRLOIN (CHOPS), BONE-IN, LN&FAT, CKD, BRSD	245	25.36	0	5.56
10058	PORK, FRSH, LOIN, SIRLOIN (CHOPS), BONE-IN, LN, CKD, BRLD	213	28.46	0	3.61
10057	PORK, FRSH, LOIN, SIRLOIN (CHOPS), BONE-IN, LN, CKD, BRSD	197	27	0	3.2
10213	PORK, FRSH, LOIN, SIRLOIN (ROASTS), BNLESS, LN&FAT, CKD, RSTD	207	28.5	0	3.42
10217	PORK, FRSH, LOIN, SIRLOIN (ROASTS), BNLESS, LN, CKD, RSTD	198	28.85	0	2.97
10055	PORK, FRSH, LOIN, SIRLOIN (ROASTS), BONE-IN, LN&FAT, CKD, RSTD	261	27.24	0	5.69
10059	PORK, FRSH, LOIN, SIRLOIN (ROASTS), BONE-IN, LN, CKD, RSTD	216	28.81	0	3.62
10221	PORK, FRSH, LOIN, TENDERLOIN, LN&FAT, CKD, BRLD	201	29.86	0	2.93
10222	PORK, FRSH, LOIN, TENDERLOIN, LN&FAT, CKD, RSTD	173	27.81	0	2.14
10218	PORK, FRSH, LOIN, TENDERLOIN, LN&FAT, RAW	136	20.54	0	1.87
10223	PORK, FRSH, LOIN, TENDERLOIN, LN, CKD, BRLD	187	30.42	0	2.24
10061	PORK, FRSH, LOIN, TENDERLOIN, LN, CKD, RSTD	164	28.14	0	1.66
10060	PORK, FRSH, LOIN, TENDERLOIN, LN, RAW	120	20.99	0	1.18
10064	PORK, FRSH, LOIN, TOP LOIN (CHOPS), BNLESS, LN&FAT, CKD, BRLD	229	29.96	0	3.95
10063	PORK, FRSH, LOIN, TOP LOIN (CHOPS), BNLESS, LN&FAT, CKD, BRSD	233	27.82	0	4.71
10186	PORK, FRSH, LOIN, TOP LOIN (CHOPS), BNLESS, LN&FAT, CKD, PAN-	257	29	0	5.3
10062	PORK, FRSH, LOIN, TOP LOIN (CHOPS), BNLESS, LN&FAT, RAW	185	20.42	0	3.75
10068	PORK, FRSH, LOIN, TOP LOIN (CHOPS), BNLESS, LN, CKD, BRLD	203	31.14	0	2.72
10067	PORK, FRSH, LOIN, TOP LOIN (CHOPS), BNLESS, LN, CKD, BRSD	202	29.07	0	3.13
10181	PORK, FRSH, LOIN, TOP LOIN (CHOPS), BNLESS, LN, CKD, PAN-FRIED	225	30.48	0	3.6

NDB #	Food Description (100 gram portions = 3½ ounces = 20 tsp = ½ cup approx.	Calories	Protein	Carbs	Sat Fat
10066	PORK, FRSH, LOIN, TOP LOIN (CHOPS), BNLESS, LN, RAW	141	21.8	0	1.83
10065	PORK, FRSH, LOIN, TOP LOIN (ROASTS), BNLESS, LN&FAT, CKD, RST	226	28.81	0	4.17
10224	PORK, FRSH, LOIN, TOP LOIN (ROASTS), BNLESS, LN&FAT, RAW	191	20.24	0	4.02
10069	PORK, FRSH, LOIN, TOP LOIN (ROASTS), BNLESS, LN, CKD, RSTD	194	30.24	0	2.62
10225	PORK, FRSH, LOIN, TOP LOIN (ROASTS), BNLESS, LN, RAW	141	21.8	0	1.82
10022	PORK, FRSH, LOIN, WHL, LN&FAT, CKD, BRLD	242	27.32	0	5.23
10021	PORK, FRSH, LOIN, WHL, LN&FAT, CKD, BRSD	239	27.23	0	5.11
10023	PORK, FRSH, LOIN, WHL, LN&FAT, CKD, RSTD	248	27.09	0	5.37
10020	PORK, FRSH, LOIN, WHL, LN&FAT, RAW	198	19.74	0	4.36
10026	PORK, FRSH, LOIN, WHL, LN, CKD, BRLD	210	28.57	0	3.64
10025	PORK, FRSH, LOIN, WHL, LN, CKD, BRSD	204	28.57	0	3.38
10027	PORK, FRSH, LOIN, WHL, LN, CKD, RSTD	209	28.62	0	3.51
10024	PORK, FRSH, LOIN, WHL, LN, RAW	143	21.43	0	1.95
10075	PORK, FRSH, SHLDR, ARM PICNIC, LN&FAT, CKD, BRSD	329	27.99	0	8.49
10076	PORK, FRSH, SHLDR, ARM PICNIC, LN&FAT, CKD, RSTD	317	23.47	0	8.78
10074	PORK, FRSH, SHLDR, ARM PICNIC, LN&FAT, RAW	253	16.69	0	7
10078	PORK, FRSH, SHLDR, ARM PICNIC, LN, CKD, BRSD	248	32.26	0	4.16
10079	PORK, FRSH, SHLDR, ARM PICNIC, LN, CKD, RSTD	228	26.68	0	4.3
10077	PORK, FRSH, SHLDR, ARM PICNIC, LN, RAW	140	19.75	0	2.13
10080	PORK, FRSH, SHLDR, BLADE, BOSTON (ROASTS OR STEAKS), LN&FA	218	17.66	0	5.48
10084	PORK, FRSH, SHLDR, BLADE, BOSTON (ROASTS OR STEAKS), LN, RA	155	19.37	0	2.76
10083	PORK, FRSH, SHLDR, BLADE, BOSTON (ROASTS), LN&FAT, CKD, RST	269	23.11	0	6.97
10087	PORK, FRSH, SHLDR, BLADE, BOSTON (ROASTS), LN, CKD, RSTD	232	24.21	0	5.19
10082	PORK, FRSH, SHLDR, BLADE, BOSTON (STEAKS), LN&FAT, CKD, BRL	259	25.58	0	5.95
10081	PORK, FRSH, SHLDR, BLADE, BOSTON (STEAKS), LN&FAT, CKD, BRS	319	28.67	0	7.94
10086	PORK, FRSH, SHLDR, BLADE, BOSTON (STEAKS), LN, CKD, BRLD	227	26.74	0	4.45
10085	PORK, FRSH, SHLDR, BLADE, BOSTON (STEAKS), LN, CKD, BRSD	273	31.09	0	5.51
10071	PORK, FRSH, SHLDR, WHL, LN&FAT, CKD, RSTD	292	23.28	0	7.86
10070	PORK, FRSH, SHLDR, WHL, LN&FAT, RAW	236	17.18	0	6.24
10073	PORK, FRSH, SHLDR, WHL, LN, CKD, RSTD	230	25.33	0	4.79
10072	PORK, FRSH, SHLDR, WHL, LN, RAW	148	19.55	0	2.47
10089	PORK, FRSH, SPARERIBS, LN&FAT, CKD, BRSD	397	29.06	0	11.12
10088	PORK, FRSH, SPARERIBS, LN&FAT, RAW	286	17.09	0	8.93
10097	PORK, FRSH, VAR MEATS&BY-PRODUCTS, BRAIN, CKD, BRSD	138	12.14	0	2.15
10096	PORK, FRSH, VAR MEATS&BY-PRODUCTS, BRAIN, RAW	127	10.28	0	2.079

NDB #	Food Description (100 gram portions = 3½ ounces = 20 tsp = ½ cup approx.	Calories	Protein	Carbs	Sat Fat
10099	PORK, FRSH, VAR MEATS&BY-PRODUCTS, CHITTERLINGS, CKD, SIM	303	10.25	0	10.1
10098	PORK, FRSH, VAR MEATS&BY-PRODUCTS, CHITTERLINGS, RAW	252	10.05	0.33	7.93
10101	PORK, FRSH, VAR MEATS&BY-PRODUCTS, EARS, FRZ, CKD, SIMMRD	166	15.95	0.2	3.86
10100	PORK, FRSH, VAR MEATS&BY-PRODUCTS, EARS, FRZ, RAW	234	22.45	0.6	5.39
10173	PORK, FRSH, VAR MEATS&BY-PRODUCTS, FEET, CKD, SIMMRD	194	19.2	0	4.28
10102	PORK, FRSH, VAR MEATS&BY-PRODUCTS, FEET, RAW	264	22.07	0	6.5
10104	PORK, FRSH, VAR MEATS&BY-PRODUCTS, HEART, CKD, BRSD	148	23.6	0.4	1.34
10103	PORK, FRSH, VAR MEATS&BY-PRODUCTS, HEART, RAW	118	17.27	1.33	1.16
10105	PORK, FRSH, VAR MEATS&BY-PRODUCTS, JOWL, RAW	655	6.38	0	25.26
10107	PORK, FRSH, VAR MEATS&BY-PRODUCTS, KIDNEYS, CKD, BRSD	151	25.4	0	1.51
10106	PORK, FRSH, VAR MEATS&BY-PRODUCTS, KIDNEYS, RAW	100	16.46	0	1.04
10109	PORK, FRSH, VAR MEATS&BY-PRODUCTS, LEAF FAT, RAW	857	1.76	0	45.23
10111	PORK, FRSH, VAR MEATS&BY-PRODUCTS, LIVER, CKD, BRSD	165	26.02	3.76	1.41
10110	PORK, FRSH, VAR MEATS&BY-PRODUCTS, LIVER, RAW	134	21.39	2.47	1.17
10113	PORK, FRSH, VAR MEATS&BY-PRODUCTS, LUNGS, CKD, BRSD	99	16.6	0	1.09
10112	PORK, FRSH, VAR MEATS&BY-PRODUCTS, LUNGS, RAW	85	14.08	0	0.96
10114	PORK, FRSH, VAR MEATS&BY-PRODUCTS, MECHANICALLY SEPARAT	304	15.03	0	9.82
10116	PORK, FRSH, VAR MEATS&BY-PRODUCTS, PANCREAS, CKD, BRSD	219	28.5	0	3.73
10115	PORK, FRSH, VAR MEATS&BY-PRODUCTS, PANCREAS, RAW	199	18.56	0	4.58
10118	PORK, FRSH, VAR MEATS&BY-PRODUCTS, SPLEEN, CKD, BRSD	149	28.2	0	1.06
10117	PORK, FRSH, VAR MEATS&BY-PRODUCTS, SPLEEN, RAW	100	17.86	0	0.86
10119	PORK, FRSH, VAR MEATS&BY-PRODUCTS, STOMACH, RAW	157	16.5	0	3.4
10175	PORK, FRSH, VAR MEATS&BY-PRODUCTS, TAIL, CKD, SIMMRD	396	17	0	12.45
10174	PORK, FRSH, VAR MEATS&BY-PRODUCTS, TAIL, RAW	378	17.75	0	11.64
10122	PORK, FRSH, VAR MEATS&BY-PRODUCTS, TONGUE, CKD, BRSD	271	24.1	0	6.449
10121	PORK, FRSH, VAR MEATS&BY-PRODUCTS, TONGUE, RAW	225	16.3	0	5.96
19042	POTATO CHIPS, BARBECUE-FLAVOR	491	7.7	52.8	8.05
19421	POTATO CHIPS, CHEESE-FLAVOR	496	8.5	57.7	8.6
19046	POTATO CHIPS, MADE FR DRIED POTATOES, SOUR-CREAM&ONION-	547	6.6	51.3	9.47
19412	POTATO CHIPS, MADE FROM DRIED POTATOES, CHEESE-FLAVOR	551	7	50.6	9.57
19045	POTATO CHIPS, MADE FROM DRIED POTATOES, LT	501	5.6	64.9	5.13
19410	POTATO CHIPS, MADE FROM DRIED POTATOES, PLN	558	5.9	51	9.45
19411	POTATO CHIPS, PLAIN, SALTED	536	7	52.9	10.96
19809	POTATO CHIPS, PLN, MADE W/PART HYDR SOYBN OIL, SALTED	536	7	52.9	5.43
19810	POTATO CHIPS, PLN, MADE W/PART HYDR SOYBN OIL, UNSALTED	536	7	52.9	5.43

NDB #	Food Description (100 gram portions = 3½ ounces = 20 tsp = ½ cup approx.	Calories	Protein	Carbs	Sat Fat
19811	POTATO CHIPS, PLN, UNSALTED	536	7	52.9	10.96
19043	POTATO CHIPS, SOUR-CREAM-AND-ONION-FLAVOR	531	8.1	51.5	8.89
11413	POTATO FLOUR	357	6.9	83.08	0.09
11672	POTATO PANCAKES, HOME-PREPARED	272	6.16	28.64	3.044
11399	POTATO PUFFS, FRZ, PREP	222	3.35	30.48	5.095
11398	POTATO PUFFS, FRZ, UNPREP	177	2.67	24.31	4.063
11414	POTATO SALAD, HOME-PREPARED	143	2.68	11.17	1.429
19415	POTATO STICKS	522	6.7	53.3	8.88
11674	POTATO, BKD, FLESH & SKN, WO/ SALT	93	2.5	21.15	0.035
11352	POTATO, FLESH & SKN, RAW	77	2.02	17.47	0.026
11385	POTATOES, AU GRATIN, DRY MIX, PREP W/H2O, WHL MILK&BUTTER	93	2.3	12.84	2.586
11384	POTATOES, AU GRATIN, DRY MIX, UNPREP	314	8.9	74.31	2.323
11373	POTATOES, AU GRATIN, HOME-PREPARED FROM RECIPE USING BUT	132	5.06	11.27	4.733
11843	POTATOES, AU GRATIN, HOME-PREPARED FROM RECIPE USING MA	132	5.06	11.27	3.53
11828	POTATOES, BKD, FLESH&SKN, W/SALT	93	2.5	21.15	0.035
11829	POTATOES, BKD, FLESH, W/SALT	93	1.96	21.56	0.026
11363	POTATOES, BKD, FLESH, WO/SALT	93	1.96	21.56	0.026
11830	POTATOES, BKD, SKN, W/SALT	198	4.29	46.07	0.026
11364	POTATOES, BKD, SKN, WO/SALT	198	4.29	46.07	0.026
11831	POTATOES, BLD, CKD IN SKN, FLESH, W/SALT	87	1.87	20.13	0.026
11365	POTATOES, BLD, CKD IN SKN, FLESH, WO/SALT	87	1.87	20.13	0.026
11832	POTATOES, BLD, CKD IN SKN, SKN, W/SALT	78	2.86	17.21	0.026
11366	POTATOES, BLD, CKD IN SKN, SKN, WO/SALT	78	2.86	17.21	0.026
11833	POTATOES, BLD, CKD WO/ SKN, FLESH, W/ SALT	86	1.71	20.01	0.026
11367	POTATOES, BLD, CKD WO/ SKN, FLESH, WO/ SALT	86	1.71	20.01	0.026
11376	POTATOES, CND, DRND SOL	60	1.41	13.61	0.054
11374	POTATOES, CND, SOL&LIQUIDS	44	1.2	9.89	0.029
11838	POTATOES, FRENCH FR, FRZ, HOME-PREPARED, HTD IN OVEN, W/SA	200	3.17	31.19	1.262
11403	POTATOES, FRENCH FR, FRZ, HOME-PREPARED, HTD IN OVEN, WO/	200	3.17	31.19	1.262
11402	POTATOES, FRENCH FR, FRZ, UNPREP	156	2.47	24.33	0.985
11840	POTATOES, FRZ, FRCH FR, PAR FR, CTTGE-CUT, PREP, HTD OVEN, W	218	3.44	34.04	3.894
11407	POTATOES, FRZ, FRCH FR, PAR FR, CTTGE-CUT, PREP, HTD OVEN, W	218	3.44	34.04	3.894
11409	POTATOES, FRZ, FRCH FR, PAR FR, EXTRUDED, PREP, HTD OVEN, W	333	3.55	39.68	5.96
11406	POTATOES, FRZ, FRENCH FR, PAR FR, COTTAGE-CUT, UNPREP	153	2.42	23.98	2.743
11408	POTATOES, FRZ, FRENCH FR, PAR FR, EXTRUDED, UNPREP	260	2.83	30.15	4.544

NDB #	Food Description (100 gram portions = 3½ ounces = 20 tsp = ½ cup approx.	Calories	Protein	Carbs	Sat Fat
11837	POTATOES, FRZ, WHL, CKD, BLD, DRND, W/SALT	65	1.98	14.52	0.034
11401	POTATOES, FRZ, WHL, CKD, BLD, DRND, WO/SALT	65	1.98	14.52	0.034
11400	POTATOES, FRZ, WHL, UNPREP	78	2.38	17.48	0.041
11391	POTATOES, HASHED BROWN, FRZ, PLN, PREP	218	3.16	28.1	4.493
11390	POTATOES, HASHED BROWN, FRZ, PLN, UNPREP	82	2.06	17.72	0.163
11393	POTATOES, HASHED BROWN, FRZ, W/BUTTER SAU, PREP	178	2.46	24.13	3.373
11392	POTATOES, HASHED BROWN, FRZ, W/BUTTER SAU, UNPREP	135	1.87	18.28	2.556
11370	POTATOES, HASHED BROWN, HOME-PREPARED	209	2.42	21.32	5.433
11675	POTATOES, MICROWAVED, CKD IN SKN, FLESH&SKN, WO/SALT	105	2.44	24.13	0.026
11835	POTATOES, MICROWAVED, CKD IN SKN, FLESH, W/SALT	100	2.1	23.28	0.026
11368	POTATOES, MICROWAVED, CKD IN SKN, FLESH, WO/SALT	100	2.1	23.28	0.026
11369	POTATOES, MICROWAVED, CKD IN SKN, SKN, WO/SALT	132	4.39	29.63	0.026
11834	POTATOES, MICROWAVED, CKD, IN SKN, FLESH&SKN, W/SALT	105	2.44	24.13	0.026
11836	POTATOES, MICROWAVED, CKD, IN SKN, SKN W/SALT	132	4.39	29.63	0.026
11378	POTATOES, MSHD, DEHYD, FLAKES WO/MILK, DRY FORM	354	8.35	81.21	0.1
11382	POTATOES, MSHD, DEHYD, GRANULES W/MILK, DRY FORM	358	10.9	77.7	0.461
11380	POTATOES, MSHD, DEHYD, GRANULES WO/MILK, DRY FORM	372	8.22	85.51	0.138
11379	POTATOES, MSHD, DEHYD, PREP FR FLKS WO/MILK, WHL MILK&BUT	113	1.9	15.02	3.434
11381	POTATOES, MSHD, DEHYD, PREP FR GRNLS WO/MILK, WHL MILK&B	108	2.05	14.36	3.056
11383	POTATOES, MSHD, DEHYD, PREP FROM GRANULES W/MILK, H2O&M	79	2	13.1	0.679
11657	POTATOES, MSHD, HOME-PREPARED, WHL MILK	77	1.94	17.55	0.333
11934	POTATOES, MSHD, HOME-PREPARED, WHL MILK&BUTTER	106	1.88	16.71	2.77
11371	POTATOES, MSHD, HOME-PREPARED, WHL MILK&MARGARINE	106	1.88	16.71	1.035
11930	POTATOES, MSHD, PREP FROM FLAKES, WO/MILK, WHL MILK&MARG	113	1.9	15.02	1.46
11929	POTATOES, MSHD, PREP FROM GRANULES, WO/MILK, WHL MILK&M	108	2.05	14.4	1.284
11397	POTATOES, O'BRIEN, FRZ, PREP	204	2.22	21.86	3.313
11396	POTATOES, O'BRIEN, FRZ, UNPREP	76	1.83	17.47	0.032
11671	POTATOES, O'BRIEN, HOME-PREPARED	81	2.35	15.47	0.797
11362	POTATOES, RAW, SKIN	58	2.57	12.44	0.026
11358	POTATOES, RED, FLESH & SKN, BKD	89	2.3	19.59	0.026
11355	POTATOES, RED, FLESH & SKN, RAW	72	1.89	15.9	0.026
11356	POTATOES, RUSSET, FLESH & SKN, BKD	97	2.63	21.44	
11353	POTATOES, RUSSET, FLESH & SKN, RAW	82	2.14	18.07	0.02
11387	POTATOES, SCALLPD, DRY MIX, PREP W/H2O, WHL MILK&BUTTER	93	2.12	12.77	2.633
11386	POTATOES, SCALLPD, DRY MIX, UNPREP	358	7.77	73.93	1.2

NDB #	Food Description (100 gram portions = 3½ ounces = 20 tsp = ½ cup approx.	Calories	Protein	Carbs	Sat Fat
11372	POTATOES, SCALLPD, HOME-PREPARED W/BUTTER	86	2.87	10.78	2.255
11844	POTATOES, SCALLPD, HOME-PREPARED W/MARGARINE	86	2.87	10.78	1.377
11357	POTATOES, WHITE, FLESH & SKN, BKD	94	2.1	21.08	0.022
11354	POTATOES, WHITE, FLESH & SKN, RAW	70	1.68	15.71	0.026
05306	POULTRY FD PRODUCTS, GROUND TURKEY, CKD	235	27.36	0	3.39
05305	POULTRY FD PRODUCTS, GROUND TURKEY, RAW	149	17.46	0	2.25
07067	POULTRY SALAD SNDWCH SPRD	200	11.64	7.41	3.45
02034	POULTRY SEASONING	307	9.59	65.59	3.29
05301	POULTRY, MECHANICALLY DEBONED, FROM BACKS&NECKS W/SKN,	272	11.39	0	7.45
05302	POULTRY, MECHANICALLY DEBONED, FROM BACKS&NECKS WO/SK	199	13.79	0	4.71
05303	POULTRY, MECHANICALLY DEBONED, FROM MATURE HENS, RAW	243	14.72	0	4.73
15206	POUT, OCEAN, CKD, DRY HEAT	102	21.33	0	0.41
15059	POUT, OCEAN, RAW	79	16.64	0	0.32
19048	PRETZELS, HARD, CONFECTIONER'S COATING, CHOCOLATE-FLAVO	458	7.5	70.9	7.68
19812	PRETZELS, HARD, PLN, MADE W/UNENR FLR, SALTED	381	9.1	79.2	0.75
19813	PRETZELS, HARD, PLN, MADE W/UNENR FLR, UNSALTED	381	9.1	79.2	0.75
19047	PRETZELS, HARD, PLN, SALTED	381	9.1	79.2	0.75
19050	PRETZELS, HARD, WHOLE-WHEAT	362	11.1	81.2	0.56
09287	PRICKLY PEARS, RAW	41	0.73	9.57	0.067
09294	PRUNE JUICE, CANNED	71	0.61	17.45	0.003
09423	PRUNE PUREE	257	2.1	65.1	0.016
09288	PRUNES, CND, HVY SYRUP PK, SOL&LIQUIDS	105	0.87	27.8	0.016
09290	PRUNES, DEHYD (LOW-MOISTURE), STWD	113	1.23	29.7	0.02
09289	PRUNES, DEHYD (LOW-MOISTURE), UNCKD	339	3.7	89.07	0.059
09293	PRUNES, DRIED, STWD, W/ SUGAR	124	1.09	32.88	0.017
09292	PRUNES, DRIED, STWD, WO/ SUGAR	107	1.17	28.08	0.019
09291	PRUNES, DRIED, UNCOOKED	239	2.61	62.73	0.041
19318	PUDDINGS, BANANA, DRY MIX, INST	367	0	92.7	0.09
19121	PUDDINGS, BANANA, DRY MIX, INST, PREP W/ 2% MILK	105	2.76	19.74	0.971
19319	PUDDINGS, BANANA, DRY MIX, INST, PREP W/ WHL MILK	115	2.73	19.63	1.679
19705	PUDDINGS, BANANA, DRY MIX, INST, W/ ADDED OIL	386	0	89	0.79
19320	PUDDINGS, BANANA, DRY MIX, REG	376	0	92.9	0.09
19122	PUDDINGS, BANANA, DRY MIX, REG, PREP W/ 2% MILK	101	2.9	18.43	1.015
19321	PUDDINGS, BANANA, DRY MIX, REG, PREP W/ WHL MILK	111	2.86	18.31	1.757
19706	PUDDINGS, BANANA, DRY MIX, REG, W/ ADDED OIL	387	0	88.4	0.9

NDB #	Food Description (100 gram portions = 3½ ounces = 20 tsp = ½ cup approx.	Calories	Protein	Carbs	Sat Fat
19311	PUDDINGS, BANANA, RTE	127	2.4	21.2	0.56
19184	PUDDINGS, CHOC, DRY MIX, INST	355	2.3	87.7	0.64
19123	PUDDINGS, CHOC, DRY MIX, INST, PREP W/ 2% MILK	105	3.15	18.89	1.064
19185	PUDDINGS, CHOC, DRY MIX, INST, PREP W/ WHL MILK	111	3.1	18.8	1.83
19188	PUDDINGS, CHOC, DRY MIX, REG	361	2.6	89	1.21
19190	PUDDINGS, CHOC, DRY MIX, REG, PREP W/ 2% MILK	109	3.28	19.55	1.189
19189	PUDDINGS, CHOC, DRY MIX, REG, PREP W/ WHL MILK	111	3.2	18	2.09
19183	PUDDINGS, CHOC, RTE	133	2.7	22.8	0.71
19235	PUDDINGS, CHOC, RTE, FAT FREE	95	2.5	20.3	0.3
19322	PUDDINGS, COCNT CRM, DRY MIX, INST	387	0.9	89.4	2.2
19191	PUDDINGS, COCNT CRM, DRY MIX, INST, PREP W/ 2% MILK	107	2.9	19.2	1.37
19323	PUDDINGS, COCNT CRM, DRY MIX, INST, PREP W/ WHL MILK	117	2.9	19.1	2.1
19324	PUDDINGS, COCNT CRM, DRY MIX, REG	392	1	87.7	4.86
19219	PUDDINGS, COCNT CRM, DRY MIX, REG, PREP W/ 2% MILK	104	3.1	17.8	1.8
19325	PUDDINGS, COCNT CRM, DRY MIX, REG, PREP W/ WHL MILK	114	3	17.7	2.57
19288	PUDDINGS, KRAFT, JELL-O BRAND FAT FREE PUDD SNACKS CHOC,	90	2.5	20.1	0.3
19289	PUDDINGS, KRAFT, JELL-O BRAND FAT FREE PUDD SNACKS VANILL	92	2.1	20.5	0.2
19284	PUDDINGS, KRAFT, JELL-O BRAND INST PUDD & PIE FILLING CHOC,	355	1.5	89.6	0.5
19285	PUDDINGS, KRAFT, JELL-O BRAND INST PUDD & PIE FILLING VAN, P	375	0.1	93.5	0.2
19330	PUDDINGS, LEMON, DRY MIX, INST	378	0	95.4	0.1
19204	PUDDINGS, LEMON, DRY MIX, INST, PREP W/ 2% MILK	107	2.76	20.2	0.974
19331	PUDDINGS, LEMON, DRY MIX, INST, PREP W/ WHL MILK	115	2.7	20.1	1.74
19332	PUDDINGS, LEMON, DRY MIX, REG	363	0.1	91.8	
19333	PUDDINGS, LEMON, DRY MIX, REG, PREP W/ SUGAR, EGG YOLK & H2	113	0.7	24.64	0.39
19708	PUDDINGS, LEMON, DRY MIX, REG, W/ ADDED OIL, K, NA	366	0.1	90.3	0.27
19380	PUDDINGS, LEMON, RTE	125	0.1	25	0.45
19194	PUDDINGS, RICE, DRY MIX	376	2.7	91.2	
19208	PUDDINGS, RICE, DRY MIX, PREP W/ 2% MILK	111	3.29	20.81	0.967
19195	PUDDINGS, RICE, DRY MIX, PREP W/ WHL MILK	121	3.25	20.68	1.682
19193	PUDDINGS, RICE, RTE	163	2	22	1.17
19198	PUDDINGS, TAPIOCA, DRY MIX	369	0.1	94.3	
19209	PUDDINGS, TAPIOCA, DRY MIX, PREP W/ 2% MILK	105	2.88	19.56	0.991
19199	PUDDINGS, TAPIOCA, DRY MIX, PREP W/ WHL MILK	115	2.84	19.43	1.724
19709	PUDDINGS, TAPIOCA, DRY MIX, W/ NO ADDED SALT	369	0.1	94.3	
19218	PUDDINGS, TAPIOCA, RTE	119	2	19.4	0.6

NDB #	Food Description (100 gram portions = 3½ ounces = 20 tsp = ½ cup approx.	Calories	Protein	Carbs	Sat Fat
19234	PUDDINGS, TAPIOCA, RTE, FAT FREE	87	1.8	20.4	0.061
19202	PUDDINGS, VANILLA, DRY MIX, INST	368	0	92.9	0.1
19203	PUDDINGS, VANILLA, DRY MIX, INST, PREP W/ WHL MILK	114	2.7	19.7	1.74
19206	PUDDINGS, VANILLA, DRY MIX, REG	369	0.3	93.5	0.09
19212	PUDDINGS, VANILLA, DRY MIX, REG, PREP W/ 2% MILK	101	2.94	18.53	1.017
19207	PUDDINGS, VANILLA, DRY MIX, REG, PREP W/ WHL MILK	111	2.9	18.5	1.83
19710	PUDDINGS, VANILLA, DRY MIX, REG, W/ ADDED OIL	369	0.3	92.4	0.2
19201	PUDDINGS, VANILLA, RTE	130	2.3	21.9	0.57
19233	PUDDINGS, VANILLA, RTE, FAT FREE	93	2.1	20.8	0.072
18337	PUFF PASTRY, FRZ, RTB	551	7.3	45.1	9.643
18211	PUFF PASTRY, FRZ, RTB, BKD	558	7.4	45.7	5.502
09295	PUMMELO, RAW	38	0.76	9.62	
11417	PUMPKIN FLOWERS, CKD, BLD, DRND, WO/SALT	15	1.09	3.3	0.041
11416	PUMPKIN FLOWERS, RAW	15	1.03	3.28	0.036
11419	PUMPKIN LEAVES, CKD, BLD, DRND, WO/SALT	21	2.72	3.39	0.114
11418	PUMPKIN LEAVES, RAW	19	3.15	2.33	0.207
11426	PUMPKIN PIE MIX, CANNED	104	1.09	26.39	0.065
02035	PUMPKIN PIE SPICE	342	5.76	69.28	6.53
12014	PUMPKIN&SQUASH SD KRNLS, DRIED	541	24.54	17.81	8.674
12516	PUMPKIN&SQUASH SD KRNLS, RSTD, W/SALT	522	32.97	13.43	7.97
12016	PUMPKIN&SQUASH SD KRNLS, RSTD, WO/SALT	522	32.97	13.43	7.97
12663	PUMPKIN&SQUASH SEEDS, WHL, RSTD, W/SALT	446	18.55	53.75	3.67
12163	PUMPKIN&SQUASH SEEDS, WHL, RSTD, WO/SALT	446	18.55	53.75	3.67
11846	PUMPKIN, CANNED, WITH SALT	34	1.1	8.08	0.146
11845	PUMPKIN, CKD, BLD, DRND, W/SALT	20	0.72	4.89	0.037
11423	PUMPKIN, CKD, BLD, DRND, WO/SALT	20	0.72	4.89	0.037
11424	PUMPKIN, CND, WO/SALT	34	1.1	8.08	0.146
11847	PUMPKIN, FLOWERS, CKD, BLD, DRND, W/SALT	15	1.09	3.3	0.041
11848	PUMPKIN, LEAVES, CKD, BLD, DRND, W/SALT	21	2.72	3.39	0.114
11422	PUMPKIN, RAW	26	1	6.5	0.052
11849	PURSLANE, CKD, BLD, DRND, W/SALT	18	1.49	3.55	
11428	PURSLANE, CKD, BLD, DRND, WO/SALT	18	1.49	3.55	
11427	PURSLANE, RAW	16	1.3	3.43	
05159	QUAIL, BREAST, MEAT ONLY, RAW	123	22.59	0	0.87
05157	QUAIL, MEAT AND SKIN, RAW	192	19.63	0	3.38

NDB #	Food Description (100 gram portions = 3½ ounces = 20 tsp = ½ cup approx.	Calories	Protein	Carbs	Sat Fat
05158	QUAIL, MEAT ONLY, RAW	134	21.76	0	1.32
18643	QUAKER OATS, AUNT JEMIMA ORIGINAL WAFFLES, FRZ	273	7.1	42.3	2.19
09296	QUINCES, RAW	57	0.4	15.3	0.01
20035	QUINOA	374	13.1	68.9	0.59
11952	RADICCHIO, RAW	23	1.43	4.48	0.06
11676	RADISH SEEDS, SPROUTED, RAW	43	3.81	3.6	0.767
11850	RADISHES, ORIENTAL, CKD, BLD, DRND, W/SALT	17	0.67	3.43	0.073
11431	RADISHES, ORIENTAL, CKD, BLD, DRND, WO/SALT	17	0.67	3.43	0.073
11432	RADISHES, ORIENTAL, DRIED	271	7.9	63.37	0.218
11430	RADISHES, ORIENTAL, RAW	18	0.6	4.11	0.03
11429	RADISHES, RAW	20	0.6	3.59	0.03
11637	RADISHES, WHITE ICICLE, RAW	14	1.1	2.63	0.03
09297	RAISINS, GOLDEN SEEDLESS	302	3.39	79.52	0.151
09299	RAISINS, SEEDED	296	2.52	78.47	0.178
09298	RAISINS, SEEDLESS	300	3.22	79.13	0.15
09301	RAMBUTAN, CND, SYRUP PK	82	0.65	20.87	
09304	RASPBERRIES, CND, RED, HVY SYRUP PK, SOL&LIQUIDS	91	0.83	23.36	0.005
09306	RASPBERRIES, FRZ, RED, SWTND	103	0.7	26.16	0.005
09302	RASPBERRIES, RAW	49	0.91	11.57	0.019
22549	RED BARON PEPPERONI PIZZA, FRZ	287	11.7	23.4	5.87
22551	RED BARON PREMIUM DEEP DISH SINGLES, PEPPERONI PIZZA, FRZ	286	9.5	28.5	4.88
22540	RED BARON PREMIUM POCKETS, ORIGINAL HAM&CHS, FRZ	268	11.2	27.2	4.66
22550	RED BARON SPL DELUXE PIZZA, TWO CHS, SAUSAGE, PEPPRONI&O	261	9.3	24.8	4.86
22598	RED BARON SUPREME PIZZA, SAUSAGE, MUSHROOMS, PEPPERONI,	253	10	23.4	4.48
16103	REFRIED BEANS, CANNED (INCL USDA COMMODITY)	94	5.49	15.53	0.474
19213	RENNIN, CHOC, DRY MIX, PREP W/ 2% MILK	85	3.24	13.47	1.231
19221	RENNIN, CHOC, DRY MIX, PREP W/ WHL MILK	96	3.2	13.34	1.999
19214	RENNIN, VANILLA, DRY MIX, PREP W/ 2% MILK	77	3.06	12.34	1.061
19223	RENNIN, VANILLA, DRY MIX, PREP W/ WHL MILK	89	3.03	12.21	1.846
09309	RHUBARB, FROZEN, UNCOOKED	21	0.55	5.1	0.029
09310	RHUBARB, FRZ, CKD, W/SUGAR	116	0.39	31.2	0.014
09307	RHUBARB, RAW	21	0.9	4.54	0.053
14342	RICE BEV, RICE DREAM, CND	49	0.17	10.14	0.068
20060	RICE BRAN, CRUDE	316	13.35	49.69	4.171
19052	RICE CAKES, BROWN RICE, BUCKWHEAT	380	9	80.1	0.64

NDB #	Food Description (100 gram portions = 3½ ounces = 20 tsp = ½ cup approx.	Calories	Protein	Carbs	Sat Fat
20053	RICE, WHITE, SHORT-GRAIN, CKD	130	2.36	28.73	0.051
20453	RICE, WHITE, SHORT-GRAIN, CKD, UNENR	130	2.36	28.73	0.051
20052	RICE, WHITE, SHORT-GRAIN, RAW	358	6.5	79.15	0.14
20452	RICE, WHITE, SHORT-GRAIN, RAW, UNENR	358	6.5	79.15	0.14
20057	RICE, WHITE, W/PASTA, CKD	122	2.54	21.43	0.541
20056	RICE, WHITE, WITH PASTA, DRY	368	9.37	75.32	0.44
07912	ROAST BF SPRD	223	15.27	3.73	6.4
15071	ROCKFISH, PACIFIC, MXD SP, CKD, DRY HEAT	121	24.04	0	0.474
15070	ROCKFISH, PACIFIC, MXD SP, RAW	94	18.75	0	0.37
15072	ROE, MIXED SPECIES, RAW	140	22.32	1.5	1.456
15207	ROE, MXD SP, CKD, DRY HEAT	204	28.62	1.92	1.866
18344	ROLLS, DINNER, EGG	307	9.5	52	1.577
18345	ROLLS, DINNER, OAT BRAN	236	9.5	40.2	0.619
18342	ROLLS, DINNER, PLN, COMMLY PREP (INCL BROWN-AND-SERVE)	300	8.4	50.4	1.753
18396	ROLLS, DINNER, PLN, PREP FROM RECIPE, MADE W/LOFAT (2%) MIL	316	8.5	53.4	1.795
18346	ROLLS, DINNER, RYE	286	10.3	53.1	0.605
18347	ROLLS, DINNER, WHEAT	273	8.6	46	1.497
18348	ROLLS, DINNER, WHOLE-WHEAT	266	8.7	51.1	0.836
18349	ROLLS, FRENCH	277	8.6	50.2	0.962
18351	ROLLS, HAMBURGER OR HOTDOG, MIXED-GRAIN	263	9.6	44.6	1.39
18350	ROLLS, HAMBURGER OR HOTDOG, PLN	286	8.5	50.3	1.201
18352	ROLLS, HAMBURGER OR HOTDOG, RED-CAL	196	8.3	42.1	0.325
18353	ROLLS, HARD (INCL KAISER)	293	9.9	52.7	0.606
09312	ROSE-APPLES, RAW	25	0.6	5.7	
09311	ROSELLE, RAW	49	0.96	11.31	
02036	ROSEMARY, DRIED	331	4.88	64.06	7.371
02063	ROSEMARY, FRESH	131	3.31	20.7	2.838
15232	ROUGHY, ORANGE, CKD, DRY HEAT	89	18.85	0	0.023
15073	ROUGHY, ORANGE, RAW	69	14.7	0	0.018
09428	ROWAL, RAW	111	2.3	23.9	0.245
11851	RUTABAGAS, CKD, BLD, DRND, W/SALT	39	1.29	8.74	0.029
11436	RUTABAGAS, CKD, BLD, DRND, WO/SALT	39	1.29	8.74	0.029
11435	RUTABAGAS, RAW	36	1.2	8.13	0.027
20062	RYE	335	14.76	69.76	0.287
20063	RYE FLOUR, DARK	324	14.03	68.74	0.309

NDB #	Food Description (100 gram portions = 3½ ounces = 20 tsp = ½ cup approx.	Calories	Protein	Carbs	Sat Fat
20053	RICE, WHITE, SHORT-GRAIN, CKD	130	2.36	28.73	0.051
20453	RICE, WHITE, SHORT-GRAIN, CKD, UNENR	130	2.36	28.73	0.051
20052	RICE, WHITE, SHORT-GRAIN, RAW	358	6.5	79.15	0.14
20452	RICE, WHITE, SHORT-GRAIN, RAW, UNENR	358	6.5	79.15	0.14
20057	RICE, WHITE, W/PASTA, CKD	122	2.54	21.43	0.541
20056	RICE, WHITE, WITH PASTA, DRY	368	9.37	75.32	0.44
07912	ROAST BF SPRD	223	15.27	3.73	6.4
15071	ROCKFISH, PACIFIC, MXD SP, CKD, DRY HEAT	121	24.04	0	0.474
15070	ROCKFISH, PACIFIC, MXD SP, RAW	94	18.75	0	0.37
15072	ROE, MIXED SPECIES, RAW	140	22.32	1.5	1.456
15207	ROE, MXD SP, CKD, DRY HEAT	204	28.62	1.92	1.866
18344	ROLLS, DINNER, EGG	307	9.5	52	1.577
18345	ROLLS, DINNER, OAT BRAN	236	9.5	40.2	0.619
18342	ROLLS, DINNER, PLN, COMMLY PREP (INCL BROWN-AND-SERVE)	300	8.4	50.4	1.753
18396	ROLLS, DINNER, PLN, PREP FROM RECIPE, MADE W/LOFAT (2%) MIL	316	8.5	53.4	1.795
18346	ROLLS, DINNER, RYE	286	10.3	53.1	0.605
18347	ROLLS, DINNER, WHEAT	273	8.6	46	1.497
18348	ROLLS, DINNER, WHOLE-WHEAT	266	8.7	51.1	0.836
18349	ROLLS, FRENCH	277	8.6	50.2	0.962
18351	ROLLS, HAMBURGER OR HOTDOG, MIXED-GRAIN	263	9.6	44.6	1.39
18350	ROLLS, HAMBURGER OR HOTDOG, PLN	286	8.5	50.3	1.201
18352	ROLLS, HAMBURGER OR HOTDOG, RED-CAL	196	8.3	42.1	0.325
18353	ROLLS, HARD (INCL KAISER)	293	9.9	52.7	0.606
09312	ROSE-APPLES, RAW	25	0.6	5.7	
09311	ROSELLE, RAW	49	0.96	11.31	
02036	ROSEMARY, DRIED	331	4.88	64.06	7.371
02063	ROSEMARY, FRESH	131	3.31	20.7	2.838
15232	ROUGHY, ORANGE, CKD, DRY HEAT	89	18.85	0	0.023
15073	ROUGHY, ORANGE, RAW	69	14.7	0	0.018
09428	ROWAL, RAW	111	2.3	23.9	0.245
11851	RUTABAGAS, CKD, BLD, DRND, W/SALT	39	1.29	8.74	0.029
11436	RUTABAGAS, CKD, BLD, DRND, WO/SALT	39	1.29	8.74	0.029
11435	RUTABAGAS, RAW	36	1.2	8.13	0.027
20062	RYE	335	14.76	69.76	0.287
20063	RYE FLOUR, DARK	324	14.03	68.74	0.309

NDB #	Food Description (100 gram portions = 3½ ounces = 20 tsp = ½ cup approx.	Calories	Protein	Carbs	Sat Fat
20065	RYE FLOUR, LIGHT	367	8.39	80.23	0.145
20064	RYE FLOUR, MEDIUM	354	9.39	77.49	0.198
15208	SABLEFISH, COOKED, DRY HEAT	250	17.19	0	4.099
15074	SABLEFISH, RAW	195	13.41	0	3.201
15075	SABLEFISH, SMOKED	257	17.65	0	4.213
12021	SAFFLOWER SD KRNLS, DRIED	517	16.18	34.29	3.682
12022	SAFFLOWER SD MEAL, PART DEFATTED	342	35.62	48.73	0.207
02037	SAFFRON	310	11.43	65.37	1.586
02038	SAGE, GROUND	315	10.63	60.73	7.03
04017	SALAD DRSNG, 1000 ISLAND, COMM, REG, W/SALT	377	0.9	15.2	6
04023	SALAD DRSNG, 1000 ISLAND, DIET, LO CAL, 10 CAL PER TSP, W/SALT	159	0.8	16.2	1.6
04140	SALAD DRSNG, BLUE + ROQUEFORT CHS, COMM, REG, WO/SALT	504	4.8	7.4	9.9
04539	SALAD DRSNG, BLUE OR ROQUEFORT CHS, COMM, REG, W/SALT	504	4.8	7.4	9.9
04120	SALAD DRSNG, FRENCH, COMM, REG, W/SALT	430	0.6	17.5	9.5
04141	SALAD DRSNG, FRENCH, COMM, REG, WO/SALT	430	0.6	17.5	9.5
04146	SALAD DRSNG, FRENCH, CTTNSD, OIL, HOME RECIPE	631	0.1	3.4	18.2
04020	SALAD DRSNG, FRENCH, DIET, LOFAT, 5 CAL PER TSP, W/SALT	134	0.2	21.7	0.8
04142	SALAD DRSNG, FRENCH, DIET, LOFAT, 5 CAL PER TSP, WO/SALT	134	0.2	21.7	0.8
04133	SALAD DRSNG, FRENCH, HOME RECIPE	631	0.1	3.4	12.6
04134	SALAD DRSNG, HOME RECIPE, CKD	157	4.2	14.9	2.9
04135	SALAD DRSNG, HOME RECIPE, VINEGAR&OIL	449	0	2.5	9.1
04021	SALAD DRSNG, ITALIAN, COMM, DIET, 2 CAL PER TSP, W/SALT	105	0.1	4.9	1.3
04144	SALAD DRSNG, ITALIAN, COMM, DIET, 2 CAL PER TSP, WO/SALT	105	0.1	4.9	1.3
04114	SALAD DRSNG, ITALIAN, COMM, REG, W/SALT	467	0.7	10.2	7
04143	SALAD DRSNG, ITALIAN, COMM, REG, WO/SALT	467	0.7	10.2	7
04121	SALAD DRSNG, KRAFT FREE FAT FREE ITALIAN DRSNG	62	1.4	11	0.5
04119	SALAD DRSNG, KRAFT FREE FAT FREE RANCH DRSNG	138	0.7	30.6	0.2
04118	SALAD DRSNG, KRAFT LT DONE RIGHT! ITALIAN DRSNG	170	1.1	8	1.3
04117	SALAD DRSNG, KRAFT LT DONE RIGHT! RANCH DRSNG	256	1.2	10.5	1.9
04013	SALAD DRSNG, KRAFT MAYO FAT FREE MAYO DRSNG	70	0.2	12.4	0.5
04011	SALAD DRSNG, KRAFT MAYO LT MAYO	334	0.6	8.5	5
04014	SALAD DRSNG, KRAFT MIRACLE WHIP FREE NONFAT DRSNG	84	0.2	15.5	0.6
04012	SALAD DRSNG, KRAFT MIRACLE WHIP LT DRSNG	231	0.6	14.4	2.9
04115	SALAD DRSNG, KRAFT RANCH DRSNG	510	1.4	4.6	8.2
04116	SALAD DRSNG, KRAFT ZESTY ITALIAN DRSNG	351	0.3	5.7	4

NDB #	Food Description (100 gram portions = 3½ ounces = 20 tsp = ½ cup approx.	Calories	Protein	Carbs	Sat Fat
04018	SALAD DRSNG, MAYO TYPE, REG, W/SALT	390	0.9	23.9	4.9
04028	SALAD DRSNG, MAYO, IMITN, MILK CRM	97	2.1	11.1	2.8
04027	SALAD DRSNG, MAYO, IMITN, SOYBN	232	0.3	16	3.3
04029	SALAD DRSNG, MAYO, IMITN, SOYBN WO/CHOL	482	0.1	15.8	7.5
04025	SALAD DRSNG, MAYO, SOYBN OIL, W/SALT	717	1.1	2.7	11.8
04145	SALAD DRSNG, MAYO, SOYBN OIL, WO/SALT	717	1.1	2.7	11.8
04026	SALAD DRSNG, MAYO, SOYBN&SAFFLOWER OIL, W/SALT	717	1.1	2.7	8.6
04022	SALAD DRSNG, RUSSIAN, LO CAL, W/SALT	141	0.5	27.6	0.6
04015	SALAD DRSNG, RUSSIAN, W/SALT	494	1.6	10.4	7.3
04016	SALAD DRSNG, SESAME SD	443	3.1	8.6	6.2
07068	SALAMI CKD BF	365	18.5	0.6	8.65
07926	SALAMI ITALIAN PORK	425	21.7	1.2	13.1
07941	SALAMI ITALIAN PORK & BF DRY SLICED 50% LESS NA	350	21.8	6.4	9.75
07913	SALAMI PORK BF LESS NA	396	15.01	15.38	10.58
07069	SALAMI, CKD, BF&PORK	250	13.92	2.25	8.09
07070	SALAMI, COOKED, TURKEY	196	16.37	0.55	4.02
07071	SALAMI, DRY OR HARD, PORK	407	22.58	1.6	11.89
07072	SALAMI, DRY OR HARD, PORK, BF	418	22.86	2.59	12.2
15237	SALMON, ATLANTIC, FARMED, CKD, DRY HEAT	206	22.1	0	2.504
15236	SALMON, ATLANTIC, FARMED, RAW	183	19.9	0	2.183
15209	SALMON, ATLANTIC, WILD, CKD, DRY HEAT	182	25.44	0	1.257
15076	SALMON, ATLANTIC, WILD, RAW	142	19.84	0	0.981
15210	SALMON, CHINOOK, CKD, DRY HEAT	231	25.72	0	3.214
15078	SALMON, CHINOOK, RAW	180	20.06	0	2.507
15077	SALMON, CHINOOK, SMOKED	117	18.28	0	0.929
15179	SALMON, CHINOOK, SMOKED, (LOX), REG	117	18.28	0	0.929
15211	SALMON, CHUM, CKD, DRY HEAT	154	25.82	0	1.077
15180	SALMON, CHUM, CND, WO/SALT, DRND SOL W/BONE	141	21.43	0	1.486
15080	SALMON, CHUM, DRND SOL W/BONE	141	21.43	0	1.486
15079	SALMON, CHUM, RAW	120	20.14	0	0.84
15239	SALMON, COHO, FARMED, CKD, DRY HEAT	178	24.3	0	1.944
15238	SALMON, COHO, FARMED, RAW	160	21.27	0	1.816
15247	SALMON, COHO, WILD, CKD, DRY HEAT	139	23.45	0	1.054
15082	SALMON, COHO, WILD, CKD, MOIST HEAT	184	27.36	0	1.595
15081	SALMON, COHO, WILD, RAW	146	21.62	0	1.26

NDB #	Food Description (100 gram portions = 3½ ounces = 20 tsp = ½ cup approx.	Calories	Protein	Carbs	Sat Fat
15212	SALMON, PINK, CKD, DRY HEAT	149	25.56	0	0.715
15084	SALMON, PINK, CND, SOL W/BONE&LIQ	139	19.78	0	1.535
15181	SALMON, PINK, CND, WO/SALT, SOL W/BONE&LIQ	139	19.78	0	1.535
15083	SALMON, PINK, RAW	116	19.94	0	0.558
15086	SALMON, SOCKEYE, CKD, DRY HEAT	216	27.31	0	1.917
15087	SALMON, SOCKEYE, CND, DRND SOL W/BONE	153	20.47	0	1.644
15182	SALMON, SOCKEYE, CND, WO/SALT, DRND SOL W/BONE	153	20.47	0	1.644
15085	SALMON, SOCKEYE, RAW	168	21.3	0	1.495
11437	SALSIFY, (VEG OYSTER), RAW	82	3.3	18.6	
11852	SALSIFY, CKD, BLD, DRND, W/SALT	68	2.73	15.37	
11438	SALSIFY, CKD, BLD, DRND, WO/SALT	68	2.73	15.37	0.041
02047	SALT, TABLE	0	0	0	0
04030	SANDWICH SPRD, W/CHOPD PICKLE, REG, UNSPEC OILS	389	0.9	22.4	5.1
07073	SANDWICH SPREAD, PORK, BEEF	235	7.66	11.94	5.99
21096	SANDWICHES&BURGERS, CHEESEBURGER, LRG, SINGLE MEAT PAT	329	16.29	25.63	8.024
21089	SANDWICHES&BURGERS, CHEESEBURGER, REG, SINGLE MEAT PAT	313	14.48	31.13	6.34
21097	SANDWICHES&BURGERS, CHSBURGER, LRG, SNGLE PATTY, W/BAC	312	16.41	19.04	8.33
21112	SANDWICHES&BURGERS, HAMBURGER, LRG, SINGLE MEAT PATTY,	311	16.51	23.16	6.12
21113	SANDWICHES&BURGERS, HAMBURGER, LRG, SINGLE PATTY, W/CO	235	11.85	18.35	4.78
21122	SANDWICHES&BURGERS, RST BF SNDWCH W/CHS	269	18.31	25.78	5.13
21123	SANDWICHES&BURGERS, STEAK SNDWCH	225	14.87	25.47	1.87
09313	SAPODILLA, RAW	83	0.44	19.96	0.194
09314	SAPOTES, (MARMALADE PLUM), RAW	134	2.12	33.76	
15088	SARDINE, ATLANTIC, CND IN OIL, DRND SOL W/BONE	208	24.62	0	1.528
15089	SARDINE, PACIFIC, CND IN TOMATO SAU, DRND SOL W/BONE	178	16.35	0	3.087
06150	SAUCE, BARBECUE SAUCE	75	1.8	12.8	0.27
06102	SAUCE, BEARNAISE, DEHYD, DRY	362	14.06	59.74	1.34
06720	SAUCE, CHS SAU MIX, DRY	438	7.68	60.52	8.44
06103	SAUCE, CHS, DEHYD, DRY	448	22.69	33.66	12.05
06930	SAUCE, CHS, RTS	174	6.71	6.83	6.01
06721	SAUCE, CPC, KNORR ALFREDO SAU, DRY MIX	412	14.8	47.5	11.05
06104	SAUCE, CURRY, DEHYD, DRY	427	9.38	50.62	3.44
06710	SAUCE, CUSTOM FOODS, RED LABEL ALLPURP ITALIAN SAU MIX, DR	346	2.86	75.69	0.309
06716	SAUCE, CUSTOM FOODS, SUPERB INST CHEDDAR CHS SAU MIX, DR	423	7.94	56.51	10.627
06715	SAUCE, CUSTOM FOODS, SUPERB INST NACHO CHS SAU MIX, DRY	420	7.99	55.93	10.315

NDB #	Food Description (100 gram portions = 3½ ounces = 20 tsp = ½ cup approx.	Calories	Protein	Carbs	Sat Fat
06179	SAUCE, FISH, READY-TO-SERVE	35	5.06	3.64	0.003
06175	SAUCE, HOISIN, RTS	220	3.31	44.08	0.568
06155	SAUCE, HOLLANDAISE, W/BUTTER FAT, DEHYD, DRY	554	11	32.1	27.05
06154	SAUCE, HOLLANDAISE, W/VEG OIL, DEHYD, DRY	374	13.75	62.45	1.93
06166	SAUCE, HOMEMADE, WHITE, MED	147	3.84	9.17	2.854
06167	SAUCE, HOMEMADE, WHITE, THICK	186	3.99	11.61	3.416
06165	SAUCE, HOMEMADE, WHITE, THIN	105	3.77	7.4	2.152
06308	SAUCE, KRAFT BARBECUE SAU HICKORY SMOKE	116	0.5	26.2	0
06307	SAUCE, KRAFT BARBECUE SAU ORIGINAL	116	0.5	26.1	0
06277	SAUCE, LA VICTORIA, CHEDDAR CHS SAU	161	1.86	9.07	3.459
06273	SAUCE, LA VICTORIA, GRN SALSA JALAPENA	32	0.92	4.7	
06139	SAUCE, LA VICTORIA, LA VICTORIA CHUNKY CHILI DIP, SALSA, CND	31	0.79	6.54	
06275	SAUCE, LA VICTORIA, LA VICTORIA ENCHILADA SAU	33	0.32	4.62	
06269	SAUCE, LA VICTORIA, LA VICTORIA GRN CHILE SALSA, MILD	25	1.3	4.3	
06260	SAUCE, LA VICTORIA, LA VICTORIA GRN TACO SAU, MED	30	0.79	5.82	
06259	SAUCE, LA VICTORIA, LA VICTORIA GRN TACO SAU, MILD	30	0.79	5.82	
06258	SAUCE, LA VICTORIA, LA VICTORIA RED TACO SAU, MED	42	1.34	8.21	
06257	SAUCE, LA VICTORIA, LA VICTORIA RED TACO SAU, MILD	42	1.34	8.21	
06266	SAUCE, LA VICTORIA, LA VICTORIA SALSA PICANTE, MED	28	1.22	4.97	
06265	SAUCE, LA VICTORIA, LA VICTORIA SALSA PICANTE, MILD	27	1.19	4.82	
06263	SAUCE, LA VICTORIA, LA VICTORIA SALSA RANCHERA, HOT	30	1.29	5.44	
06268	SAUCE, LA VICTORIA, LA VICTORIA SALSA SUPREMA, MED	26	1.16	4.65	
06267	SAUCE, LA VICTORIA, LA VICTORIA SALSA SUPREMA, MILD	27	0.79	5.4	
06262	SAUCE, LA VICTORIA, LA VICTORIA SALSA VICTORIA, HOT	24	0.92	4.43	
06272	SAUCE, LA VICTORIA, LA VICTORIA THICK 'N CHUNKY SALSA, HOT	28	1.53	4.63	
06271	SAUCE, LA VICTORIA, LA VICTORIA THICK 'N CHUNKY SALSA, MED	25	1.19	4.39	
06270	SAUCE, LA VICTORIA, LA VICTORIA THICK 'N CHUNKY SALSA, MILD	26	0.88	4.88	
06276	SAUCE, LA VICTORIA, MOLE POBLANO	421	14.5	49.82	
06278	SAUCE, LA VICTORIA, NACHO CHS SAU W/JALAPENO PEPPERS, MED	170	1.82	10.26	3.739
06274	SAUCE, LA VICTORIA, RED SALSA JALAPENA	40	1.45	7.24	
06261	SAUCE, LA VICTORIA, SALSA BRAVA, HOT	40	1.36	6.16	
06933	SAUCE, LIPTON, RAGU OLD WORLD STYLE SMOOTH PASTA SAU, TR	64	1.5	9.69	0.29
06137	SAUCE, MOLE POBLANO, DRY MIX, SINGLE BRAND	571	7.48	41.7	
06136	SAUCE, MOLE POBLANO, PREP FROM RECIPE	164	3.54	12.94	
06106	SAUCE, MUSHROOM, DEHYD, DRY	349	14.38	54.72	1.42

NDB #	Food Description (100 gram portions = 3½ ounces = 20 tsp = ½ cup approx.	Calories	Protein	Carbs	Sat Fat
06921	SAUCE, NESTLE, CHEF-MATE BASIC CHEDDAR CHS SAU, RTS	132	2.9	12.93	2.54
06908	SAUCE, NESTLE, CHEF-MATE GOLDEN CHS SAU, RTS	220	10.65	3.65	8.84
06156	SAUCE, NESTLE, CHEF-MATE HOT DOG CHILI SAU, RTS	110	4.27	14.65	1.54
06907	SAUCE, NESTLE, CHEF-MATE SHARP CHEDDAR CHS SAU, READY-T	211	8.66	2.9	7.25
06130	SAUCE, NESTLE, LJ MINOR ALLPURP STIR FRY SAU, RTS	108	1.53	15.66	0.616
06903	SAUCE, NESTLE, LJ MINOR CREOLE SAU, RTS	40	1.49	5.98	0.108
06181	SAUCE, NESTLE, LJ MINOR ITALIAN SAU, RTS	98	1.68	18.49	0.26
06905	SAUCE, NESTLE, LJ MINOR LEMON SAU, RTS	134	0.22	31.92	0.072
06131	SAUCE, NESTLE, LJ MINOR SWT N' SOUR GLAZE, RTS	158	0.46	38.93	0.005
06132	SAUCE, NESTLE, LJ MINOR SWT N' SOUR SAU, RTS	122	0.48	24.79	0.37
06129	SAUCE, NESTLE, LJ MINOR TERIYAKI SAU, RTS	130	0.93	23.37	0.361
06153	SAUCE, NESTLE, ORTEGA ENCHILADA SAUCE, RTS	50	1.45	6.71	0.29
06909	SAUCE, NESTLE, ORTEGA MILD NACHO CHS SAU, RTS	189	7.17	4	6.71
06910	SAUCE, NESTLE, ORTEGA NACHO CHS SAU, RTS	203	8.32	6.38	9.2
06157	SAUCE, NESTLE, ORTEGA PICANTE SAUCE, RTS	34	1.22	6.66	0.021
06922	SAUCE, NESTLE, QUE BUENO JALAPENO CHS SAU, RTS	129	3.19	12.3	2.87
06711	SAUCE, NESTLE, TRIO ALFREDO SAU MIX, DRY	535	15.32	36.52	13.18
06713	SAUCE, NESTLE, TRIO CHS SAU MIX, DRY	446	7.38	60.91	6.67
06714	SAUCE, NESTLE, TRIO NACHO CHS SAU MIX, DRY	428	8.95	63.06	6.66
06176	SAUCE, OYSTER, RTS	51	1.35	10.92	0.043
06931	SAUCE, PASTA, SPAGHETTI/MARINARA, RTS	57	1.42	8.22	0.295
06151	SAUCE, PLUM, READY-TO-SERVE	184	0.89	42.81	0.153
06932	SAUCE, PREGO 100% NAT SPAGHETTI SAU, TRADITIONAL, JAR	105	1.7	16	0.87
06140	SAUCE, RIDG'S, BULLS-EYE ORIGINAL BARBECUE SAU	175	1.2	42.1	
06168	SAUCE, RTS, PEPPER OR HOT	11	0.51	1.75	0.052
06169	SAUCE, RTS, PEPPER, TABASCO	12	1.29	0.8	0.106
06164	SAUCE, RTS, SALSA	28	1.27	6.24	0.03
06142	SAUCE, SOFRITO, PREP FROM RECIPE	237	12.8	5.46	
06148	SAUCE, SOUR CRM, DEHYD, DRY	512	15.7	48.31	15.65
06108	SAUCE, SPAGHETTI W/MUSHROOMS, DEHYD, DRY	304	10	49	5.73
06107	SAUCE, SPAGHETTI, DEHYD, DRY	281	6	64.26	0.64
06109	SAUCE, STROGANOFF, DEHYD, DRY	351	12.1	57.66	6.19
06110	SAUCE, SWT&SOUR, DEHYD, DRY	389	1	96.13	0.01
06111	SAUCE, TERIYAKI, DEHYD, DRY	283	9	60	0.29
06112	SAUCE, TERIYAKI, RTS	84	5.93	15.95	0

NDB #	Food Description (100 gram portions = 3½ ounces = 20 tsp = ½ cup approx.	Calories	Protein	Carbs	Sat Fat
06141	SAUCE, TEXAS BEST BARBECUE SAU ORIGINAL RECIPE	131	2.02	12.61	1.837
06113	SAUCE, WHITE, DEHYD, DRY	463	10.94	50.56	6.68
11439	SAUERKRAUT, CND, SOL&LIQUIDS	19	0.91	4.28	0.035
07004	SAUSAGE BERLINER PORK BF	230	15.27	2.59	6.08
07928	SAUSAGE CHICK BF PORK SKINLESS SMOKED	216	13.6	8.2	4.8
07914	SAUSAGE ITALIAN SWT LINKS	149	16.13	2.1	3.257
07927	SAUSAGE ITALIAN TURKEY SMOKED	158	15.05	4.65	3.77
07915	SAUSAGE POLISH BF W/ CHICK HOT	259	17.6	3.6	8.01
07916	SAUSAGE POLISH PORK & BF SMOKED	313	12.07	2.56	11.54
07917	SAUSAGE PORK & BF W/ CHEDDAR CHS SMOKED	293	12.89	2.13	10.47
07918	SAUSAGE SMMR PORK & BF STKS W/ CHEDDAR CHS	426	19.43	1.82	10.47
07919	SAUSAGE TURKEY BRKFST LINKS MILD	231	15.42	1.56	3.77
07929	SAUSAGE TURKEY HOT SMOKED	158	15.05	4.65	3.77
22902	SAUSAGE&PEPPERONI PIZZA, FRZ	264	10.8	24.78	4.34
07089	SAUSAGE, ITALIAN, PORK, CKD	323	20.03	1.5	9.07
07036	SAUSAGE, ITALIAN, PORK, RAW	346	14.25	0.65	11.27
16107	SAUSAGE, MEATLESS	256	18.53	9.85	2.926
02039	SAVORY, GROUND	272	6.73	68.73	3.26
15172	SCALLOP, MIXED SPECIES, RAW	88	16.78	2.36	0.079
15173	SCALLOP, MXD SP, CKD, BREADED&FRIED	215	18.07	10.13	2.669
15174	SCALLOP, MXD SP, IMITN, MADE FROM SURIMI	99	12.77	10.62	0.08
22595	SCRAMBLED EGGS&SAUSAGE W/HASHED BROWN POTATOES, FRZ	204	7.1	9.7	4.15
15213	SCUP, COOKED, DRY HEAT	135	24.21	0	
15090	SCUP, RAW	105	18.88	0	0.64
15092	SEA BASS, MXD SP, CKD, DRY HEAT	124	23.63	0	0.655
15091	SEA BASS, MXD SP, RAW	97	18.43	0	0.511
15214	SEATROUT, MXD SP, CKD, DRY HEAT	133	21.46	0	1.293
15093	SEATROUT, MXD SP, RAW	104	16.74	0	1.009
11663	SEAWEED, AGAR, DRIED	306	6.21	80.89	0.061
11442	SEAWEED, AGAR, RAW	26	0.54	6.75	0.006
11444	SEAWEED, IRISHMOSS, RAW	49	1.51	12.29	0.033
11445	SEAWEED, KELP, RAW	43	1.68	9.57	0.247
11446	SEAWEED, LAVER, RAW	35	5.81	5.11	0.061
11667	SEAWEED, SPIRULINA, DRIED	290	57.47	23.9	2.65
11666	SEAWEED, SPIRULINA, RAW	26	5.92	2.42	0.135

NDB #	Food Description (100 gram portions = 3½ ounces = 20 tsp = ½ cup approx.	Calories	Protein	Carbs	Sat Fat
11669	SEAWEED, WAKAME, RAW	45	3.03	9.14	0.13
12220	SEEDS, FLAXSEED	492	19.5	34.25	3.196
20066	SEMOLINA, ENRICHED	360	12.68	72.83	0.15
20466	SEMOLINA, UNENRICHED	360	12.68	72.83	0.15
12169	SESAME BUTTER, PASTE	595	18.08	25.45	7.124
12198	SESAME BUTTER, TAHINI, FROM RAW&STONE GROUND KRNLS	570	17.81	26.19	6.722
12166	SESAME BUTTER, TAHINI, FROM RSTD&TSTD KRNLS (MOST COMMO	595	17	21.19	7.529
12171	SESAME BUTTER, TAHINI, FROM UNROASTED KRNLS	607	17.95	17.89	7.904
12698	SESAME BUTTER, TAHINI, KRNLS UNSPEC	592	17.4	21.5	7.423
12170	SESAME FLOUR, HIGH-FAT	526	30.78	26.62	5.196
12033	SESAME FLOUR, LOW-FAT	333	50.14	35.51	0.201
12032	SESAME FLR, PART DEFATTED	382	40.32	35.14	1.634
12034	SESAME MEAL, PART DEFATTED	567	16.96	26.04	6.722
12201	SESAME SD KRNLS, DRIED (DECORT)	588	26.38	9.39	7.672
12529	SESAME SD KRNLS, TSTD, W/SALT (DECORT)	567	16.96	26.04	6.722
12029	SESAME SD KRNLS, TSTD, WO/SALT (DECORT)	567	16.96	26.04	6.722
12024	SESAME SEEDS, WHL, RSTD&TSTD	565	16.96	25.74	6.722
12023	SESAME SEEDS, WHOLE, DRIED	573	17.73	23.45	6.957
19418	SESAME STKS, WHEAT-BASED, SALTED	541	10.9	46.5	6.48
19820	SESAME STKS, WHEAT-BASED, UNSALTED	541	10.9	46.5	6.48
11922	SESBANIA FLOWER, CKD, STMD, W/SALT	22	1.14	5.23	
11448	SESBANIA FLOWER, CKD, STMD, WO/SALT	22	1.14	5.23	
11447	SESBANIA FLOWER, RAW	27	1.28	6.73	
15215	SHAD, AMERICAN, CKD, DRY HEAT	252	21.71	0	
15094	SHAD, AMERICAN, RAW	197	16.93	0	3.126
14428	SHAKE, FAST FD, STRAWBERRY	113	3.4	18.9	1.734
14346	SHAKE, FAST FOOD, CHOCOLATE	127	3.4	20.5	2.313
14347	SHAKE, FAST FOOD, VANILLA	111	3.5	17.9	1.858
11640	SHALLOTS, FREEZE-DRIED	348	12.3	80.7	0.084
11677	SHALLOTS, RAW	72	2.5	16.8	0.017
15095	SHARK, MIXED SPECIES, RAW	130	20.98	0	0.925
15096	SHARK, MXD SP, CKD, BATTER-DIPPED&FRIED	228	18.62	6.39	3.205
15098	SHEEPSHEAD, CKD, DRY HEAT	126	26.02	0	0.36
15097	SHEEPSHEAD, RAW	108	20.21	0	0.609
19097	SHERBET, ORANGE	138	1.1	30.4	1.16

NDB #	Food Description (100 gram portions = 3½ ounces = 20 tsp = ½ cup approx.	Calories	Protein	Carbs	Sat Fat
04546	SHORTENING BREAD, SOYBN (HYDR)&CTTNSD	884	0	0	22
04548	SHORTENING CAKE MIX, SOYBN (HYDR)&CTTNSD (HYDR)	884	0	0	27.2
04551	SHORTENING CONFECTIONERY, COCNT (HYDR)&OR PALM KERNEL (	884	0	0	91.3
04550	SHORTENING FRYING (HVY DUTY), BF TALLOW&CTTNSD	900	0	0	44.9
04556	SHORTENING FRYING (HVY DUTY), PALM (HYDR)	884	0	0	47.5
04547	SHORTENING FRYING (REG), SOYBN (HYDR)&CTTNSD (HYDR)	884	0	0	15.4
04560	SHORTENING FRYING HVY DUTY, SOYBN HYDR, LINOLEIC (LESS THA	884	0	0	21.1
04552	SHORTENING FRYING HVY DUTY, SOYBN HYDR, LINOLEIC 30% W/SILI	884	0	0	18.4
04559	SHORTENING HOUSEHOLD SOYBN (HYDR)&PALM	884	0	0	25.02
04549	SHORTENING INDUSTRIAL, LARD&VEG OIL	900	0	0	35.7
04554	SHORTENING INDUSTRIAL, SOYBN (HYDR)&CTTNSD	884	0	0	25.6
04570	SHORTENING, CONFECTIONERY, FRACTIONATED PALM	884	0	0	65.5
04544	SHORTENING, HOUSEHOLD, LARD&VEG OIL	900	0	0	40.3
04031	SHORTENING, HOUSEHOLD, SOYBN (HYDR) -COTTONSEED (HYDR)	884	0	0	25
04595	SHORTENING, MULTIPURPOSE, SOYBN (HYDR)&PALM (HYDR)	884	0	0	30.423
04587	SHORTENING, SPL PURPOSE FOR BAKING, SOYBN (HYDR) PALM&CT	884	0	0	28.843
04586	SHORTENING, SPL PURPOSE FOR CAKES&FROSTINGS, SOYBN (HYD	884	0	0	20.001
15149	SHRIMP, MIXED SPECIES, RAW	106	20.31	0.91	0.328
15150	SHRIMP, MXD SP, CKD, BREADED&FRIED	242	21.39	11.47	2.087
15151	SHRIMP, MXD SP, CKD, MOIST HEAT	99	20.91	0	0.289
15152	SHRIMP, MXD SP, CND	120	23.08	1.03	0.373
15153	SHRIMP, MXD SP, IMITN, MADE FROM SURIMI	101	12.39	9.13	0.29
21140	SIDE DISHES, POTATO SALAD	114	1.53	13.53	1.03
12193	SISYMBRIUM SP. SEEDS, WHL, DRIED	318	12.14	58.26	0.902
15100	SMELT, RAINBOW, CKD, DRY HEAT	124	22.6	0	0.579
15099	SMELT, RAINBOW, RAW	97	17.63	0	0.452
07074	SMOKED LINK SAUSAGE, PORK	389	22.2	2.1	11.32
07075	SMOKED LINK SAUSAGE, PORK&BF	336	13.4	1.43	10.62
07076	SMOKED LINK SAUSAGE, PORK&BF, FLR&NONFAT DRY MILK	268	13.97	3.97	7.82
07077	SMOKED LINK SAUSAGE, PORK&BF, NONFAT DRY MILK	313	13.28	1.92	9.72
19407	SNACKS, BF STKS, SMOKED	550	21.5	5.4	20.8
19804	SNACKS, CORN-BASE, EXTRUD, CHIPS, BARBECUE-FLAVOR, W/ENR	523	7	56.2	4.46
19802	SNACKS, CORN-BASED, EXTRDD, PUFFS OR TWISTS, CHEESE-FLAV	554	7.6	53.8	6.59
19272	SNACKS, FARLEY CANDY, FARLEY FRUIT SNACKS, W/VITAMINS A, C,	341	4.4	80.9	
19269	SNACKS, GENERAL MILLS, BETTY CROCKER FRT RL UPS, BRY FLV,	373	0.1	85.2	0.99

NDB #	Food Description (100 gram portions = 3½ ounces = 20 tsp = ½ cup approx.	Calories	Protein	Carbs	Sat Fat
19441	SNACKS, KELLOGG, KELLOGG'S NUTRI-GRAIN CRL BARS, FRUIT	368	4.4	72.9	1.5
19438	SNACKS, KELLOGG, KELLOGG'S RICE KRISPIES TREATS SQUARES	414	3.4	80.5	1.4
19439	SNACKS, KELLOGG'S LOFAT GRANOLA BAR, CRUNCHY ALMD/BRN S	390	8	78	1.1
19049	SNACKS, M&M MARS, COMBOS SNACKS CHEDDAR CHS PRETZEL	463	9.85	66.5	
19440	SNACKS, M&M MARS, KUDOS WHL GRAIN BARS, CHOC CHIP	437	5.76	67.69	9.45
19422	SNACKS, POTATO CHIPS, RED FAT	471	7.1	66.9	4.16
19814	SNACKS, PRETZELS, HARD, PLN, MADE W/ ENR FLR, UNSALTED	381	9.1	79.2	0.75
19273	SNACKS, SUNKIST, SUNKIST FRUIT ROLL, STRAWBERRY, W/VITMNS	342	0.6	82.7	
19857	SNACKS, TORTILLA CHIPS, NACHO-FLAVOR, MADE W/ENR MASA FLR	498	7.8	62.4	4.9
19424	SNACKS, TORTILLA CHIPS, NACHO-FLAVOR, RED FAT	445	8.7	71.6	2.91
15101	SNAPPER, MIXED SPECIES, RAW	100	20.51	0	0.285
15102	SNAPPER, MXD SP, CKD, DRY HEAT	128	26.3	0	0.365
14123	SNAPPLE, SNAPPLE KIWI STRAWBERRY COCKTAIL, RTD	48	0.1	11.8	
19251	SOKOL, SOLO POPPY SD FILLING	332	4.8	58.1	1.03
20067	SORGHUM	339	11.3	74.63	0.457
06731	SOUP, BEAN W/BACON, COND, SINGLE BRAND	117	6.5	18	0.601
06074	SOUP, BEAN W/BACON, DEHYD, DRY MIX	370	19.38	57.72	3.38
06474	SOUP, BEAN W/BACON, DEHYD, PREP W/H2O	40	2.07	6.18	0.36
06006	SOUP, BEAN W/FRANKFURTERS, CND, COND, COMM	142	7.6	16.75	1.61
06406	SOUP, BEAN W/FRANKFURTERS, CND, PREP W/EQ VOLUME H2O, CO	75	3.99	8.8	0.85
06007	SOUP, BEAN W/HAM, CND, CHUNKY, RTS, COMM	95	5.19	11.16	1.37
06004	SOUP, BEAN W/PORK, CND, COND, COMM	129	5.88	16.97	1.14
06404	SOUP, BEAN W/PORK, CND, PREP W/EQ VOLUME H2O, COMM	68	3.12	9.01	0.6
06076	SOUP, BEEF BROTH, CUBED, DRY	170	17.3	16.1	1.99
06032	SOUP, BF BROTH BOUILLON&CONSOMME, CND, COND, COMM	24	4.37	1.44	0
06008	SOUP, BF BROTH OR BOUILLON CND, RTS	7	1.14	0.04	0.11
06075	SOUP, BF BROTH OR BOUILLON, PDR, DRY	238	15.97	23.65	4.32
06475	SOUP, BF BROTH OR BOUILLON, PDR, PREP W/H2O	8	0.52	0.77	0.141
06432	SOUP, BF BROTH, BOUILLON, CONSOMME, PREP W/EQ VOLUME H2	12	2.22	0.73	0
06732	SOUP, BF BROTH, CND, COND, SINGLE BRAND	18	2.6	0	
06476	SOUP, BF BROTH, CUBED, PREP W/H2O	3	0.35	0.33	0.04
06147	SOUP, BF MUSHROOM, CND, COND, COMM	61	4.6	5.2	1.2
06547	SOUP, BF MUSHROOM, CND, PREP W/EQ VOLUME H2O, COMM	30	2.37	2.6	0.61
06077	SOUP, BF NOODLE MIX, DEHYD, DRY FORM	330	17.93	48.64	2.07
06009	SOUP, BF NOODLE, CND, COND, COMM	67	3.85	7.16	0.91

NDB #	Food Description (100 gram portions = 3½ ounces = 20 tsp = ½ cup approx.	Calories	Protein	Carbs	Sat Fat
06409	SOUP, BF NOODLE, CND, PREP W/EQ VOLUME H2O, COMM	34	1.98	3.68	0.47
06477	SOUP, BF NOODLE, DEHYD, PREP W/H2O	16	0.88	2.4	0.1
06749	SOUP, BF W/COUNTRY VEG, CHUNKY, RTS, SINGLE BRAND	63	5.1	6.6	0.539
06733	SOUP, BF W/VEG&BARLEY, CND, COND, SINGLE BRAND	61	3.9	8.2	0.48
06070	SOUP, BF, CND, CHUNKY, RTS	71	4.89	8.15	1.06
06002	SOUP, BLACK BEAN, CND, COND, COMM	91	4.83	15.42	0.34
06402	SOUP, BLACK BEAN, CND, PREP W/EQ VOLUME H2O, COMM	47	2.28	8.02	0.16
06059	SOUP, CAMPBELL'S CHICK NOODLE, CND, COND	51	2.6	6.9	0.5
06078	SOUP, CAULIFLOWER, DEHYD, DRY MIX	360	15.31	56.59	1.36
06478	SOUP, CAULIFLOWER, DEHYD, PREP W/H2O	27	1.13	4.19	0.1
06081	SOUP, CHICK BROTH CUBES, DEHYD, DRY	198	14.6	23.5	1.25
06481	SOUP, CHICK BROTH CUBES, DEHYD, PREP W/H2O	5	0.39	0.62	0.03
06080	SOUP, CHICK BROTH OR BOUILLON, DEHYD, DRY	267	16.66	18.01	3.43
06480	SOUP, CHICK BROTH OR BOUILLON, DEHYD, PREP W/H2O	9	0.55	0.59	0.11
06013	SOUP, CHICK BROTH, CND, COND, COMM	31	4.42	0.75	0.31
06413	SOUP, CHICK BROTH, CND, PREP W/EQ VOLUME H2O, COMM	16	2.02	0.38	0.16
06725	SOUP, CHICK CORN CHOWDER, CHUNKY, RTS, SINGLE BRAND	99	3.1	7.5	1.75
06017	SOUP, CHICK GUMBO, CND, COND, COMM	45	2.1	6.67	0.26
06417	SOUP, CHICK GUMBO, CND, PREP W/EQ VOLUME H2O, COMM	23	1.08	3.43	0.13
06726	SOUP, CHICK MUSHROOM CHOWDER, CHUNKY, RTS, SINGLE BRAN	80	3	7.1	1.15
06149	SOUP, CHICK MUSHROOM, CND, COND, COMM	109	3.5	7.6	1.92
06549	SOUP, CHICK MUSHROOM, CND, PREP W/EQ VOLUME H2O, COMM	54	1.8	3.8	0.98
06128	SOUP, CHICK NOODLE MIX, DEHYD, DRY FORM	385	13.88	60.44	2.008
06741	SOUP, CHICK NOODLE W/CELERY&CARROTS, HOMESTYLE, RTS, SIN	31	2.1	3.1	0.283
06727	SOUP, CHICK NOODLE, CHUNKY, RTS, SINGLE BRAND	47	3.2	5.7	0.321
06018	SOUP, CHICK NOODLE, CND, CHUNKY, RTS	73	5.3	7.1	0.58
06019	SOUP, CHICK NOODLE, CND, COND, COMM	61	3.23	7.62	0.49
06419	SOUP, CHICK NOODLE, CND, PREP W/EQ VOLUME H2O, COMM	31	1.68	3.88	0.27
06528	SOUP, CHICK NOODLE, DEHYD, PREP W/H2O	23	0.84	3.67	0.122
06021	SOUP, CHICK NOODLE, W/MEATBALLS, CND, CHUNKY, RTS	40	3.27	3.37	0.43
06085	SOUP, CHICK RICE MIX, DEHYD, DRY FORM	369	15.07	57.09	1.99
06022	SOUP, CHICK RICE, CND, CHUNKY, RTS	53	5.11	5.41	0.4
06485	SOUP, CHICK RICE, DEHYD, PREP W/H2O	24	0.97	3.66	0.13
06740	SOUP, CHICK VEG, CHUNKY, RED FAT, RED NA, RTS, SINGLE BRAND	40	2.7	6.3	0.121
06024	SOUP, CHICK VEG, CND, CHUNKY, RTS	69	5.13	7.87	0.6

NDB #	Food Description (100 gram portions = 3½ ounces = 20 tsp = ½ cup approx.	Calories	Protein	Carbs	Sat Fat
06025	SOUP, CHICK VEG, CND, COND, COMM	61	2.94	7.01	0.69
06425	SOUP, CHICK VEG, CND, PREP W/EQ VOLUME H2O, COMM	31	1.5	3.56	0.35
06086	SOUP, CHICK VEG, DEHYD, DRY	346	18.98	55.04	1.29
06486	SOUP, CHICK VEG, DEHYD, PREP W/H2O	20	1.07	3.11	0.07
06012	SOUP, CHICK W/DUMPLINGS, CND, COND, COMM	79	4.58	4.93	1.07
06412	SOUP, CHICK W/DUMPLINGS, CND, PREP W/EQ VOLUME H2O, COMM	40	2.33	2.51	0.54
06023	SOUP, CHICK W/RICE, CND, COND, COMM	49	2.89	5.84	0.37
06423	SOUP, CHICK W/RICE, CND, PREP W/EQ VOLUME H2O, COMM	25	1.47	2.97	0.19
06734	SOUP, CHICK W/STAR-SHAPED PASTA, CND, COND, SINGLE BRAND	50	2.3	7.1	0.342
06015	SOUP, CHICK, CND, CHUNKY, RTS, COMM	71	5.06	6.88	0.79
06026	SOUP, CHILI BF, CND, COND, COMM	129	5.09	16.33	2.51
06426	SOUP, CHILI BF, CND, PREP W/EQ VOLUME H2O, COMM	68	2.68	8.58	1.34
06011	SOUP, CHS, CND, COND, COMM	121	4.22	8.19	5.19
06411	SOUP, CHS, CND, PREP W/EQ VOLUME H2O, COMM	63	2.19	4.26	2.7
06211	SOUP, CHS, CND, PREP W/EQ VOLUME MILK, COMM	92	3.77	6.47	3.63
06027	SOUP, CLAM CHOWDER, MANHATTAN STYLE, CND, CHUNKY, RTS	56	3.02	7.84	0.88
06087	SOUP, CLAM CHOWDER, MANHATTAN STYLE, DEHYD, DRY	345	10.94	57.46	1.39
06028	SOUP, CLAM CHOWDER, MANHATTAN, CND, COND, COMM	61	1.74	9.74	0.305
06428	SOUP, CLAM CHOWDER, MANHATTAN, CND, PREP W/EQ VOLUME H2	32	0.9	5.01	0.157
06030	SOUP, CLAM CHOWDER, NEW ENGLAND, CND, COND, COMM	70	4.33	8.69	0.3
06430	SOUP, CLAM CHOWDER, NEW ENGLAND, CND, PREP W/EQ VOLUME	39	1.97	5.09	0.17
06230	SOUP, CLAM CHOWDER, NEW ENGLAND, CND, PREP W/EQ VOLUME	66	3.82	6.7	1.19
06088	SOUP, CLAM CHOWDER, NEW ENGLAND, DEHYD, DRY	418	12.29	56.74	2.73
06089	SOUP, CONSOMME W/GELATIN, DEHYD, DRY	137	17.19	16.3	0.02
06489	SOUP, CONSOMME W/GELATIN, DEHYD, PREP W/H2O	7	0.87	0.83	0
06034	SOUP, CRAB, CND, RTS	31	2.25	4.22	0.16
06001	SOUP, CRM OF ASPARAGUS, CND, COND, COMM	69	1.82	8.52	0.82
06401	SOUP, CRM OF ASPARAGUS, CND, PREP W/EQ VOLUME H2O, COMM	35	0.94	4.38	0.43
06201	SOUP, CRM OF ASPARAGUS, CND, PREP W/EQ VOLUME MILK, COMM	65	2.55	6.61	1.34
06073	SOUP, CRM OF ASPARAGUS, DEHYD, DRY MIX	366	13.75	55.75	1.61
06473	SOUP, CRM OF ASPARAGUS, DEHYD, PREP W/H2O	23	0.88	3.57	0.02
06010	SOUP, CRM OF CELERY, CND, COND, COMM	72	1.32	7.03	1.12
06410	SOUP, CRM OF CELERY, CND, PREP W/EQ VOLUME H2O, COMM	37	0.68	3.62	0.58
06210	SOUP, CRM OF CELERY, CND, PREP W/EQ VOLUME MILK, COMM	66	2.29	5.86	1.59
06079	SOUP, CRM OF CELERY, DEHYD, DRY	358	15	55.9	1.39

NDB #	Food Description (100 gram portions = 3½ ounces = 20 tsp = ½ cup approx.	Calories	Protein	Carbs	Sat Fat
06479	SOUP, CRM OF CELERY, DEHYD, PREP W/H2O	25	1.03	3.84	0.1
06016	SOUP, CRM OF CHICK, CND, COND, COMM	93	2.73	7.38	1.66
06736	SOUP, CRM OF CHICK, CND, COND, SINGLE BRAND	99	2.4	7.7	1.61
06416	SOUP, CRM OF CHICK, CND, PREP W/EQ VOLUME H2O, COMM	48	1.41	3.8	0.85
06083	SOUP, CRM OF CHICK, DEHYD, DRY	436	7.25	54.34	13.78
06483	SOUP, CRM OF CHICK, DEHYD, PREP W/H2O	41	0.68	5.11	1.3
06216	SOUP, CRM OF CHICK, PREP W/EQ VOLUME MILK, COMM	77	3.01	6.04	1.87
06043	SOUP, CRM OF MUSHROOM, CND, COND, COMM	103	1.61	7.4	2.05
06443	SOUP, CRM OF MUSHROOM, CND, PREP W/EQ VOLUME H2O, COMM	53	0.95	3.81	1
06243	SOUP, CRM OF MUSHROOM, CND, PREP W/EQ VOLUME MILK, COMM	82	2.44	6.05	2.07
06046	SOUP, CRM OF ONION, CND, COND, COMM	88	2.2	10.4	1.17
06446	SOUP, CRM OF ONION, CND, PREP W/EQ VOLUME H2O, COMM	44	1.13	5.2	0.6
06246	SOUP, CRM OF ONION, CND, PREP W/EQ VOLUME MILK, COMM	75	2.74	7.4	1.63
06053	SOUP, CRM OF POTATO, CND, COND	59	1.39	9.14	0.97
06453	SOUP, CRM OF POTATO, CND, PREP W/EQ VOLUME H2O, COMM	30	0.72	4.7	0.5
06253	SOUP, CRM OF POTATO, CND, PREP W/EQ VOLUME MILK, COMM	60	2.33	6.92	1.52
06056	SOUP, CRM OF SHRIMP, CND, COND	72	2.22	6.53	2.58
06456	SOUP, CRM OF SHRIMP, CND, PREP W/EQ VOLUME H2O, COMM	37	1.14	3.36	1.33
06256	SOUP, CRM OF SHRIMP, CND, PREP W/EQ VOLUME MILK, COMM	66	2.75	5.61	2.33
06101	SOUP, CRM OF VEG, DEHYD, DRY	446	8	52.1	6.03
06501	SOUP, CRM OF VEG, DEHYD, PREP W/H2O	41	0.73	4.73	0.55
06035	SOUP, ESCAROLE, CND, RTS	11	0.62	0.72	0.22
06036	SOUP, GAZPACHO, CND, RTS	19	2.9	1.8	0.01
06490	SOUP, LEEK, DEHYD, PREP W/H2O	28	0.83	4.5	0.4
06090	SOUP, LEEK, DEHYDRATED, DRY	377	11.25	60.78	5.43
06037	SOUP, LENTIL W/HAM, CND, RTS	56	3.74	8.16	0.45
06286	SOUP, LIPTON, CUP-A-SOUP BROCCOLI&CHS, MIX, DRY	418	11.35	55.64	4.974
06291	SOUP, LIPTON, CUP-A-SOUP CHICK FLAVOR VEG	374	9.87	68.85	2.551
06289	SOUP, LIPTON, CUP-A-SOUP CHICK NOODLE W/MEAT	381	15.76	61.85	2.917
06290	SOUP, LIPTON, CUP-A-SOUP CRM OF CHICK, MIX, DRY	401	4.52	68.67	1.916
06295	SOUP, LIPTON, CUP-A-SOUP CRM OF MUSHROOM, MIX, DRY	399	5.15	65.23	2.083
06294	SOUP, LIPTON, CUP-A-SOUP GRN PEA, MIX, DRY	358	21.2	58.61	0.862
06288	SOUP, LIPTON, CUP-A-SOUP HEARTY CHICK NOODLE, MIX, DRY	384	16.07	63.53	2.667
06287	SOUP, LIPTON, CUP-A-SOUP HEARTY CHICK SUPREME, MIX, DRY	429	5.02	64.87	6.623
06292	SOUP, LIPTON, CUP-A-SOUP RING NOODLE, MIX, DRY	381	11.09	66.68	2.722

NDB #	Food Description (100 gram portions = 3½ ounces = 20 tsp = ½ cup approx.	Calories	Protein	Carbs	Sat Fat
06296	SOUP, LIPTON, CUP-A-SOUP SPRING VEG, MIX, DRY	361	13.26	63.32	1.632
06293	SOUP, LIPTON, CUP-A-SOUP TOMATO, MIX, DRY	366	8.84	76.79	1.629
06297	SOUP, LIPTON, FAT FREE CUP-A-SOUP CHICK BROTH, MIX, DRY	307	20.1	54.02	0.427
06298	SOUP, LIPTON, FAT FREE CUP-A-SOUP CHICKEN/PASTA, MIX, DRY	340	16.3	64	0.363
06300	SOUP, LIPTON, KETTLE CREATIONS CHICK W/PASTA&BEAN, MIX, DR	353	15.57	64.71	0.924
06299	SOUP, LIPTON, KETTLE CREATIONS HOMESTYLE LENTIL, MIX, DRY	354	20.71	62.49	0.384
06031	SOUP, LIPTON, KETTLE CREATIONS PASTA&BEAN, MIX, DRY	358	16.34	65.3	0.923
06722	SOUP, LIPTON, RECIPE SECRETS BEEFY MUSHROOM, MIX, DRY	298	7.76	60.22	0.485
06724	SOUP, LIPTON, RECIPE SECRETS BEEFY ONION, MIX, DRY	314	6.47	58.53	1.801
06723	SOUP, LIPTON, RECIPE SECRETS FIESTA HERB W/RED, MIX, DRY	322	10.66	64.44	0.637
06302	SOUP, LIPTON, RECIPE SECRETS ONION MUSHROOM, MIX, DRY	322	8.42	57.45	1.069
06033	SOUP, LIPTON, RECIPE SECRETS ONION, MIX, DRY	263	6.58	61.55	0.34
06305	SOUP, LIPTON, RECIPE SECRETS SAVORY HERB W/GARLIC, MIX, DRY	343	10.54	67.09	1.06
06301	SOUP, LIPTON, RECIPE SECRETS VEG, MIX, DRY	276	8.11	64.71	0.395
06281	SOUP, LIPTON, SOUP SECRETS CHICK NOODLE, MIX, DRY	385	17.31	56.52	2.936
06279	SOUP, LIPTON, SOUP SECRETS EX NOODLE, MIX, DRY	374	14.06	65.1	2.479
06283	SOUP, LIPTON, SOUP SECRETS GIGGLE NOODLE, MIX, DRY	387	13.28	60.34	3.624
06284	SOUP, LIPTON, SOUP SECRETS NOODLE W/REAL CHICK BROTH, MIX	388	12.83	57.37	3.878
06282	SOUP, LIPTON, SOUP SECRETS RING-O-NOODLE	388	12.96	58.28	3.761
06280	SOUP, LIPTON, SOUP SECRETS SPIRAL PASTA SOUP, MIX, DRY	353	12.22	63.63	1.6
06039	SOUP, MINESTRONE, CND, CHUNKY, RTS	53	2.13	8.64	0.62
06040	SOUP, MINESTRONE, CND, COND, COMM	68	3.48	9.17	0.44
06440	SOUP, MINESTRONE, CND, PREP W/EQ VOLUME H2O, COMM	34	1.77	4.66	0.23
06092	SOUP, MINESTRONE, DEHYD, DRY	358	20	53.6	3.68
06492	SOUP, MINESTRONE, DEHYD, PREP W/H2O	31	1.75	4.69	0.32
06042	SOUP, MUSHROOM BARLEY, CND, COND, COMM	61	1.5	9.6	0.35
06442	SOUP, MUSHROOM BARLEY, CND, PREP W/EQ VOLUME H2O, COMM	30	0.77	4.8	0.18
06044	SOUP, MUSHROOM W/BF STOCK, CND, COND, COMM	68	2.51	7.41	1.24
06444	SOUP, MUSHROOM W/BF STOCK, CND, PREP W/EQ VOLUME H2O, C	35	1.29	3.81	0.64
06093	SOUP, MUSHROOM, DEHYD, DRY	441	10.18	51.18	3.78
06493	SOUP, MUSHROOM, DEHYD, PREP W/H2O	38	0.88	4.4	0.32
06582	SOUP, NISSIN, CUP NOODLES, RAMEN NOODLE, CHICK FLAVOR, DRY	463	8.7	57.5	9.77
06094	SOUP, ONION MIX, DEHYD, DRY FORM	294	11.6	53.51	1.38
06045	SOUP, ONION, CND, COND, COMM	46	3.06	6.68	0.21
06445	SOUP, ONION, CND, PREP W/EQ VOLUME H2O, COMM	24	1.56	3.39	0.11

NDB #	Food Description (100 gram portions = 3½ ounces = 20 tsp = ½ cup approx.	Calories	Protein	Carbs	Sat Fat
06494	SOUP, ONION, DEHYD, PREP W/H2O	11	0.45	2.06	0.05
06581	SOUP, OODLES OF NOODLES RAMEN NOODLE ORIENTAL FLAVOR,	453	9.3	65.5	7.63
06095	SOUP, OXTAIL, DEHYD, DRY	377	15	47.9	6.77
06495	SOUP, OXTAIL, DEHYD, PREP W/H2O	28	1.11	3.54	0.5
06048	SOUP, OYSTER STEW, CND, COND, COMM	48	1.72	3.32	2.04
06448	SOUP, OYSTER STEW, CND, PREP W/EQ VOLUME H2O, COMM	24	0.87	1.69	1.04
06248	SOUP, OYSTER STEW, CND, PREP W/EQ VOLUME MILK, COMM	55	2.51	3.99	2.06
06049	SOUP, PEA, GRN, CND, COND, COMM	125	6.54	20.18	1.07
06449	SOUP, PEA, GRN, CND, PREP W/EQ VOLUME H2O, COMM	66	3.44	10.6	0.56
06249	SOUP, PEA, GRN, CND, PREP W/EQ VOLUME MILK, COMM	94	4.97	12.69	1.58
06096	SOUP, PEA, GRN, MIX, DEHYD, DRY FORM	356	20.49	60.68	1.54
06496	SOUP, PEA, GRN, MIX, DEHYD, PREP W/H2O	49	2.83	8.37	0.16
06050	SOUP, PEA, SPLIT W/HAM, CND, CHUNKY, RTS	77	4.62	11.17	0.66
06051	SOUP, PEA, SPLIT W/HAM, CND, COND, COMM	141	7.68	20.81	1.31
06451	SOUP, PEA, SPLIT W/HAM, CND, PREP W/EQ VOLUME H2O, COMM	75	4.08	11.05	0.7
06052	SOUP, PEPPERPOT, CND, COND, COMM	84	5.19	7.66	1.68
06452	SOUP, PEPPERPOT, CND, PREP W/EQ VOLUME H2O, COMM	43	2.64	3.89	0.85
06728	SOUP, POTATO HAM CHOWDER, CHUNKY, RTS, SINGLE BRAND	80	2.7	5.6	1.62
06205	SOUP, PROG HEALTHY CLASSICS NEW ENGLAND CLAM CHOWDER,	48	2.13	8.11	0.21
06747	SOUP, PROGRESSO CHICK&WILD RICE W/VEG	39	2.5	5	0.25
06748	SOUP, PROGRESSO HEALTHY CLASSICS BF BARLEY, 99% FAT FREE	57	5.1	7.1	0.29
06199	SOUP, PROGRESSO HEALTHY CLASSICS BF BARLEY, CND, RTS	59	4.7	8.3	0.31
06198	SOUP, PROGRESSO HEALTHY CLASSICS BF VEG, CND, RTS	64	4.18	10.25	0.25
06200	SOUP, PROGRESSO HEALTHY CLASSICS CHICK NOODLE, CND, RTS	32	2.42	3.98	0.176
06202	SOUP, PROGRESSO HEALTHY CLASSICS CHICK RICE W/VEG, CND, R	37	2.62	5.23	0.18
06203	SOUP, PROGRESSO HEALTHY CLASSICS CRM OF BROCCOLI, CND, R	36	0.97	5.46	0.27
06197	SOUP, PROGRESSO HEALTHY CLASSICS GARLIC&PASTA, CND, RTS	41	1.81	7.33	0.13
06204	SOUP, PROGRESSO HEALTHY CLASSICS LENTIL, CND, RTS	52	3.22	8.39	0.11
06206	SOUP, PROGRESSO HEALTHY CLASSICS MINESTRONE, CND, RTS	51	1.98	8.44	0.17
06192	SOUP, PROGRESSO HEALTHY CLASSICS SPLIT PEA, CND, RTS	71	3.85	11.83	0.3
06191	SOUP, PROGRESSO HEALTHY CLASSICS TOMATO GARDEN, CND, RT	40	1.42	7.77	0.07
06207	SOUP, PROGRESSO HEALTHY CLASSICS VEG, CND, RTS	34	1.76	5.56	0.14
06055	SOUP, SCOTCH BROTH, CND, COND, COMM	66	4.05	7.73	0.91
06455	SOUP, SCOTCH BROTH, CND, PREP W/EQ VOLUME H2O, COMM	33	2.06	3.93	0.46
06180	SOUP, SHARK FIN, REST-PREP	46	3.2	3.8	0.501

NDB #	Food Description (100 gram portions = 3½ ounces = 20 tsp = ½ cup approx.	Calories	Protein	Carbs	Sat Fat
06729	SOUP, SIRLOIN BURGER W/VEG, RTS, SINGLE BRAND	77	4.2	6.8	1.33
06730	SOUP, SPLIT PEA W/ HAM, CHUNKY, RED FAT, RED NA, RTS, SINGLE	76	5.2	11.3	0.3
06738	SOUP, SPLIT PEA W/HAM&BACON, CND, COND, SINGLE BRAND	140	8.6	21.2	0.676
06174	SOUP, STOCK, FISH, HOME-PREPARED	17	2.26	0	0.203
06060	SOUP, STOCKPOT, CND, COND, COMM	78	3.79	8.95	0.67
06460	SOUP, STOCKPOT, CND, PREP W/EQ VOLUME H2O, COMM	40	1.97	4.65	0.35
06061	SOUP, TOMATO BF W/NOODLE, CND, COND, COMM	112	3.55	16.87	1.27
06461	SOUP, TOMATO BF W/NOODLE, CND, PREP W/EQ VOLUME H2O, COM	57	1.83	8.67	0.65
06158	SOUP, TOMATO BISQUE, CND, COND, COMM	96	1.76	18.47	0.42
06558	SOUP, TOMATO BISQUE, CND, PREP W/EQ VOLUME H2O, COMM	50	0.92	9.6	0.22
06358	SOUP, TOMATO BISQUE, CND, PREP W/EQ VOLUME MILK, COMM	79	2.51	11.73	1.25
06063	SOUP, TOMATO RICE, CND, COND, COMM	93	1.64	17.08	0.4
06463	SOUP, TOMATO RICE, CND, PREP W/EQ VOLUME H2O, COMM	48	0.85	8.88	0.21
06099	SOUP, TOMATO VEG MIX, DEHYD, DRY FORM	325	11.73	59.9	2.32
06499	SOUP, TOMATO VEG, DEHYD, PREP W/H2O	22	0.79	4.04	0.15
06159	SOUP, TOMATO, CND, COND, COMM	68	1.64	13.22	0.29
06559	SOUP, TOMATO, CND, PREP W/EQ VOLUME H2O, COMM	35	0.84	6.8	0.15
06359	SOUP, TOMATO, CND, PREP W/EQ VOLUME MILK, COMM	65	2.46	8.99	1.17
06098	SOUP, TOMATO, DEHYD, DRY	360	8.63	68.3	3.81
06498	SOUP, TOMATO, DEHYD, PREP W/H2O	39	0.93	7.32	0.41
06065	SOUP, TURKEY NOODLE, CND, COND, COMM	55	3.11	6.88	0.44
06465	SOUP, TURKEY NOODLE, CND, PREP W/EQ VOLUME H2O, COMM	28	1.6	3.54	0.23
06066	SOUP, TURKEY VEG, CND, COND, COMM	60	2.52	7.05	0.73
06466	SOUP, TURKEY VEG, CND, PREP W/EQ VOLUME H2O, COMM	30	1.28	3.58	0.37
06064	SOUP, TURKEY, CHUNKY, RTS	57	4.33	5.96	0.52
06071	SOUP, VEG BF, CND, COND, COMM	63	4.45	8.11	0.68
06739	SOUP, VEG BF, CND, COND, SINGLE BRAND	53	3.8	7.7	0.231
06100	SOUP, VEG BF, DEHYD, DRY	344	18.91	51.74	3.59
06500	SOUP, VEG BF, DEHYD, PREP W/H2O	21	1.16	3.17	0.22
06742	SOUP, VEG BF, MICROWAVABLE, RTS, SINGLE BRAND	44	6.2	3.3	0.221
06471	SOUP, VEG BF, PREP W/EQ VOLUME H2O, COMM	32	2.29	4.17	0.35
06072	SOUP, VEG W/BF BROTH, CND, COND, COMM	66	2.42	10.7	0.36
06472	SOUP, VEG W/BF BROTH, CND, PREP W/EQ VOLUME H2O, COMM	34	1.23	5.44	0.18
06067	SOUP, VEG, CND, CHUNKY, RTS, COMM	51	1.46	7.92	0.23
06068	SOUP, VEGETARIAN VEG, CND, COND, COMM	59	1.72	9.78	0.24

NDB #	Food Description (100 gram portions = 3½ ounces = 20 tsp = ½ cup approx.	Calories	Protein	Carbs	Sat Fat
06468	SOUP, VEGETARIAN VEG, CND, PREP W/EQ VOLUME H2O, COMM	30	0.87	4.97	0.12
01074	SOUR CRM, IMITN, CULTURED	208	2.4	6.63	17.791
01058	SOUR DRSNG, NON-BUTTERFAT, CULTURED, FILLED CREAM-TYPE	178	3.25	4.68	13.272
09315	SOURSOP, RAW	66	1	16.84	0.051
16117	SOY FLOUR, DEFATTED	329	47.01	38.37	0.136
16115	SOY FLOUR, FULL-FAT, RAW	436	34.54	35.2	2.987
16118	SOY FLOUR, LOW-FAT	372	46.53	37.98	0.969
16417	SOY FLR, DEFATTED, CRUDE PROT BASIS (N X 6.25)	327	51.46	33.93	0.136
16415	SOY FLR, FULL-FAT, RAW, CRUDE PROT BASIS (N X 6.25)	434	37.8	31.93	2.987
16116	SOY FLR, FULL-FAT, RSTD	441	34.8	33.67	3.162
16416	SOY FLR, FULL-FAT, RSTD, CRUDE PROT BASIS (N X 6.25)	439	38.09	30.38	3.162
16418	SOY FLR, LOW-FAT, CRUDE PROT BASIS (N x 6.25)	369	50.93	33.58	0.969
16119	SOY MEAL, DEFATTED, RAW	339	44.95	40.14	0.268
16419	SOY MEAL, DEFATTED, RAW, CRUDE PROT BASIS (N X 6.25)	337	49.2	35.89	0.268
16120	SOY MILK, FLUID	33	2.75	1.81	0.214
16421	SOY PROT CONC, CRUDE PROT BASIS (N X 6.25), ACID WASH	328	63.63	25.41	0.052
16420	SOY PROT CONC, PRODUCED BY ACID WASH	332	58.13	31.21	0.052
16121	SOY PROT CONC, PRODUCED BY ALCOHOL EXTRACTION	332	58.13	31.21	0.052
16422	SOY PROT ISOLATE, K TYPE	338	80.69	7.36	0.422
16423	SOY PROT ISOLATE, K TYPE, CRUDE PROT BASIS	321	88.32	2.59	0.066
16176	SOY PROT ISOLATE, PROT TECHNOLOGIES INTERNATIONAL, PROPL	380	86	0	0.4
16175	SOY PROT ISOLATE, PROT TECHNOLOGIES INTERNATIONAL, SUPRO	388	87.75	0	0.871
16122	SOY PROTEIN ISOLATE	338	80.69	7.36	0.422
16125	SOY SAU MADE FROM HYDROLYZED VEG PROT	41	2.43	7.73	0.006
16124	SOY SAU MADE FROM SOY (TAMARI)	60	10.51	5.57	0.011
16123	SOY SAU MADE FROM SOY&WHEAT (SHOYU)	53	5.17	8.51	0.01
16424	SOY SAU MADE FROM SOY&WHEAT (SHOYU), LO NA	53	5.17	8.51	0.01
11450	SOYBEANS, GREEN, RAW	147	12.95	11.05	0.786
11853	SOYBEANS, GRN, CKD, BLD, DRND, W/SALT	141	12.35	11.05	0.74
11451	SOYBEANS, GRN, CKD, BLD, DRND, WO/SALT	141	12.35	11.05	0.74
16109	SOYBEANS, MATURE CKD, BLD, WO/SALT	173	16.64	9.92	1.297
16409	SOYBEANS, MATURE SEEDS, CKD, BLD, W/SALT	173	16.64	9.92	1.297
16111	SOYBEANS, MATURE SEEDS, DRY RSTD	450	39.58	32.72	3.127
16108	SOYBEANS, MATURE SEEDS, RAW	416	36.49	30.16	2.884
16110	SOYBEANS, MATURE SEEDS, RSTD, SALTED	471	35.22	33.56	3.674

NDB #	Food Description (100 gram portions = 3½ ounces = 20 tsp = ½ cup approx.	Calories	Protein	Carbs	Sat Fat
16410	SOYBEANS, MATURE SEEDS, RSTED, NO SALT ADDED	471	35.22	33.56	3.674
11454	SOYBEANS, MATURE SEEDS, SPROUTED, CKD, STIR-FRIED	125	13.1	9.4	0.985
11924	SOYBEANS, MATURE SEEDS, SPROUTED, CKD, STIR-FRIED, W/SALT	125	13.1	9.4	
11453	SOYBEANS, MATURE SEEDS, SPROUTED, CKD, STMD	81	8.47	6.53	0.617
11923	SOYBEANS, MATURE SEEDS, SPROUTED, CKD, STMD, W/SALT	81	8.47	6.53	0.617
11452	SOYBEANS, MATURE SEEDS, SPROUTED, RAW	122	13.09	9.57	0.929
20321	SPAGHETTI, CKD, ENR, W/ SALT	141	4.77	28.34	0.095
20121	SPAGHETTI, CKD, ENR, WO/ SALT	141	4.77	28.34	0.095
20521	SPAGHETTI, CKD, UNENR, W/ SALT	141	4.77	28.34	0.095
20421	SPAGHETTI, CKD, UNENR, WO/ SALT	141	4.77	28.34	0.095
20120	SPAGHETTI, DRY, ENRICHED	371	12.78	74.69	0.225
20420	SPAGHETTI, DRY, UNENRICHED	371	12.78	74.69	0.225
20123	SPAGHETTI, PROTEIN-FORTIFIED, CKD, ENR (N X 5.70)	164	8.08	31.66	0.032
20523	SPAGHETTI, PROTEIN-FORTIFIED, CKD, ENR (N X 6.25)	164	8.86	30.88	0.032
20122	SPAGHETTI, PROTEIN-FORTIFIED, DRY, ENR (N X 5.70)	375	19.86	67.56	0.328
20622	SPAGHETTI, PROTEIN-FORTIFIED, DRY, ENR (N X 6.25)	374	21.78	65.65	0.328
20127	SPAGHETTI, SPINACH, COOKED	130	4.58	26.15	0.091
20126	SPAGHETTI, SPINACH, DRY	372	13.35	74.81	0.226
20125	SPAGHETTI, WHOLE-WHEAT, CKD	124	5.33	26.54	0.099
20124	SPAGHETTI, WHOLE-WHEAT, DRY	348	14.63	75.03	0.258
02066	SPEARMINT, DRIED	285	19.93	52.04	1.577
02065	SPEARMINT, FRESH	44	3.29	8.41	0.191
02003	SPICES, BASIL, DRIED	251	14.37	60.96	0.24
02004	SPICES, BAY LEAF	313	7.61	74.97	2.28
02006	SPICES, CARDAMOM	311	10.76	68.47	0.68
02041	SPICES, TARRAGON, DRIED	295	22.77	50.22	1.881
02042	SPICES, THYME, DRIED	276	9.11	63.94	2.73
11658	SPINACH SOUFFLE, HOME-PREPARED	161	8.08	2.08	5.256
11854	SPINACH, CKD, BLD, DRND, W/SALT	23	2.97	3.75	0.042
11458	SPINACH, CKD, BLD, DRND, WO/SALT	23	2.97	3.75	0.042
11461	SPINACH, CND, DRND SOL	23	2.81	3.4	0.081
11855	SPINACH, CND, NO SALT, SOL&LIQUIDS	19	2.11	2.92	0.06
11459	SPINACH, CND, REG PK, SOL&LIQUIDS	19	2.11	2.92	0.06
11856	SPINACH, FRZ, CHOPD OR LEAF, CKD, BLD, DRND, W/SALT	28	3.14	5.34	0.033
11464	SPINACH, FRZ, CHOPD OR LEAF, CKD, BLD, DRND, WO/SALT	28	3.14	5.34	0.033

NDB #	Food Description (100 gram portions = 3½ ounces = 20 tsp = ½ cup approx.	Calories	Protein	Carbs	Sat Fat
11463	SPINACH, FRZ, CHOPD OR LEAF, UNPREP	24	2.92	4	0.051
11457	SPINACH, RAW	22	2.86	3.5	0.056
15228	SPINY LOBSTER, MXD SP, CKD, MOIST HEAT	143	26.41	3.12	0.303
15154	SPINY LOBSTER, MXD SP, RAW	112	20.6	2.43	0.237
15216	SPOT, COOKED, DRY HEAT	158	23.73	0	1.859
15103	SPOT, RAW	123	18.51	0	1.45
05162	SQUAB, (PIGEON), LT MEAT WO/SKN, RAW	134	21.76	0	1.18
05161	SQUAB, (PIGEON), MEAT ONLY, RAW	142	17.5	0	1.96
05160	SQUAB, (PIGEON), MEAT&SKN, RAW	294	18.47	0	8.43
11857	SQUASH, SMMR, ALL VAR, CKD, BLD, DRND, W/SALT	20	0.91	4.31	0.064
11642	SQUASH, SMMR, ALL VAR, CKD, BLD, DRND, WO/SALT	20	0.91	4.31	0.064
11641	SQUASH, SMMR, ALL VAR, RAW	20	1.18	4.35	0.044
11858	SQUASH, SMMR, CROOKNECK&STRAIGHTNECK, CKD, BLD, DRND, W	20	0.91	4.31	0.064
11468	SQUASH, SMMR, CROOKNECK&STRAIGHTNECK, CKD, BLD, DRND, W	20	0.91	4.31	0.064
11471	SQUASH, SMMR, CROOKNECK&STRAIGHTNECK, CND, DRND, SOLID,	13	0.61	2.96	0.015
11859	SQUASH, SMMR, CROOKNECK&STRAIGHTNECK, FRZ, CKD, BLD, DRN	25	1.28	5.54	0.04
11474	SQUASH, SMMR, CROOKNECK&STRAIGHTNECK, FRZ, CKD, BLD, DRN	25	1.28	5.54	0.04
11473	SQUASH, SMMR, CROOKNECK&STRAIGHTNECK, FRZ, UNPREP	20	0.83	4.8	0.029
11467	SQUASH, SMMR, CROOKNECK&STRAIGHTNECK, RAW	19	0.94	4.04	0.049
11860	SQUASH, SMMR, SCALLOP, CKD, BLD, DRND, W/SALT	16	1.03	3.3	0.035
11476	SQUASH, SMMR, SCALLOP, CKD, BLD, DRND, WO/SALT	16	1.03	3.3	0.035
11861	SQUASH, SMMR, ZUCCHINI, INCL SKN, CKD, BLD, DRND, W/SALT	16	0.64	3.93	0.01
11478	SQUASH, SMMR, ZUCCHINI, INCL SKN, CKD, BLD, DRND, WO/SALT	16	0.64	3.93	0.01
11862	SQUASH, SMMR, ZUCCHINI, INCL SKN, FRZ, CKD, BLD, DRND, W/SALT	17	1.15	3.56	0.027
11480	SQUASH, SMMR, ZUCCHINI, INCL SKN, FRZ, CKD, BLD, DRND, WO/SA	17	1.15	3.56	0.027
11479	SQUASH, SMMR, ZUCCHINI, INCL SKN, FRZ, UNPREP	17	1.16	3.59	0.027
11477	SQUASH, SMMR, ZUCCHINI, INCL SKN, RAW	14	1.16	2.9	0.029
11481	SQUASH, SMMR, ZUCCHINI, ITALIAN STYLE, CND	29	1.03	6.85	0.023
11475	SQUASH, SUMMER, SCALLOP, RAW	18	1.2	3.84	0.041
11482	SQUASH, WINTER, ACORN, RAW	40	0.8	10.42	0.021
11489	SQUASH, WINTER, HUBBARD, RAW	40	2	8.7	0.103
11864	SQUASH, WNTR, ACORN, CKD, BKD, W/SALT	56	1.12	14.58	0.029
11483	SQUASH, WNTR, ACORN, CKD, BKD, WO/SALT	56	1.12	14.58	0.029
11865	SQUASH, WNTR, ACORN, CKD, BLD, MSHD, W/SALT	34	0.67	8.78	0.017
11484	SQUASH, WNTR, ACORN, CKD, BLD, MSHD, WO/SALT	34	0.67	8.78	0.017

NDB #	Food Description (100 gram portions = 3½ ounces = 20 tsp = ½ cup approx.	Calories	Protein	Carbs	Sat Fat
11863	SQUASH, WNTR, ALL VAR, CKD, BKD, W/SALT	39	0.89	8.75	0.13
11644	SQUASH, WNTR, ALL VAR, CKD, BKD, WO/SALT	39	0.89	8.75	0.13
11643	SQUASH, WNTR, ALL VAR, RAW	37	1.45	8.8	0.046
11866	SQUASH, WNTR, BUTTERNUT, CKD, BKD, W/SALT	40	0.9	10.49	0.019
11486	SQUASH, WNTR, BUTTERNUT, CKD, BKD, WO/SALT	40	0.9	10.49	0.019
11867	SQUASH, WNTR, BUTTERNUT, FRZ, CKD, BLD, W/SALT	39	1.23	10.05	0.014
11488	SQUASH, WNTR, BUTTERNUT, FRZ, CKD, BLD, WO/SALT	39	1.23	10.05	0.014
11487	SQUASH, WNTR, BUTTERNUT, FRZ, UNPREP	57	1.76	14.41	0.021
11485	SQUASH, WNTR, BUTTERNUT, RAW	45	1	11.69	0.021
11868	SQUASH, WNTR, HUBBARD, CKD, BKD, W/SALT	50	2.48	10.81	0.128
11490	SQUASH, WNTR, HUBBARD, CKD, BKD, WO/SALT	50	2.48	10.81	0.128
11869	SQUASH, WNTR, HUBBARD, CKD, BLD, MSHD, W/SALT	30	1.48	6.45	0.076
11491	SQUASH, WNTR, HUBBARD, CKD, BLD, MSHD, WO/SALT	30	1.48	6.45	0.076
11870	SQUASH, WNTR, SPAGHETTI, CKD, BLD, DRND, OR BKD, W/SALT	27	0.66	6.46	0.062
11493	SQUASH, WNTR, SPAGHETTI, CKD, BLD, DRND, OR BKD, WO/SALT	27	0.66	6.46	0.062
11492	SQUASH, WNTR, SPAGHETTI, RAW	31	0.64	6.91	0.117
11953	SQUASH, ZUCCHINI, BABY, RAW	21	2.71	3.1	0.083
15175	SQUID, MIXED SPECIES, RAW	92	15.58	3.08	0.358
15176	SQUID, MXD SP, CKD, FRIED	175	17.94	7.79	1.878
22716	STAGG CLASSIC CHILI W/BNS, CND ENTREE	131	6.97	11.83	2.71
22717	STAGG COUNTRY CHILI W/BNS, CND ENTREE	129	6.27	11.74	2.77
22714	STAGG DYNAMITE CHILI W/BNS, CND ENTREE	135	7.4	12.44	2.29
22715	STAGG RANCHHOUSE CHILI W/BNS, CND ENTREE	115	7.78	12.78	1.06
22718	STAGG SILVERADO CHILI W/BNS, CND ENTREE	92	7.29	13.39	0.39
22615	STOUFFER'S CHICK ENCHLDA&MEX RICE, MONT JACK CHS SAU, FRZ	133	4.4	17.1	1.19
22527	STOUFFER'S CHICK PIE, FRZ ENTREE	202	8.2	12.9	3.79
22579	STOUFFER'S CRMD CHIPPED BF, FRZ ENTREE	140	7.9	5.7	4.03
22554	STOUFFER'S DELUX FRENCH BREAD PIZZA W/SSG, PEPRONI&MUSH	245	9.2	25.4	3.64
22614	STOUFFER'S ESCALLOPED CHICK&NOODLES, FRZ ENTREE	148	6	11.1	2.32
22553	STOUFFER'S FRENCH BREAD PIZZA W/SAUSAGE&PEPPERONI, FRZ	253	10	24.6	4.03
22583	STOUFFER'S HOMESTYLE SALSBRY STK, GRAVY&MACRONI&CHS, F	142	8.3	9.7	2.94
22570	STOUFFER'S LASAGNA W/MEAT&SAU, FRZ ENTREE	129	8.7	12.3	2.19
22581	STOUFFER'S LN CUISINE CHICK A L'ORANGE W/SAU, BROC&RICE, FR	105	9.6	15.1	0.164
22577	STOUFFER'S LN CUISINE CHICK&VEG W/VERMICELLI, FRZ ENTREE	85	6.3	10.8	0.346
22585	STOUFFER'S LN CUISINE HOMESTY STUFF CABGE, MT, TOM SAU, PO	74	4.3	9.6	0.625

NDB #	Food Description (100 gram portions = 3½ ounces = 20 tsp = ½ cup approx.	Calories	Protein	Carbs	Sat Fat
22578	STOUFFER'S LN CUISINE HOMESTYLE BF POT RST, WHIP POT, FRZ E	81	6.8	8.8	0.512
22609	STOUFFER'S LN CUISINE LUNCH EXP RICE&CHICK STIR-FRY, FRZ EN	106	4.6	15.5	0.364
22576	STOUFFER'S LN CUISINE MACARONI&BF IN TOMATO SAU, FRZ ENTR	88	4.9	12.9	0.578
22582	STOUFFER'S LN CUISINE ORIENTAL BF W/VEG&RICE, FRZ MEAL	95	5.3	14.2	0.714
22580	STOUFFER'S LN CUISINE SPAGHETTI W/MEAT SAU, FRZ ENTREE	96	4.4	15.5	0.415
22572	STOUFFER'S LN CUISINE SPAGHETTI W/MEATBALLS&SAU, FRZ ENTR	111	6.7	14.7	0.767
22573	STOUFFER'S LN CUISINE SWEDISH MEATBALLS W/PASTA, FRZ ENTR	107	8.4	12.1	0.939
22611	STOUFFER'S LN CUISN CHICK ENCHLDA SUIZA, SAU&MEX-STY RICE,	117	4.5	20.4	0.57
22610	STOUFFER'S LUNCH EXPRS CHICK ALFREDO W/FETUCINI&VEG, FRZ	137	7	12	2.57
22569	STOUFFER'S STUFFED PEPPERS W/BF IN TOMATO SAU, FRZ ENTREE	86	3.6	9.5	1.24
22602	STOUFFER'S, CRMD SPINACH, FRZ	135	2.8	7.2	2.96
09317	STRAWBERRIES, CND, HVY SYRUP PK, SOL&LIQUIDS	92	0.56	23.53	0.014
09320	STRAWBERRIES, FRZ, SWTND, SLICED	96	0.53	25.92	0.007
09319	STRAWBERRIES, FRZ, SWTND, WHL	78	0.52	21	0.007
09318	STRAWBERRIES, FRZ, UNSWTND	35	0.43	9.13	0.006
09316	STRAWBERRIES, RAW	30	0.61	7.02	0.02
14350	STRAWBERRY-FLAVOR BEV MIX, PDR	387	0.1	99.1	0.035
14351	STRAWBERRY-FLAVOR BEV MIX, PDR, PREP W/ WHL MILK	88	3	12.3	1.91
18354	STRUDEL, APPLE	274	3.3	41.1	2.044
15105	STURGEON, MXD SP, CKD, DRY HEAT	135	20.7	0	1.173
15104	STURGEON, MXD SP, RAW	105	16.14	0	0.915
15106	STURGEON, MXD SP, SMOKED	173	31.2	0	1.037
11871	SUCCOTASH, (CORN&LIMAS), CKD, BLD, DRND, W/SALT	115	5.07	24.38	0.148
11496	SUCCOTASH, (CORN&LIMAS), CKD, BLD, DRND, WO/SALT	115	5.07	24.38	0.148
11497	SUCCOTASH, (CORN&LIMAS), CND, W/CRM STYLE CORN	77	2.64	17.61	0.101
11499	SUCCOTASH, (CORN&LIMAS), CND, W/WHL KERNEL CORN, SOL&LIQ	63	2.6	13.98	0.092
11872	SUCCOTASH, (CORN&LIMAS), FRZ, CKD, BLD, DRND, W/SALT	93	4.31	19.95	0.166
11502	SUCCOTASH, (CORN&LIMAS), FRZ, CKD, BLD, DRND, WO/SALT	93	4.31	19.95	0.166
11501	SUCCOTASH, (CORN&LIMAS), FRZ, UNPREP	93	4.31	19.94	0.166
11495	SUCCOTASH, (CORN&LIMAS), RAW	99	5.03	19.59	0.19
15217	SUCKER, WHITE, CKD, DRY HEAT	119	21.49	0	0.579
15107	SUCKER, WHITE, RAW	92	16.76	0	0.452
09321	SUGAR-APPLES, (SWEETSOP), RAW	94	2.06	23.64	0.048
19334	SUGARS, BROWN	376	0	97.3	0
19335	SUGARS, GRANULATED	387	0	99.9	0

NDB #	Food Description (100 gram portions = 3½ ounces = 20 tsp = ½ cup approx.	Calories	Protein	Carbs	Sat Fat
19340	SUGARS, MAPLE	354	0.1	90.9	0.036
19336	SUGARS, POWDERED	389	0	99.5	0.018
15218	SUNFISH, PUMPKIN SD, CKD, DRY HEAT	114	24.87	0	0.178
15108	SUNFISH, PUMPKIN SEED, RAW	89	19.4	0	0.139
12540	SUNFLOWER SD BUTTER, W/SALT	579	19.66	27.42	5.002
12040	SUNFLOWER SD BUTTER, WO/SALT	579	19.66	27.42	5.002
12041	SUNFLOWER SD FLR, PART DEFATTED	326	48.06	35.83	0.138
12036	SUNFLOWER SD KRNLS, DRIED	570	22.78	18.76	5.195
12537	SUNFLOWER SD KRNLS, DRY RSTD, W/SALT	582	19.33	24.07	5.219
12037	SUNFLOWER SD KRNLS, DRY RSTD, WO/SALT	582	19.33	24.07	5.219
12538	SUNFLOWER SD KRNLS, OIL RSTD, W/SALT	615	21.36	14.73	6.021
12038	SUNFLOWER SD KRNLS, OIL RSTD, WO/SALT	615	21.36	14.73	6.021
12539	SUNFLOWER SD KRNLS, TSTD, W/SALT	619	17.21	20.59	5.953
12039	SUNFLOWER SD KRNLS, TSTD, WO/SALT	619	17.21	20.59	5.953
22363	SUNNY FRSH, BRKFST "STUFF-ITS", PRE-COOKED FRZ EGG&CHS PO	230	10.63	22.99	4.79
22362	SUNNY FRSH, FRZ BAGEL FRENCH TOAST W/MAPLE SYRUP	268	19.75	29.6	1.769
22360	SUNNY FRSH, PRE-COOKED FRZ EGG&CHS BISCUIT SNDWCH	226	9.97	24.83	2.375
22361	SUNNY FRSH, PRE-COOKED FRZ EGG, HAM&CHS BISCUIT SNDWCH	202	10.17	20.94	2.187
15109	SURIMI	99	15.18	6.85	0.18
11503	SWAMP CABBAGE, (SKUNK CABBAGE), RAW	19	2.6	3.14	
11873	SWAMP CABBAGE, CKD, BLD, DRND, W/SALT	20	2.08	3.71	
11504	SWAMP CABBAGE, CKD, BLD, DRND, WO/SALT	20	2.08	3.71	0.039
18355	SWEET ROLLS, CHEESE	360	7.1	43.7	6.059
18356	SWEET ROLLS, CINN, COMMLY PREP W/RAISINS	372	6.2	50.9	3.079
18357	SWEET ROLLS, CINN, REFR DOUGH W/FRSTNG	333	5	51.6	3.081
18358	SWEET ROLLS, CINN, REFR DOUGH W/FRSTNG, BKD	362	5.4	56.1	3.348
22703	SWEET SUE CHICK&DUMPLINGS, CND	91	6.3	9.5	0.748
19337	SWEETENERS, EQ	352	2.18	85.54	0.03
43158	SWEETNER, SACCHARIN	364	0	94	0
11874	SWEETPOTATO LEAVES, CKD, STMD, W/SALT	34	2.32	7.32	0.065
11506	SWEETPOTATO LEAVES, CKD, STMD, WO/SALT	34	2.32	7.32	0.065
11505	SWEETPOTATO LEAVES, RAW	35	4	6.38	0.065
11514	SWEETPOTATO, CANNED, MASHED	101	1.98	23.2	0.043
11875	SWEETPOTATO, CKD, BKD IN SKN, W/SALT	103	1.72	24.27	0.024
11508	SWEETPOTATO, CKD, BKD IN SKN, WO/SALT	103	1.72	24.27	0.024

NDB #	Food Description (100 gram portions = 3½ ounces = 20 tsp = ½ cup approx.	Calories	Protein	Carbs	Sat Fat
11876	SWEETPOTATO, CKD, BLD, WO/SKN, W/SALT	105	1.65	24.28	0.064
11510	SWEETPOTATO, CKD, BLD, WO/SKN, WO/SALT	105	1.65	24.28	0.064
11659	SWEETPOTATO, CKD, CANDIED, HOME-PREPARED	137	0.87	27.86	1.35
11647	SWEETPOTATO, CND, SYRUP PK, DRND SOL	108	1.28	25.36	0.069
11645	SWEETPOTATO, CND, SYRUP PK, SOL&LIQUIDS	89	0.98	20.93	0.043
11512	SWEETPOTATO, CND, VACUUM PK	91	1.65	21.13	0.043
11877	SWEETPOTATO, FRZ, CKD, BKD, W/SALT	100	1.71	23.4	0.026
11517	SWEETPOTATO, FRZ, CKD, BKD, WO/SALT	100	1.71	23.4	0.026
11516	SWEETPOTATO, FRZ, UNPREP	96	1.71	22.22	0.039
11507	SWEETPOTATO, RAW	105	1.65	24.28	0.064
07920	SWISSWURST PORK & BF W/ SWISS CHS SMOKED	306	12.69	2.29	10.47
15111	SWORDFISH, COOKED, DRY HEAT	155	25.39	0	1.406
15110	SWORDFISH, RAW	121	19.8	0	1.097
19348	SYRUPS, CHOC, FUDGE-TYPE	350	4.6	62.9	3.98
19345	SYRUPS, CHOC, HERSHEY'S GENUINE CHOC FLAV LITE SYRUP	146	0.72	34.52	0
19349	SYRUPS, CORN, DARK	282	0	76.6	0
19351	SYRUPS, CORN, HIGH-FRUCTOSE	281	0	76	0
19350	SYRUPS, CORN, LIGHT	282	0	76.6	0
19352	SYRUPS, MALT	318	6.2	71.3	0
19353	SYRUPS, MAPLE	262	0	67.2	0.036
19355	SYRUPS, SORGHUM	290	0	74.9	0
19361	SYRUPS, TABLE BLENDS, CANE&15% MAPLE	279	0.1	75.2	0.018
19362	SYRUPS, TABLE BLENDS, CORN, REFINER, &SUGAR	319	0	83.9	0
19129	SYRUPS, TABLE BLENDS, PANCAKE	287	0	75.7	0
19128	SYRUPS, TABLE BLENDS, PANCAKE, RED-CAL	164	0	44.3	0
19360	SYRUPS, TABLE BLENDS, PANCAKE, W/2% MAPLE	265	0	69.6	0.018
19720	SYRUPS, TABLE BLENDS, PANCAKE, W/2% MAPLE, W/ K	265	0	69.6	0
19113	SYRUPS, TABLE BLENDS, PANCAKE, W/BUTTER	296	0	74.1	1.01
14133	TABASCO TOMATO COCKTAIL, BLOODY MARY MIX, MILD, RTD	23	0.9	4.9	
18360	TACO SHELLS, BAKED	468	7.2	62.4	3.245
18448	TACO SHELLS, BKD, WO/ SALT	468	7.2	62.4	3.245
09322	TAMARINDS, RAW	239	2.8	62.5	0.272
09223	TANGERINE JUC, CND, SWTND	50	0.5	12	0.013
09225	TANGERINE JUC, FRZ CONC, SWTND, DIL W/3 VOLUME H2O	46	0.43	11.06	0.007
09224	TANGERINE JUC, FRZ CONC, SWTND, UNDIL	161	1.5	38.85	0.026

NDB #	Food Description (100 gram portions = 3½ ounces = 20 tsp = ½ cup approx.	Calories	Protein	Carbs	Sat Fat
09221	TANGERINE JUICE, RAW	43	0.5	10.1	0.024
09219	TANGERINES, (MANDARIN ORANGES), CND, JUC PK	37	0.62	9.57	0.003
09220	TANGERINES, (MANDARIN ORANGES), CND, LT SYRUP PK	61	0.45	16.19	0.012
09218	TANGERINES, (MANDARIN ORANGES), RAW	44	0.63	11.19	0.022
20068	TAPIOCA, PEARL, DRY	358	0.19	88.69	0.005
19524	TARO CHIPS	498	2.3	68.1	6.43
11521	TARO LEAVES, CKD, STMD, WO/SALT	24	2.72	4.02	0.083
11520	TARO LEAVES, RAW	42	4.98	6.71	0.151
11523	TARO SHOOTS, CKD, WO/SALT	14	0.73	3.2	0.016
11522	TARO SHOOTS, RAW	11	0.92	2.32	0.018
11878	TARO, COOKED, WITH SALT	142	0.52	34.6	0.023
11519	TARO, COOKED, WITHOUT SALT	142	0.52	34.6	0.023
11879	TARO, LEAVES, CKD, STMD, W/SALT	24	2.72	4.02	0.083
11518	TARO, RAW	112	1.5	26.46	0.041
11880	TARO, SHOOTS, CKD, W/SALT	14	0.73	3.2	0.016
11881	TARO, TAHITIAN, CKD, W/SALT	44	4.16	6.85	0.139
11526	TARO, TAHITIAN, CKD, WO/SALT	44	4.16	6.85	0.139
11525	TARO, TAHITIAN, RAW	44	2.79	6.91	0.197
14544	TEA, BREWED, PREP W/DISTILLED H2O	1	0	0.3	0.002
14355	TEA, BREWED, PREP W/TAP H2O	1	0	0.3	0.002
14352	TEA, BREWED, PREP W/TAP H2O, DECAFFEINATED	1	0	0.3	0.002
14545	TEA, HERB, CHAMOMILE, BREWED	1	0	0.2	0.002
14381	TEA, HERB, OTHER THAN CHAMOMILE, BREWED	1	0	0.2	0.002
14356	TEA, INST, SWTND W/NA SACCHARIN, LEMON-FLAV, PDR, DECAFFEI	332	7.24	81.3	0.074
14375	TEA, INST, SWTND W/NA SACCHARIN, LEMON-FLAVORED, PDR	332	3.3	81.4	0.074
14376	TEA, INST, SWTND W/NA SACCHARIN, LEMON-FLAVORED, PREP	2	0	0.5	0
14357	TEA, INST, SWTND W/SUGAR, LEMN-FLAV, WO/ VIT C, PDR, DECAFFEI	385	0.6	97.6	0.037
14548	TEA, INST, SWTND W/SUGAR, LEMON-FLAVORED, W/ VIT C, PDR	385	0.6	97.6	0.037
14549	TEA, INST, SWTND W/SUGAR, LEMON-FLAVORED, W/ VIT C, PDR, PRE	34	0.1	8.5	0.003
14370	TEA, INST, SWTND W/SUGAR, LEMON-FLAVORED, WO/ VIT C, PDR	385	0.6	97.6	0.037
14371	TEA, INST, SWTND W/SUGAR, LEMON-FLAVORED, WO/ VIT C, PDR, P	34	0.1	8.5	0.003
14368	TEA, INST, UNSWTND, LEMON-FLAVORED, PDR	297	7.4	75.1	0.05
14369	TEA, INST, UNSWTND, LEMON-FLAVORED, PDR, PREP	2	0	0.4	0
14366	TEA, INST, UNSWTND, PDR	256	11.7	57	0.05
14353	TEA, INST, UNSWTND, PDR, DECAFFEINATED	256	19.8	57.1	0.05

NDB #	Food Description (100 gram portions = 3½ ounces = 20 tsp = ½ cup approx.	Calories	Protein	Carbs	Sat Fat
14367	TEA, INST, UNSWTND, PDR, PREP	1	0	0.2	0
16114	TEMPEH	193	18.54	9.39	2.22
16174	TEMPEH, CKD	197	18.19	9.35	3.4
22673	THE BUDGET GOURMET ITALIAN SAUSAGE LASAGNA, FRZ ENTREE	153	6.9	13.4	2.74
22603	THE BUDGET GOURMET, SPINACH AU GRATIN, FRZ	143	4.3	7.4	4.9
14382	THIRST QUENCHER DRK, BTLD	25	0	6.3	0
07078	THURINGER, CERVELAT, SMMR SAUSAGE, BF, PORK	335	15.78	0.26	12.03
02049	THYME, FRESH	101	5.56	24.45	0.467
15113	TILEFISH, COOKED, DRY HEAT	147	24.49	0	0.868
15112	TILEFISH, RAW	96	17.5	0	0.441
18361	TOASTER PASTRIES, BROWN-SUGAR-CINNAMON	412	5.1	68.1	3.639
18362	TOASTER PASTRIES, FRUIT	393	4.7	71.1	1.518
18483	TOASTER PASTRIES, KELLOGG, KELLOG POP TARTS, FRSTD CHOC	391	5	70.84	1.94
18475	TOASTER PASTRIES, KELLOGG, KELLOGG'S POP TARTS, APPL CINN	395	4.4	72.02	1.69
18476	TOASTER PASTRIES, KELLOGG, KELLOGG'S POP TARTS, BLUEBERR	408	4.6	68.38	2.02
18478	TOASTER PASTRIES, KELLOGG, KELLOGG'S POP TARTS, BRWN SUG	438	5.4	64.4	2.08
18477	TOASTER PASTRIES, KELLOGG, KELLOGG'S POP TARTS, FRSTD BLU	391	4.6	71.77	1.98
18481	TOASTER PASTRIES, KELLOGG, KELLOGG'S POP TARTS, FRSTD CHE	393	4.2	71.96	1.94
18482	TOASTER PASTRIES, KELLOGG, KELLOGG'S POP TARTS, FRSTD CH	387	5.1	71.8	1.9
18484	TOASTER PASTRIES, KELLOGG, KELLOGG'S POP TARTS, FRSTD GRA	391	4.4	72.25	1.73
18486	TOASTER PASTRIES, KELLOGG, KELLOGG'S POP TARTS, FRSTD RAS	395	4.2	71.54	1.88
18490	TOASTER PASTRIES, KELLOGG, KELLOGG'S POP TARTS, FRSTD WL	388	4.3	72.9	2.6
18485	TOASTER PASTRIES, KELLOGG, KELLOGG'S POP TARTS, MILK CHOC	395	6.5	68.5	2.9
18487	TOASTER PASTRIES, KELLOGG, KELLOGG'S POP TARTS, S'MORES	392	6.2	69.6	2.8
18488	TOASTER PASTRIES, KELLOGG, KELLOGG'S POP TARTS, STRAWBER	394	4.7	71	2.9
18479	TOASTER PASTRIES, KELLOGG, KELLOGG'S POP TRTS, FRSTD BR S	422	5	68.32	2.26
18480	TOASTER PASTRIES, KELLOGG, KELLOGG'S POPTARTS, CHERRY	393	4.6	71.19	1.67
18489	TOASTER PASTRIES, KELLOGG, KELLOG'S POP TARTS, FRSTD STRA	390	4.4	72.4	2.6
03930	TODDLER FORMULA, MEAD JOHNSON NEXT STEP SOY, PREP FROM	66	2.1	7.8	1.25
03932	TODDLER FORMULA, MEAD JOHNSON NEXT STEP SOY, PRP FROM L	66	1.9	6.6	1.5
16128	TOFU, DRIED-FROZEN (KOYADOFU)	480	47.94	14.56	4.388
16428	TOFU, DRIED-FROZEN (KOYADOFU), PREP W/CA SULFATE	480	47.94	14.56	4.388
16159	TOFU, EX FIRM, PREP W/NIGARI	96	10.41	1.96	0.898
16126	TOFU, FIRM, PREP W/CA SULFATE&MAGNESIUM CHLORIDE (NIGARI)	77	8.04	2.97	0.646
16129	TOFU, FRIED	271	17.19	10.5	2.918

NDB #	Food Description (100 gram portions = 3½ ounces = 20 tsp = ½ cup approx.	Calories	Protein	Carbs	Sat Fat
16429	TOFU, FRIED, PREP W/CA SULFATE	271	17.19	10.5	2.918
16160	TOFU, HARD, PREP W/NIGARI	146	12.68	4.39	1.445
16130	TOFU, OKARA	77	3.22	12.54	0.193
16426	TOFU, RAW, FIRM, PREP W/CA SULFATE	145	15.78	4.28	1.261
16427	TOFU, RAW, REG, PREP W/CA SULFATE	76	8.08	1.88	0.691
16132	TOFU, SALTED&FERMENTED (FUYU)	116	8.15	5.15	1.157
16432	TOFU, SALTED&FERMENTED (FUYU), PREP W/CA SULFATE	116	8.15	5.15	1.157
16127	TOFU, SOFT, PREP W/CA SULFATE&MAGNESIUM CHLORIDE (NIGARI)	61	6.55	1.8	0.533
11954	TOMATILLOS, RAW	32	0.96	5.83	0.139
11540	TOMATO JUC, CND, W/SALT	17	0.76	4.23	0.008
11886	TOMATO JUC, CND, WO/SALT	17	0.76	4.23	0.008
11548	TOMATO POWDER	302	12.91	74.68	0.062
11887	TOMATO PRODUCTS, CND, PASTE, W/SALT	82	3.67	19.3	0.078
11546	TOMATO PRODUCTS, CND, PASTE, WO/SALT	82	3.67	19.3	0.078
11888	TOMATO PRODUCTS, CND, PUREE, W/SALT	40	1.69	9.56	0.021
11547	TOMATO PRODUCTS, CND, PUREE, WO/SALT	40	1.69	9.56	0.021
11549	TOMATO PRODUCTS, CND, SAU	30	1.33	7.18	0.024
11649	TOMATO PRODUCTS, CND, SAU, SPANISH STYLE	33	1.44	7.24	0.038
11555	TOMATO PRODUCTS, CND, SAU, W/HERBS&CHS	59	2.13	10.24	0.627
11551	TOMATO PRODUCTS, CND, SAU, W/MUSHROOMS	35	1.45	8.43	0.017
11553	TOMATO PRODUCTS, CND, SAU, W/ONIONS	42	1.56	9.94	0.03
11557	TOMATO PRODUCTS, CND, SAU, W/ONIONS, GRN PEPPERS, &CELER	41	0.94	8.76	0.133
11559	TOMATO PRODUCTS, CND, SAU, W/TOMATO TIDBITS	32	1.32	7.09	0.055
11693	TOMATOES, CRUSHED, CANNED	32	1.64	7.29	0.04
11527	TOMATOES, GREEN, RAW	24	1.2	5.1	0.028
11695	TOMATOES, ORANGE, RAW	16	1.16	3.18	0.025
11884	TOMATOES, RED, RIPE, CKD, BLD, W/SALT	27	1.07	5.83	0.057
11530	TOMATOES, RED, RIPE, CKD, BLD, WO/SALT	27	1.07	5.83	0.057
11660	TOMATOES, RED, RIPE, CKD, STWD	79	1.96	13.05	0.521
11533	TOMATOES, RED, RIPE, CND, STWD	28	0.95	6.78	0.019
11537	TOMATOES, RED, RIPE, CND, W/GRN CHILIES	15	0.69	3.62	0.011
11535	TOMATOES, RED, RIPE, CND, WEDGES IN TOMATO JUC	26	0.79	6.31	0.023
11885	TOMATOES, RED, RIPE, CND, WHL, NO SALT	19	0.92	4.37	0.019
11531	TOMATOES, RED, RIPE, CND, WHL, REG PK	19	0.92	4.37	0.019
11883	TOMATOES, RED, RIPE, RAW, JUNE THRU OCTOBER AVERAGE	21	0.85	4.64	0.045

NDB #	Food Description (100 gram portions = 3½ ounces = 20 tsp = ½ cup approx.	Calories	Protein	Carbs	Sat Fat
11882	TOMATOES, RED, RIPE, RAW, NOVEMBER THRU MAY AVERAGE	21	0.85	4.64	0.045
11529	TOMATOES, RED, RIPE, RAW, YEAR RND AVERAGE	21	0.85	4.64	0.045
11955	TOMATOES, SUN-DRIED	258	14.11	55.76	0.426
11956	TOMATOES, SUN-DRIED, PACKED IN OIL, DRND	213	5.06	23.33	1.893
11696	TOMATOES, YELLOW, RAW	15	0.98	2.98	0.036
22556	TOMBSTONE ORIGINAL PEPPERONI PIZZA, FRZ, 12 INCH	276	12.8	25	5.31
22555	TOMBSTONE ORIGINAL PEPPERONI PIZZA, FRZ, 9 INCH	272	11.7	25.4	5.16
22560	TOMBSTONE ORIGINAL PEPPERONI&SAUSAGE PIZZA, FRZ	269	11.3	23.1	5.34
22557	TOMBSTONE ORIGINAL SAUSAGE&MUSHROOM PIZZA, FRZ	232	10.9	23.6	3.84
22559	TOMBSTONE ORIGINAL SAUSAGE&PEPPERONI PIZZA, FRZ	262	11.5	24.5	4.87
22565	TONY'S D'PRIMO DEEP DISH SAUSAGE PIZZA, FRZ	277	8.8	28.8	4.07
22562	TONY'S PEPPERONI PIZZA W/ITALIAN STYLE PASTRY CRUST, FRZ	294	10.8	26.3	5.53
22563	TONY'S SAUSAGE&PEPPERONI PIZZA W/ITAL STYLE PASTRY CRUST,	295	10.2	28.2	4.67
22561	TONY'S SUPREME PIZZA, SSG, PEPRONI, MSHRM, GRN&RED PEP, ON,	258	10.2	25.2	4.44
22564	TONY'S TACO STY PIZZA, MEX STY SSG&TACO SAU, CORN STY CRST,	284	9.3	27.8	5.03
19125	TOPPING, CHOCOLATE-FLAVORED HAZELNUT SPRD	498	5.89	61.29	4.275
19364	TOPPINGS, BUTTERSCOTCH OR CARAMEL	252	1.5	65.9	0.11
19365	TOPPINGS, MARSHMLLW CRM	322	0.8	79	0.056
19367	TOPPINGS, NUTS IN SYRUP	408	4.5	53.4	1.96
19366	TOPPINGS, PINEAPPLE	253	0.1	66.4	0.018
19137	TOPPINGS, STRAWBERRY	254	0.2	66.3	0.005
19057	TORTILLA CHIPS, NACHO-FLAVOR	498	7.8	62.4	4.9
19056	TORTILLA CHIPS, PLAIN	501	7	62.9	5.02
19058	TORTILLA CHIPS, RANCH-FLAVOR	490	7.6	64.6	4.56
19063	TORTILLA CHIPS, TACO-FLAVOR	480	7.9	63.1	4.64
18363	TORTILLAS, RTB OR -FRY, CORN	222	5.7	46.6	0.334
18449	TORTILLAS, RTB OR -FRY, CORN, WO/ SALT	222	5.7	46.6	0.334
18364	TORTILLAS, RTB OR -FRY, FLR	325	8.7	55.6	1.745
18450	TORTILLAS, RTB OR -FRY, FLR, WO/ CA	325	8.7	55.6	1.745
21088	TOSTADA WITH GUACAMOLE	138	4.78	12.27	3.78
22566	TOTINO'S PARTY PIZZA CRISP CRUST COMB SSG&PEPRONI PIZZA, FR	253	9.3	23.7	2.91
22568	TOTINO'S PARTY PIZZA CRISP CRUST PEPPERONI, FRZ	251	8.8	23.8	2.62
22531	TOTINO'S PIZZA ROLLS PIZZA SNACKS, HAMBURGER, FRZ	272	11	31.1	
22533	TOTINO'S PIZZA ROLLS PIZZA SNACKS, PEPPERONI. FRZ	273	10.2	28	3.54
22532	TOTINO'S PIZZA ROLLS PIZZA SNACKS, SAUSAGE, FRZ	249	10	28.5	2.45

NDB #	Food Description (100 gram portions = 3½ ounces = 20 tsp = ½ cup approx.	Calories	Protein	Carbs	Sat Fat
19821	TRAIL MIX, REG, UNSALTED	462	13.8	44.9	5.55
19062	TRAIL MIX, REG, W/CHOC CHIPS, SALTED NUTS&SEEDS	484	14.2	44.9	6.1
19822	TRAIL MIX, REG, W/CHOC CHIPS, UNSALTED NUTS&SEEDS	484	14.2	44.9	6.1
19059	TRAIL MIX, REGULAR	462	13.8	44.9	5.55
19061	TRAIL MIX, TROPICAL	407	6.3	65.6	8.48
11928	TREE FERN, CKD, W/SALT	40	0.29	10.98	
11563	TREE FERN, CKD, WO/SALT	40	0.29	10.98	0.009
20069	TRITICALE	336	13.05	72.13	0.366
20070	TRITICALE FLR, WHOLE-GRAIN	338	13.18	73.14	0.318
14139	TROPICANA TWISTER ORANGE STRAWBERRY BANANA DRK, FRZ CO	191	0.4	46.5	
15114	TROUT, MIXED SPECIES, RAW	148	20.77	0	1.149
15219	TROUT, MXD SP, CKD, DRY HEAT	190	26.63	0	1.474
15241	TROUT, RAINBOW, FARMED, CKD, DRY HEAT	169	24.27	0	2.105
15240	TROUT, RAINBOW, FARMED, RAW	138	20.87	0	1.554
15116	TROUT, RAINBOW, WILD, CKD, DRY HEAT	150	22.92	0	1.619
15115	TROUT, RAINBOW, WILD, RAW	119	20.48	0	0.722
15128	TUNA SALAD	187	16.04	9.41	1.544
15117	TUNA, FRESH, BLUEFIN, RAW	144	23.33	0	1.257
15123	TUNA, FRESH, SKIPJACK, RAW	103	22	0	0.328
15127	TUNA, FRESH, YELLOWFIN, RAW	108	23.38	0	0.235
15118	TUNA, FRSH, BLUEFIN, CKD, DRY HEAT	184	29.91	0	1.612
15121	TUNA, LT, CND IN H2O, DRND SOL	116	25.51	0	0.234
15184	TUNA, LT, CND IN H2O, WO/SALT, DRND SOL	116	25.51	0	0.234
15119	TUNA, LT, CND IN OIL, DRND SOL	198	29.13	0	1.534
15183	TUNA, LT, CND IN OIL, WO/SALT, DRND SOL	198	29.13	0	1.534
15220	TUNA, SKIPJACK, FRSH, CKD, DRY HEAT	132	28.21	0	0.42
15126	TUNA, WHITE, CND IN H2O, DRND SOL	128	23.62	0	0.792
15186	TUNA, WHITE, CND IN H2O, WO/SALT, DRND SOL	128	23.62	0	0.792
15124	TUNA, WHITE, CND IN OIL, DRND SOL	186	26.53	0	1.65
15185	TUNA, WHITE, CND IN OIL, WO/SALT, DRND SOL	186	26.53	0	1.65
15221	TUNA, YELLOWFIN, FRSH, CKD, DRY HEAT	139	29.97	0	0.301
15222	TURBOT, EUROPEAN, CKD, DRY HEAT	122	20.58	0	
15129	TURBOT, EUROPEAN, RAW	95	16.05	0	0.75
07944	TURKEY WHITE ROTISSERIE DELI CUT	112	13.5	7.7	0.91
05286	TURKEY AND GRAVY, FROZEN	67	5.88	4.61	0.85

NDB #	Food Description (100 gram portions = 3½ ounces = 20 tsp = ½ cup approx.	Calories	Protein	Carbs	Sat Fat
07079	TURKEY BREAST MEAT	110	22.5	0	0.48
05293	TURKEY BREAST, PRE-BASTED, MEAT&SKN, CKD, RSTD	126	22.16	0	0.98
07080	TURKEY HAM, CURED TURKEY THIGH MEAT	128	18.93	0.37	1.7
05292	TURKEY PATTIES, BREADED, BATTERED, FRIED	283	14	15.7	4.69
22528	TURKEY POT PIE, FRZ ENTREE	176	6.5	17.7	2.88
07081	TURKEY ROLL, LIGHT MEAT	147	18.7	0.53	2.02
07082	TURKEY ROLL, LT&DK MEAT	149	18.14	2.13	2.04
05295	TURKEY RST, BNLESS, FRZ, SEASONED, LT&DK MEAT, RAW	120	17.6	6.4	0.73
05296	TURKEY RST, BNLESS, FRZ, SEASONED, LT&DK MEAT, RSTD	155	21.32	3.07	1.9
05300	TURKEY STKS, BREADED, BATTERED, FRIED	279	14.2	17	4.38
05294	TURKEY THIGH, PRE-BASTED, MEAT&SKN, CKD, RSTD	157	18.8	0	2.65
05190	TURKEY, ALL CLASSES, BACK, MEAT&SKN, CKD, RSTD	243	26.59	0	4.18
05189	TURKEY, ALL CLASSES, BACK, MEAT&SKN, RAW	196	18.11	0	3.66
05192	TURKEY, ALL CLASSES, BREAST, MEAT&SKN, CKD, RSTD	189	28.71	0	2.1
05191	TURKEY, ALL CLASSES, BREAST, MEAT&SKN, RAW	157	21.89	0	1.91
05188	TURKEY, ALL CLASSES, DK MEAT, CKD, RSTD	187	28.57	0	2.42
05184	TURKEY, ALL CLASSES, DK MEAT, MEAT&SKN, CKD, RSTD	221	27.49	0	3.49
05183	TURKEY, ALL CLASSES, DK MEAT, MEAT&SKN, RAW	160	18.92	0	2.58
05187	TURKEY, ALL CLASSES, DK MEAT, RAW	125	20.07	0	1.47
05172	TURKEY, ALL CLASSES, GIBLETS, CKD, SIMMRD, SOME GIBLET FAT	167	26.57	2.09	1.54
05171	TURKEY, ALL CLASSES, GIBLETS, RAW	129	19.36	2.09	1.26
05194	TURKEY, ALL CLASSES, LEG, MEAT&SKN, CKD, RSTD	208	27.87	0	3.06
05193	TURKEY, ALL CLASSES, LEG, MEAT&SKN, RAW	144	19.54	0	2.06
05186	TURKEY, ALL CLASSES, LT MEAT, CKD, RSTD	157	29.9	0	1.03
05182	TURKEY, ALL CLASSES, LT MEAT, MEAT&SKN, CKD, RSTD	197	28.57	0	2.34
05181	TURKEY, ALL CLASSES, LT MEAT, MEAT&SKN, RAW	159	21.64	0	2
05185	TURKEY, ALL CLASSES, LT MEAT, RAW	115	23.56	0	0.5
05168	TURKEY, ALL CLASSES, MEAT ONLY, CKD, RSTD	170	29.32	0	1.64
05167	TURKEY, ALL CLASSES, MEAT ONLY, RAW	119	21.77	0	0.95
05164	TURKEY, ALL CLASSES, MEAT&SKN&GIBLETS&NECK, CKD, RSTD	205	27.98	0.07	2.77
05163	TURKEY, ALL CLASSES, MEAT&SKN&GIBLETS&NECK, RAW	157	20.37	0.08	2.2
05166	TURKEY, ALL CLASSES, MEAT&SKN, CKD, RSTD	208	28.1	0	2.84
05165	TURKEY, ALL CLASSES, MEAT&SKN, RAW	160	20.42	0	2.26
05180	TURKEY, ALL CLASSES, NECK, MEAT ONLY, CKD, SIMMRD	180	26.84	0	2.44
05179	TURKEY, ALL CLASSES, NECK, MEAT ONLY, RAW	135	20.14	0	1.82

NDB #	Food Description (100 gram portions = 3½ ounces = 20 tsp = ½ cup approx.	Calories	Protein	Carbs	Sat Fat
05170	TURKEY, ALL CLASSES, SKN ONLY, CKD, RSTD	442	19.7	0	10.34
05169	TURKEY, ALL CLASSES, SKN ONLY, RAW	387	12.71	0	9.63
05196	TURKEY, ALL CLASSES, WING, MEAT&SKN, CKD, RSTD	229	27.38	0	3.39
05195	TURKEY, ALL CLASSES, WING, MEAT&SKN, RAW	197	20.22	0	3.28
07943	TURKEY, BREAST, SMOKED, LEMON PEPPER FLAVOR, 97% FAT-FRE	95	20.9	1.31	0.22
05284	TURKEY, CND, MEAT ONLY, W/BROTH	163	23.68	0	2
05285	TURKEY, DICED, LT&DK MEAT, SEASONED	138	18.7	1	1.75
05216	TURKEY, FRYER-ROASTERS, BACK, MEAT ONLY, CKD, RSTD	170	28.02	0	1.89
05215	TURKEY, FRYER-ROASTERS, BACK, MEAT ONLY, RAW	120	20.66	0	1.18
05214	TURKEY, FRYER-ROASTERS, BACK, MEAT&SKN, CKD, RSTD	204	26.15	0	2.99
05213	TURKEY, FRYER-ROASTERS, BACK, MEAT&SKN, RAW	151	19.89	0	2.12
05220	TURKEY, FRYER-ROASTERS, BREAST, MEAT ONLY, CKD, RSTD	135	30.06	0	0.24
05219	TURKEY, FRYER-ROASTERS, BREAST, MEAT ONLY, RAW	111	24.6	0	0.21
05218	TURKEY, FRYER-ROASTERS, BREAST, MEAT&SKN, CKD, RSTD	153	29.07	0	0.87
05217	TURKEY, FRYER-ROASTERS, BREAST, MEAT&SKN, RAW	125	23.76	0	0.72
05212	TURKEY, FRYER-ROASTERS, DK MEAT, MEAT ONLY, CKD, RSTD	162	28.84	0	1.45
05211	TURKEY, FRYER-ROASTERS, DK MEAT, MEAT ONLY, RAW	111	20.46	0	0.9
05208	TURKEY, FRYER-ROASTERS, DK MEAT, MEAT&SKN, CKD, RSTD	182	27.69	0	2.12
05207	TURKEY, FRYER-ROASTERS, DK MEAT, MEAT&SKN, RAW	129	20.06	0	1.43
05224	TURKEY, FRYER-ROASTERS, LEG, MEAT ONLY, CKD, RSTD	159	29.19	0	1.27
05223	TURKEY, FRYER-ROASTERS, LEG, MEAT ONLY, RAW	108	20.35	0	0.8
05222	TURKEY, FRYER-ROASTERS, LEG, MEAT&SKN, CKD, RSTD	170	28.49	0	1.67
05221	TURKEY, FRYER-ROASTERS, LEG, MEAT&SKN, RAW	118	20.13	0	1.1
05210	TURKEY, FRYER-ROASTERS, LT MEAT, MEAT ONLY, CKD, RSTD	140	30.19	0	0.38
05209	TURKEY, FRYER-ROASTERS, LT MEAT, MEAT ONLY, RAW	108	24.18	0	0.16
05206	TURKEY, FRYER-ROASTERS, LT MEAT, MEAT&SKN, CKD, RSTD	164	28.77	0	1.25
05205	TURKEY, FRYER-ROASTERS, LT MEAT, MEAT&SKN, RAW	133	23.09	0	1.02
05202	TURKEY, FRYER-ROASTERS, MEAT ONLY, CKD, RSTD	150	29.56	0	0.87
05201	TURKEY, FRYER-ROASTERS, MEAT ONLY, RAW	110	22.32	0	0.53
05198	TURKEY, FRYER-ROASTERS, MEAT&SKN&GIBLETS&NECK, CKD, RST	171	28.08	0.04	1.64
05197	TURKEY, FRYER-ROASTERS, MEAT&SKN&GIBLETS&NECK, RAW	133	22.15	0.05	1.22
05200	TURKEY, FRYER-ROASTERS, MEAT&SKN, CKD, RSTD	172	28.26	0	1.65
05199	TURKEY, FRYER-ROASTERS, MEAT&SKN, RAW	134	22.37	0	1.21
05204	TURKEY, FRYER-ROASTERS, SKN ONLY, CKD, RSTD	299	20.94	0	6.07
05203	TURKEY, FRYER-ROASTERS, SKN ONLY, RAW	283	16.6	0	6.14

NDB #	Food Description (100 gram portions = 3½ ounces = 20 tsp = ½ cup approx.	Calories	Protein	Carbs	Sat Fat
05228	TURKEY, FRYER-ROASTERS, WING, MEAT ONLY, CKD, RSTD	163	30.85	0	1.1
05227	TURKEY, FRYER-ROASTERS, WING, MEAT ONLY, RAW	106	22.49	0	0.36
05226	TURKEY, FRYER-ROASTERS, WING, MEAT&SKN, CKD, RSTD	207	27.65	0	2.71
05225	TURKEY, FRYER-ROASTERS, WING, MEAT&SKN, RAW	159	20.85	0	2.06
05174	TURKEY, GIZZARD, ALL CLASSES, CKD, SIMMRD	163	29.43	0.6	1.11
05173	TURKEY, GIZZARD, ALL CLASSES, RAW	117	19.1	0.62	1.06
05176	TURKEY, HEART, ALL CLASSES, CKD, SIMMRD	177	26.76	2.05	1.75
05175	TURKEY, HEART, ALL CLASSES, RAW	143	18.05	0.65	2.01
05178	TURKEY, LIVER, ALL CLASSES, CKD, SIMMRD	169	23.97	3.43	1.88
05177	TURKEY, LIVER, ALL CLASSES, RAW	137	20.02	4.13	1.25
05304	TURKEY, MECHANICALLY DEBONED, FROM TURKEY FRAMES, RAW	201	13.29	0	5.31
05246	TURKEY, YOUNG HEN, BACK, MEAT&SKN, CKD, RSTD	254	26.41	0	4.54
05245	TURKEY, YOUNG HEN, BACK, MEAT&SKN, RAW	218	17.51	0	4.41
05248	TURKEY, YOUNG HEN, BREAST, MEAT&SKN, CKD, RSTD	194	28.8	0	2.25
05247	TURKEY, YOUNG HEN, BREAST, MEAT&SKN, RAW	167	21.62	0	2.25
05244	TURKEY, YOUNG HEN, DK MEAT, MEAT ONLY, CKD, RSTD	192	28.42	0	2.61
05243	TURKEY, YOUNG HEN, DK MEAT, MEAT ONLY, RAW	130	20.07	0	1.64
05240	TURKEY, YOUNG HEN, DK MEAT, MEAT&SKN, CKD, RSTD	232	27.37	0	3.86
05239	TURKEY, YOUNG HEN, DK MEAT, MEAT&SKN, RAW	172	18.65	0	2.99
05250	TURKEY, YOUNG HEN, LEG, MEAT&SKN, CKD, RSTD	213	27.73	0	3.28
05249	TURKEY, YOUNG HEN, LEG, MEAT&SKN, RAW	151	19.46	0	2.29
05242	TURKEY, YOUNG HEN, LT MEAT, MEAT ONLY, CKD, RSTD	161	29.89	0	1.19
05241	TURKEY, YOUNG HEN, LT MEAT, MEAT ONLY, RAW	116	23.64	0	0.53
05238	TURKEY, YOUNG HEN, LT MEAT, MEAT&SKN, CKD, RSTD	207	28.64	0	2.65
05237	TURKEY, YOUNG HEN, LT MEAT, MEAT&SKN, RAW	165	21.51	0	2.19
05234	TURKEY, YOUNG HEN, MEAT ONLY, CKD, RSTD	175	29.25	0	1.82
05233	TURKEY, YOUNG HEN, MEAT ONLY, RAW	122	21.76	0	1.05
05230	TURKEY, YOUNG HEN, MEAT&SKN&GIBLETS&NECK, CKD, RSTD	215	28	0.07	3.1
05229	TURKEY, YOUNG HEN, MEAT&SKN&GIBLETS&NECK, RAW	166	20.15	0.11	2.49
05232	TURKEY, YOUNG HEN, MEAT&SKN, CKD, RSTD	218	28.09	0	3.18
05231	TURKEY, YOUNG HEN, MEAT&SKN, RAW	168	20.18	0	2.56
05236	TURKEY, YOUNG HEN, SKN ONLY, CKD, RSTD	482	19.03	0	11.59
05235	TURKEY, YOUNG HEN, SKN ONLY, RAW	417	11.79	0	10.6
05252	TURKEY, YOUNG HEN, WING, MEAT&SKN, CKD, RSTD	238	27.3	0	3.68
05251	TURKEY, YOUNG HEN, WING, MEAT&SKN, RAW	210	19.93	0	3.68

NDB #	Food Description (100 gram portions = 3½ ounces = 20 tsp = ½ cup approx.	Calories	Protein	Carbs	Sat Fat
05270	TURKEY, YOUNG TOM, BACK, MEAT&SKN, CKD, RSTD	238	26.8	0	3.97
05269	TURKEY, YOUNG TOM, BACK, MEAT&SKN, RAW	179	18.47	0	3.14
05272	TURKEY, YOUNG TOM, BREAST, MEAT&SKN, CKD, RSTD	189	28.61	0	2.08
05271	TURKEY, YOUNG TOM, BREAST, MEAT&SKN, RAW	151	21.96	0	1.73
05268	TURKEY, YOUNG TOM, DK MEAT, MEAT ONLY, CKD, RSTD	185	28.68	0	2.34
05267	TURKEY, YOUNG TOM, DK MEAT, MEAT ONLY, RAW	123	20.04	0	1.38
05264	TURKEY, YOUNG TOM, DK MEAT, MEAT&SKN, CKD, RSTD	216	27.58	0	3.28
05263	TURKEY, YOUNG TOM, DK MEAT, MEAT&SKN, RAW	152	19.05	0	2.32
05274	TURKEY, YOUNG TOM, LEG, MEAT&SKN, CKD, RSTD	206	27.93	0	2.99
05273	TURKEY, YOUNG TOM, LEG, MEAT&SKN, RAW	141	19.54	0	1.94
05266	TURKEY, YOUNG TOM, LT MEAT, MEAT ONLY, CKD, RSTD	154	29.88	0	0.93
05265	TURKEY, YOUNG TOM, LT MEAT, MEAT ONLY, RAW	114	23.43	0	0.5
05262	TURKEY, YOUNG TOM, LT MEAT, MEAT&SKN, CKD, RSTD	191	28.48	0	2.15
05261	TURKEY, YOUNG TOM, LT MEAT, MEAT&SKN, RAW	156	21.63	0	1.91
05258	TURKEY, YOUNG TOM, MEAT ONLY, CKD, RSTD	168	29.36	0	1.54
05257	TURKEY, YOUNG TOM, MEAT ONLY, RAW	117	21.72	0	0.89
05254	TURKEY, YOUNG TOM, MEAT&SKN&GIBLETS&NECK, CKD, RSTD	199	27.97	0.1	2.58
05253	TURKEY, YOUNG TOM, MEAT&SKN&GIBLETS&NECK, RAW	152	20.39	0.08	2.05
05256	TURKEY, YOUNG TOM, MEAT&SKN, CKD, RSTD	202	28.09	0	2.64
05255	TURKEY, YOUNG TOM, MEAT&SKN, RAW	154	20.45	0	2.1
05260	TURKEY, YOUNG TOM, SKN ONLY, CKD, RSTD	422	20.14	0	9.72
05259	TURKEY, YOUNG TOM, SKN ONLY, RAW	368	13.24	0	9.02
05276	TURKEY, YOUNG TOM, WING, MEAT&SKN, CKD, RSTD	221	27.45	0	3.13
05275	TURKEY, YOUNG TOM, WING, MEAT&SKN, RAW	188	20.45	0	2.99
02043	TURMERIC, GROUND	354	7.83	64.93	3.12
11568	TURNIP GREENS, RAW	27	1.5	5.73	0.07
11893	TURNIP GRNS&TURNIPS, FRZ, CKD, BLD, DRND, W/SALT	17	2.08	2.88	0.027
11577	TURNIP GRNS&TURNIPS, FRZ, CKD, BLD, DRND, WO/SALT	17	2.08	2.88	0.027
11576	TURNIP GRNS&TURNIPS, FRZ, UNPREP	21	2.46	3.4	0.032
11891	TURNIP GRNS, CKD, BLD, DRND, W/SALT	20	1.14	4.36	0.053
11569	TURNIP GRNS, CKD, BLD, DRND, WO/SALT	20	1.14	4.36	0.053
11570	TURNIP GRNS, CND, SOL&LIQUIDS	14	1.36	2.42	0.07
11892	TURNIP GRNS, FRZ, CKD, BLD, DRND, W/SALT	30	3.35	4.98	0.099
11575	TURNIP GRNS, FRZ, CKD, BLD, DRND, WO/SALT	30	3.35	4.98	0.099
11574	TURNIP GRNS, FRZ, UNPREP	22	2.47	3.67	0.073

NDB #	Food Description (100 gram portions = 3½ ounces = 20 tsp = ½ cup approx.	Calories	Protein	Carbs	Sat Fat
11889	TURNIPS, CKD, BLD, DRND, W/SALT	21	0.71	4.9	0.008
11565	TURNIPS, CKD, BLD, DRND, WO/SALT	21	0.71	4.9	0.008
11566	TURNIPS, FROZEN, UNPREPARED	16	1.04	2.94	0.017
11890	TURNIPS, FRZ, CKD, BLD, DRND, W/SALT	23	1.53	4.35	0.025
11567	TURNIPS, FRZ, CKD, BLD, DRND, WO/SALT	23	1.53	4.35	0.025
11564	TURNIPS, RAW	27	0.9	6.23	0.011
22686	TYSON BF STIR FRY KIT;RICE, VEGS, BEEF STRIPS, SAUCE, FRZ ENTR	107	6.37	17.48	
22687	TYSON CHICK FAJITA KIT, FRZ ENTREE, PROD CD 2266-921	121	7.49	16.24	0.78
22688	TYSON CHICK MESQ W/BBQ SAU, CORN, POTATOES AU GRATIN, FRZ	126	6.97	17.63	1.02
22712	TYSON RSTD CHICK W/GARLIC SAU, PASTA&VEG MEDLEY, FRZ ENTR	84	6.64	8.44	0.51
23501	USDA COMMODITY, BF PATTIES W/VPP, FRZ, CKD	247	15.64	7.89	6.253
23506	USDA COMMODITY, BF PATTIES W/VPP, FRZ, RAW	225	15.21	3.84	5.872
23502	USDA COMMODITY, BF, GROUND BULK/COARSE GROUND, FRZ, CKD	259	26.06	0	5.744
23508	USDA COMMODITY, BF, GROUND, BULK/COARSE GROUND, FRZ, RA	228	17.37	0	6.813
23503	USDA COMMODITY, BF, PATTIES (100%), FRZ, CKD	249	22.98	0.91	6.252
23507	USDA COMMODITY, BF, PATTIES (100%), FRZ, RAW	204	14.63	0	6.333
07907	USDA COMMODITY, PORK SAUSAGE, BULK/LINKS/PATTIES, FRZ, RA	231	14.95	0	4.968
10802	USDA COMMODITY, PORK, CURED, HAM, BNLESS, CKD, HTD	149	18.84	0	1.701
10804	USDA COMMODITY, PORK, CURED, HAM, BNLESS, CKD, UNHTD	133	17.44	0.69	1.673
10803	USDA COMMODITY, PORK, GROUND, FINE/COARSE, FRZ, CKD	265	23.55	0	5.515
10805	USDA COMMODITY, PORK, GROUND, FINE/COARSE, FRZ, RAW	221	15.41	0	6.379
07901	USDA COMMODITY, PORK, SAUSAGE, BULK/LINKS/PATTIES, FRZ, CK	267	19.76	0	5.532
11410	USDA COMMODITY, POTATO WEDGES, FRZ	123	2.7	25.5	0.55
15251	USDA COMMODITY, SALMON NUGGETS, BREADED, FRZ, HTD	212	12.69	13.96	1.57
15252	USDA COMMODITY, SALMON NUGGETS, CKD AS PURCHASED, UNHT	189	11.97	11.85	1.497
06178	USDA COMMODITY, SALSA	36	1.5	7	0.029
06143	USDA COMMODITY, SPAGHETTI SAU, MEATLESS, CND	48	1.2	8.7	0.162
05600	USDA COMMODITY, TURKEY HAM, DK MEAT, SMOKED, FRZ	118	16.3	3.1	1.2
02050	VANILLA EXTRACT	288	0.06	12.65	0.01
02051	VANILLA EXTRACT, IMITN, ALCOHOL	237	0.05	2.41	
02052	VANILLA EXTRACT, IMITN, NO ALCOHOL	56	0.03	14.4	0
17270	VEAL, BREAST, FAT, CKD	521	9.4	0	21.407
17273	VEAL, BREAST, PLATE HALF, BNLESS, LN&FAT, CKD, BRSD	282	25.93	0	7.434
17274	VEAL, BREAST, POINT HALF, BNLESS, LN&FAT, CKD, BRSD	248	28.23	0	5.489
17272	VEAL, BREAST, WHL, BNLESS, LN&FAT, CKD, BRSD	266	26.97	0	6.55

NDB #	Food Description (100 gram portions = 3½ ounces = 20 tsp = ½ cup approx.	Calories	Protein	Carbs	Sat Fat
17271	VEAL, BREAST, WHL, BNLESS, LN&FAT, RAW	208	17.47	0	5.896
17275	VEAL, BREAST, WHL, BNLESS, LN, CKD, BRSD	218	30.32	0	3.72
17093	VEAL, COMP OF RTL CUTS, FAT, CKD	642	9.42	0	32.39
17092	VEAL, COMP OF RTL CUTS, FAT, RAW	638	6.02	0	32.92
17089	VEAL, COMP OF RTL CUTS, LN&FAT, CKD	231	30.1	0	4.28
17088	VEAL, COMP OF RTL CUTS, LN&FAT, RAW	144	19.35	0	2.79
17091	VEAL, COMP OF RTL CUTS, LN, CKD	196	31.9	0	1.84
17090	VEAL, COMP OF RTL CUTS, LN, RAW	112	20.2	0	0.86
17141	VEAL, CUBED FOR STEW (LEG&SHLDR), LN, CKD, BRSD	188	34.94	0	1.3
17140	VEAL, CUBED FOR STEW (LEG&SHLDR), LN, RAW	109	20.27	0	0.75
17143	VEAL, GROUND, CKD, BRLD	172	24.38	0	3.04
17142	VEAL, GROUND, RAW	144	19.35	0	2.79
17095	VEAL, LEG (TOP RND), LN&FAT, CKD, BRSD	211	36.16	0	2.53
17096	VEAL, LEG (TOP RND), LN&FAT, CKD, PAN-FRIED, BREADED	228	27.29	9.85	3.06
17097	VEAL, LEG (TOP RND), LN&FAT, CKD, PAN-FRIED, NOT BREADED	211	31.75	0	3.16
17098	VEAL, LEG (TOP RND), LN&FAT, CKD, RSTD	160	27.7	0	1.84
17094	VEAL, LEG (TOP RND), LN&FAT, RAW	117	20.98	0	1.18
17100	VEAL, LEG (TOP RND), LN, CKD, BRSD	203	36.71	0	1.92
17101	VEAL, LEG (TOP RND), LN, CKD, PAN-FRIED, BREADED	206	28.41	9.78	1.6
17102	VEAL, LEG (TOP RND), LN, CKD, PAN-FRIED, NOT BREADED	183	33.17	0	1.29
17103	VEAL, LEG (TOP RND), LN, CKD, RSTD	150	28.07	0	1.22
17099	VEAL, LEG (TOP RND), LN, RAW	107	21.28	0	0.53
17105	VEAL, LOIN, LN&FAT, CKD, BRSD	284	30.19	0	6.73
17106	VEAL, LOIN, LN&FAT, CKD, RSTD	217	24.8	0	5.26
17104	VEAL, LOIN, LN&FAT, RAW	163	18.89	0	3.88
17108	VEAL, LOIN, LN, CKD, BRSD	226	33.57	0	2.55
17109	VEAL, LOIN, LN, CKD, RSTD	175	26.32	0	2.58
17107	VEAL, LOIN, LN, RAW	116	20.17	0	1.01
17111	VEAL, RIB, LN&FAT, CKD, BRSD	251	32.43	0	4.95
17112	VEAL, RIB, LN&FAT, CKD, RSTD	228	23.96	0	5.41
17110	VEAL, RIB, LN&FAT, RAW	162	18.86	0	3.71
17114	VEAL, RIB, LN, CKD, BRSD	218	34.44	0	2.56
17115	VEAL, RIB, LN, CKD, RSTD	177	25.76	0	2.08
17113	VEAL, RIB, LN, RAW	120	19.97	0	1.17
17277	VEAL, SHANK (FORE&HIND), LN&FAT, CKD, BRSD	191	31.54	0	2.078

NDB #	Food Description (100 gram portions = 3½ ounces = 20 tsp = ½ cup approx.	Calories	Protein	Carbs	Sat Fat
17276	VEAL, SHANK (FORE&HIND), LN&FAT, RAW	113	19.15	0	1.06
17279	VEAL, SHANK (FORE&HIND), LN, CKD, BRSD	177	32.22	0	1.14
17278	VEAL, SHANK (FORE&HIND), LN, RAW	108	19.28	0	0.738
17123	VEAL, SHLDR, ARM, LN&FAT, CKD, BRSD	236	33.63	0	3.96
17124	VEAL, SHLDR, ARM, LN&FAT, CKD, RSTD	183	25.46	0	3.51
17122	VEAL, SHLDR, ARM, LN&FAT, RAW	132	19.34	0	2.26
17126	VEAL, SHLDR, ARM, LN, CKD, BRSD	201	35.73	0	1.49
17127	VEAL, SHLDR, ARM, LN, CKD, RSTD	164	26.13	0	2.31
17125	VEAL, SHLDR, ARM, LN, RAW	105	20.04	0	0.65
17129	VEAL, SHLDR, BLADE, LN&FAT, CKD, BRSD	225	31.26	0	3.64
17130	VEAL, SHLDR, BLADE, LN&FAT, CKD, RSTD	186	25.15	0	3.46
17128	VEAL, SHLDR, BLADE, LN&FAT, RAW	129	19.23	0	1.94
17132	VEAL, SHLDR, BLADE, LN, CKD, BRSD	198	32.66	0	1.81
17133	VEAL, SHLDR, BLADE, LN, CKD, RSTD	171	25.64	0	2.57
17131	VEAL, SHLDR, BLADE, LN, RAW	113	19.64	0	0.98
17117	VEAL, SHLDR, WHL (ARM&BLD), LN&FAT, CKD, BRSD	228	32.06	0	3.75
17118	VEAL, SHLDR, WHL (ARM&BLD), LN&FAT, CKD, RSTD	184	25.32	0	3.4
17116	VEAL, SHLDR, WHL (ARM&BLD), LN&FAT, RAW	130	19.27	0	2.05
17120	VEAL, SHLDR, WHL (ARM&BLD), LN, CKD, BRSD	199	33.68	0	1.7
17121	VEAL, SHLDR, WHL (ARM&BLD), LN, CKD, RSTD	170	25.81	0	2.5
17119	VEAL, SHLDR, WHL (ARM&BLD), LN, RAW	112	19.79	0	0.9
17135	VEAL, SIRLOIN, LN&FAT, CKD, BRSD	252	31.26	0	5.18
17136	VEAL, SIRLOIN, LN&FAT, CKD, RSTD	202	25.14	0	4.51
17134	VEAL, SIRLOIN, LN&FAT, RAW	152	19.07	0	3.35
17138	VEAL, SIRLOIN, LN, CKD, BRSD	204	33.96	0	1.82
17139	VEAL, SIRLOIN, LN, CKD, RSTD	168	26.32	0	2.41
17137	VEAL, SIRLOIN, LN, RAW	110	20.2	0	0.78
17189	VEAL, VAR MEATS&BY-PRODUCTS, BRAIN, CKD, BRSD	136	11.48	0	2.18
17190	VEAL, VAR MEATS&BY-PRODUCTS, BRAIN, CKD, PAN-FRIED	213	14.48	0	3.96
17188	VEAL, VAR MEATS&BY-PRODUCTS, BRAIN, RAW	118	10.32	0	1.91
17194	VEAL, VAR MEATS&BY-PRODUCTS, HEART, CKD, BRSD	186	29.12	0.13	1.82
17193	VEAL, VAR MEATS&BY-PRODUCTS, HEART, RAW	110	17.18	0.08	1.07
17198	VEAL, VAR MEATS&BY-PRODUCTS, KIDNEYS, CKD, BRSD	163	26.32	0	1.74
17197	VEAL, VAR MEATS&BY-PRODUCTS, KIDNEYS, RAW	99	15.76	0.85	0.96
17203	VEAL, VAR MEATS&BY-PRODUCTS, LIVER, CKD, BRSD	165	21.63	2.72	2.56

NDB #	Food Description (100 gram portions = 3½ ounces = 20 tsp = ½ cup approx.	Calories	Protein	Carbs	Sat Fat
17204	VEAL, VAR MEATS&BY-PRODUCTS, LIVER, CKD, PAN-FRIED	245	29.77	3.94	4.23
17202	VEAL, VAR MEATS&BY-PRODUCTS, LIVER, RAW	134	17.86	4.59	1.63
17208	VEAL, VAR MEATS&BY-PRODUCTS, LUNGS, CKD, BRSD	104	18.74	0	0.91
17207	VEAL, VAR MEATS&BY-PRODUCTS, LUNGS, RAW	90	16.3	0	0.79
17213	VEAL, VAR MEATS&BY-PRODUCTS, PANCREAS, CKD, BRSD	256	29.1	0	5.01
17212	VEAL, VAR MEATS&BY-PRODUCTS, PANCREAS, RAW	182	15	0	4.51
17217	VEAL, VAR MEATS&BY-PRODUCTS, SPLEEN, CKD, BRSD	129	24.08	0	0.96
17216	VEAL, VAR MEATS&BY-PRODUCTS, SPLEEN, RAW	98	18.3	0	0.73
17219	VEAL, VAR MEATS&BY-PRODUCTS, THYMUS, CKD, BRSD	174	31.58	0	1.48
17218	VEAL, VAR MEATS&BY-PRODUCTS, THYMUS, RAW	99	18	0	0.84
17223	VEAL, VAR MEATS&BY-PRODUCTS, TONGUE, CKD, BRSD	202	25.85	0	4.35
17222	VEAL, VAR MEATS&BY-PRODUCTS, TONGUE, RAW	131	17.18	1.91	2.35
11578	VEGETABLE JUC COCKTAIL, CND	19	0.63	4.55	0.013
04581	VEGETABLE OIL, AVOCADO	884	0	0	11.56
04582	VEGETABLE OIL, CANOLA	884	0	0	7.1
04047	VEGETABLE OIL, COCONUT	862	0	0	86.5
04583	VEGETABLE OIL, MUSTARD	884	0	0	11.582
04588	VEGETABLE OIL, OAT	884	0	0	19.62
04513	VEGETABLE OIL, PALM KERNEL	862	0	0	81.5
04531	VEGETABLE OIL, SOYBN LECITHIN	763	0	0	15.005
04584	VEGETABLE OIL, SUNFLOWER, OLEIC (70%&OVER)	884	0	0	9.748
11581	VEGETABLES, MXD, CND, DRND SOL	47	2.59	9.26	0.051
11579	VEGETABLES, MXD, CND, SOL&LIQUIDS	36	1.42	7.12	0.051
11894	VEGETABLES, MXD, FRZ, CKD, BLD, DRND, W/SALT	59	2.86	13.09	0.031
11584	VEGETABLES, MXD, FRZ, CKD, BLD, DRND, WO/SALT	59	2.86	13.09	0.031
11583	VEGETABLES, MXD, FRZ, UNPREP	64	3.33	13.46	0.098
14122	VERYFINE APPL QUENCHERS APPL RSPBRRY CHRY JUC CKTL, RTD	52	0.1	13	
07083	VIENNA SAUSAGE, CND, BF&PORK	279	10.29	2.04	9.28
02048	VINEGAR, CIDER	14	0	5.9	0
11587	VINESPINACH, (BASELLA), RAW	19	1.8	3.4	
18365	WAFFLES, PLN, FRZ, RTH (INCL BTTRMLK)	251	5.9	38.6	1.296
18403	WAFFLES, PLN, FRZ, RTH, TSTD (INCL BTTRMLK)	264	6.2	40.7	1.439
18367	WAFFLES, PLN, PREP FROM RECIPE	291	7.9	32.9	2.866
12154	WALNUTS, BLACK, DRIED	618	24.06	9.91	3.368
12155	WALNUTS, ENGLISH	654	15.23	13.71	6.126

NDB #	Food Description (100 gram portions = 3½ ounces = 20 tsp = ½ cup approx.	Calories	Protein	Carbs	Sat Fat
11990	WASABI, ROOT, RAW	109	4.8	23.54	
14384	WATER, BTLD, PERRIER	0	0	0	0
14385	WATER, BTLD, POLAND SPRING	0	0	0	0
14429	WATER, MUNICIPAL	0	0	0	0
11588	WATERCHESTNUTS, CHINESE, (MATAI), RAW	97	1.4	23.94	0.026
11590	WATERCHESTNUTS, CHINESE, CND, SOL&LIQUIDS	50	0.88	12.43	0.016
11591	WATERCRESS, RAW	11	2.3	1.29	0.027
12174	WATERMELON SD KRNLS, DRIED	557	28.33	15.31	9.779
09326	WATERMELON, RAW	32	0.62	7.18	0.048
11895	WAXGOURD, (CHINESE PRESERVING MELON), CKD, BLD, DRND, W/S	13	0.4	3.03	0.016
11594	WAXGOURD, (CHINESE PRESERVING MELON), CKD, BLD, DRND, WO	13	0.4	3.03	0.016
11593	WAXGOURD, (CHINESE PRESERVING MELON), RAW	13	0.4	3	0.016
22671	WEIGHT WATCHERS CHICKEN ENCHILADA SUIZA, FRZ ENTREE	111	6.3	13	1.45
22680	WEIGHT WATCHERS MACARONI&BF IN TOMATO SAU, FRZ ENTREE	105	5.8	16.6	0.588
22541	WEIGHT WATCHERS ON-THE-GO CHICK, BROCLI&CHDR POCKT SND	189	9.5	28.1	1.28
22672	WEIGHT WATCHERS SMART ONES RST TURKEY&MUSHROOMS, SAU,	89	6.3	14.4	0.186
22618	WEIGHT WATCHERS ULTIMATE 200 BARBQ GLAZE CHICK, SAU, FRZ	104	9	12.4	0.476
14141	WELCH'S ORCHARD TROPICALS PASSION FRUIT DRK, FRZ CONC	198	0.3	49.3	
20077	WHEAT BRAN, CRUDE	216	15.55	64.51	0.63
20080	WHEAT FLOUR, WHOLE-GRAIN	339	13.7	72.57	0.322
20081	WHEAT FLR, WHITE, ALL-PURPOSE, ENR, BLEACHED	364	10.33	76.31	0.155
20381	WHEAT FLR, WHITE, ALL-PURPOSE, ENR, CALCIUM-FORTIFIED	364	10.33	76.31	0.155
20581	WHEAT FLR, WHITE, ALL-PURPOSE, ENR, UNBLEACHED	364	10.33	76.31	0.155
20082	WHEAT FLR, WHITE, ALL-PURPOSE, SELF-RISING, ENR	354	9.89	74.22	0.154
20481	WHEAT FLR, WHITE, ALL-PURPOSE, UNENR	364	10.33	76.31	0.155
20083	WHEAT FLR, WHITE, BREAD, ENR	361	11.98	72.53	0.244
20084	WHEAT FLR, WHITE, CAKE, ENR	362	8.2	78.03	0.127
20086	WHEAT FLR, WHITE, TORTILLA MIX, ENR	405	9.66	67.14	4.1
20078	WHEAT GERM, CRUDE	360	23.15	51.8	1.665
20076	WHEAT, DURUM	339	13.68	71.13	0.454
20071	WHEAT, HARD RED SPRING	329	15.4	68.03	0.314
20072	WHEAT, HARD RED WINTER	327	12.61	71.18	0.269
20074	WHEAT, HARD WHITE	342	11.31	75.9	0.277
20073	WHEAT, SOFT RED WINTER	331	10.35	74.24	0.289
20075	WHEAT, SOFT WHITE	340	10.69	75.36	0.368

NDB #	Food Description (100 gram portions = 3½ ounces = 20 tsp = ½ cup approx.	Calories	Protein	Carbs	Sat Fat
20087	WHEAT, SPROUTED	198	7.49	42.53	0.206
15178	WHELK, UNSPEC, CKD, MOIST HEAT	275	47.68	15.52	0.062
15177	WHELK, UNSPECIFIED, RAW	137	23.84	7.76	0.031
01113	WHEY, ACID, DRIED	339	11.73	73.45	0.342
01112	WHEY, ACID, FLUID	24	0.76	5.12	0.057
01115	WHEY, SWEET, DRIED	353	12.93	74.46	0.684
01114	WHEY, SWEET, FLUID	27	0.85	5.14	0.23
14530	WHISKEY SOUR MIX, BTLD, W/ K&NA	84	0.1	21.4	0.008
14028	WHISKEY SOUR MIX, BTLD, WO/ K&NA	84	0.1	21.4	0.008
15223	WHITEFISH, MXD SP, CKD, DRY HEAT	172	24.47	0	1.162
15130	WHITEFISH, MXD SP, RAW	134	19.09	0	0.906
15131	WHITEFISH, MXD SP, SMOKED	108	23.4	0	0.228
15132	WHITING, MIXED SPECIES, RAW	90	18.31	0	0.247
15133	WHITING, MXD SP, CKD, DRY HEAT	116	23.48	0	0.4
20089	WILD RICE, COOKED	101	3.99	21.34	0.049
20088	WILD RICE, RAW	357	14.73	74.9	0.156
14553	WINE, NON-ALCOHOLIC	6	0.5	1.1	0
11597	WINGED BEAN LEAVES, RAW	74	5.85	14.1	0.272
11599	WINGED BEAN TUBER, RAW	148	11.6	28.1	0.222
11896	WINGED BEAN, IMMAT SEEDS, CKD, BLD, DRND, W/SALT	38	5.31	3.21	0.181
11596	WINGED BNS, IMMAT SEEDS, CKD, BLD, DRND, WO/SALT	38	5.31	3.21	0.181
11595	WINGED BNS, IMMAT SEEDS, RAW	49	6.95	4.31	0.238
16436	WINGED BNS, MATURE SEEDS, CKD, BLD, W/SALT	147	10.62	14.94	0.825
16135	WINGED BNS, MATURE SEEDS, RAW	409	29.65	41.71	2.303
15224	WOLFFISH, ATLANTIC, CKD, DRY HEAT	123	22.44	0	0.468
15134	WOLFFISH, ATLANTIC, RAW	96	17.5	0	0.365
18368	WONTON WRAPPERS (INCL EGG ROLL WRAPPERS)	291	9.8	57.9	0.263
22126	WORTHINGTON FOODS, LOMA LINDA, BIG FRANKS, MEATLESS FRAN	232	23.77	2.97	1.58
22120	WORTHINGTON FOODS, MORNINGSTAR FARMS “BURGER”CRUMBLE	210	20.14	6.02	2.961
22121	WORTHINGTON FOODS, MORNINGSTAR FARMS BETTER’N BURGER	107	16.36	8.86	0.126
22122	WORTHINGTON FOODS, MORNINGSTAR FARMS BRKFST PATTIES	209	26.1	9.78	1.34
22119	WORTHINGTON FOODS, MORNINGSTAR FARMS DELI FRANKS	248	23.08	8.22	1.985
22118	WORTHINGTON FOODS, MORNINGSTAR FARMS GARDEN VEGE PAT	178	16.73	15.23	0.804
22123	WORTHINGTON FOODS, MORNINGSTAR FARMS, SPICY BLACK BEAN	147	15.11	19.49	0.23
22128	WORTHINGTON FOODS, NAT TOUCH VEGAN BURGERS, FRZ	107	16.36	8.86	0.126

NDB #	Food Description (100 gram portions = 3½ ounces = 20 tsp = ½ cup approx.	Calories	Protein	Carbs	Sat Fat
22127	WORTHINGTON FOODS, NAT TOUCH, GARDEN VEGE PATTIES, FRZ	178	16.73	15.23	0.804
07930	YACHTWURST, W/ PISTACHIO NUTS, CKD	268	14.8	1.4	7.9
11897	YAM, CKD, BLD, DRND, OR BKD, W/SALT	116	1.49	27.6	0.029
11602	YAM, CKD, BLD, DRND, OR BKD, WO/SALT	116	1.49	27.6	0.029
11601	YAM, RAW	118	1.53	27.89	0.037
11898	YAMBEAN (JICAMA), CKD, BLD, DRND, W/SALT	38	0.72	8.82	
11604	YAMBEAN (JICAMA), CKD, BLD, DRND, WO/SALT	38	0.72	8.82	
11603	YAMBEAN (JICAMA), RAW	38	0.72	8.82	0.021
11899	YARDLONG BEAN, CKD, BLD, DRND, W/SALT	47	2.53	9.18	0.026
11200	YARDLONG BEAN, CKD, BLD, DRND, WO/SALT	47	2.53	9.18	0.026
11199	YARDLONG BEAN, RAW	47	2.8	8.35	0.105
16134	YARDLONG BNS, MATURE SEEDS, CKD, BLD, WO/SALT	118	8.29	21.09	0.116
16133	YARDLONG BNS, MATURE SEEDS, RAW	347	24.33	61.91	0.339
16434	YARDLONG BNS, YARDLONG, MATURE SEEDS, CKD, BLD, W/SALT	118	8.29	21.09	0.116
11991	YAUTIA (TANNIER), RAW	98	1.46	23.68	0.082
15225	YELLOWTAIL, MXD SP, CKD, DRY HEAT	187	29.67	0	
15135	YELLOWTAIL, MXD SP, RAW	146	23.14	0	1.28
01121	YOGURT, FRUIT, LOFAT, 10 GRAMS PROT PER 8 OZ	102	4.37	19.05	0.697
01122	YOGURT, FRUIT, LOFAT, 11 GRAMS PROT PER 8 OZ	105	4.86	18.6	0.909
01120	YOGURT, FRUIT, LOFAT, 9 GRAMS PROT PER 8 OZ	99	3.98	18.64	0.742
01117	YOGURT, PLN, LOFAT, 12 GRAMS PROT PER 8 OZ	63	5.25	7.04	1
01118	YOGURT, PLN, SKIM MILK, 13 GRAMS PROT PER 8 OZ	56	5.73	7.68	0.116
01116	YOGURT, PLN, WHL MILK, 8 GRAMS PROT PER 8 OZ	61	3.47	4.66	2.096
01119	YOGURT, VANILLA, LOFAT, 11 GRAMS PROT PER 8 OZ	85	4.93	13.8	0.806
03217	ZWIEBACK	426	10.1	74.2	3.95

Index

A

active men 30
active women 30
alcohol 27
  caloric content 69
  calorie calculator 70
  one drink, defined 69
alertness 31
American Dietetic Association 43
amino acids 31, 32
animal products 32
anti-rejection medications 22
antioxidants 32
appetite 29
Asians 39

B

Bariatric surgery 96
Barry Goldwater 25
beans 32
bedtime 29
behavior change 47 – 49
biking 35
biochemistry 20
blood pressure 27
blood sugar 26, 37, 38, 40
bloodstream 11
BMI 88
  charts 89
body fat 88
body frame 88
booze 25
bound 15
brain 11
brain's fuel gauge 51
bran cereal 26
bread 26
breakfast 95
brown rice 26, 27, 39
bulgur (cracked wheat) 27
buttery spray 104

C

calcium 32
  sources of 117
calorie burning machine 36
calorie-dense 19
calories 11, 12, 28, 35
calories from protein 32
cancer 26
candy 105
canola oil 29
carbohydrates 11, 31, 36
catalyst 18
caution tape 25
cereal 26, 32
cheese 32, 33
children 30
Chinese food 37
chips 21
cholesterol 20, 36
clear tape 19
clinical 21
clogging arteries 36
Columbus Day 106
comfort food 118
comfort foods 17

D

density, foods 97
diabetes 26, 37, 43, 111
duct tape 11- 15, 25, 101

E

eggs 32
emotional crisis 63
emotional distress 110
emotional issues 57
emotional turmoil 46
energy 31
energy expenditure chart 130
equilibrium 36
everything white 26
excess body fat 25
excuse 18
exercise 32, 43
  doesn't burn fat 131
  equipment 132
  weight loss 129

F

fad diet 19, 32, 36
fad diet books 20
farding 94
fast eaters 51
fat 12, 36
  calories from 91
fat accumulation 26
fat cells 111
fat free 78
feel full 31
fiber 26, 35, 40
fish 32
fitting-room mirrors 25
food 54
  lower calorie alternatives 54
  typical male attitudes 54
food cravings 31
food diary 91
Food Guide Pyramid 39
  starches 71
food volume 97
free-radicals 32
fruits 41

G

gagged 15
gastrointestinal 26
glucose 26, 37, 38
glycemic 38
goal setting 109
graham flour 27
Greek pizza 34
ground beef 34
ground turkey 34
guy thing 44 - 47

H

Halloween 106
HDLs 115
he said/she said 47
health 21
health food 22
healthy eating 19
heart disease 26, 36
heart valve 22
herbal supplements 22
high blood pressure 22
high glycemic 26, 28, 38
high-calorie binge 28
high-density foods 97
high-fiber 20
Honeymooner's 25
hunger 37
  defined 52
hunger-inducing 28
hydrogenated 27
hydrogenated oil 79, 115
hypertension 23

I

incomplete proteins 32
insoluble fiber 26
insulin 11, 26, 28, 38
insulin resistance 37 - 38

K

K.I.S.S. 19
keep it simple, successful 135
kidney 14, 22, 31, 32, 43
kilocalorie 30

L

LDL 36 115
lean body mass 86
lifelong weight maintenance 28
lifestyle 37, 43
liver 36
long-term weight loss 19
low-carb diet 36
low-density foods 97
low-fat approach 77
lunch routine 51

M

Mae West 43
man-sized portions 50
Mardi Gras 25
meat 32
meat-protein substitute 32
medical history 31
medical/nutritional 21
men, teenage boys 30
men's health 43
methodology 21
midsection 43
milk 32
mirror 18
monounsaturated fat 27, 29, 33
motivation 18, 107
mumbo-jumbo 20
mummify 15, 19
muscles 31, 36, 57

N

New Year's Eve 106
nutrients 35
Nutrition Facts 79, 80
nuts 32

O

oat bran 20, 21
oatmeal 27
obesity 17, 37
among children 111
physical, psychological 110
U.S. percentage 71
older adults 30
orange juice 67
overfat 86
overweight 14
vs. overfat 86

P

pancreas *14*, 37
pancreas transplant 43
pasta 26, 32, 40
pearl barley 27
photograph 18
pizza 29
polyunsaturated fat 33
popcorn 11, 14, 27, 29
portion size 27, 41
marketing tool 77
misunderstood 71
potatoes 26
poultry 32
professional 21, 22, 36
protein 31
psychological issues 108

Q

questions 29
quick weight loss 35 - 36

R

red wine 11, 69
refined flour 26
refined grains 40
refined white flour 28
registered dietitian 14, 30, 31, 43
  married to 53
regularity 26
research studies 20
restaurants 7
  alternatives 121 - 122
  caloric content 125
  food cost 122 - 123
  regulars 124
  sadly boycotted 123
  strong chairs 125
revenge 15
rice 26
rocket scientists 20
roulette 35

S

salad
  "kits" 122
  w/shredded chicken 121
salad croutons 34
satisfaction 35
saturated fat 29, 36, 115
schools 111
seafood 55
sedentary men, women 30
self loathing 17
self punishment 110
self-esteem 28
self-medicating 31
self-perception 108
self-preservation 35
servings and portions 71 - 75
set point 28, 86
simple carbohydrates 28, 35, 40
simple sugars 39
small meals 52
smaller portions 97
snacking 59
  late night 61
snacks 21
  100 cal. short list 60
sodium 116
  and hypertension 116
  daily limit 117
  depletion of calcium 116
  processed foods 116
  restaurant meals 117
soft drinks 66
soluble fiber 26
sources of calcium 117
soy products 33
soy protein 32, 23
spaghetti sauce 33
special days 105
St. Patrick's 25, 106
stomach's fuel level 51
sugar 65
sugar syrup 25
super sized portions 50
supermarket 122
sweetened drinks 66 - 68

T

teenage boys 30
temptations 15
tension 17
The Duct Tape Diet 11, 58
then and now 113
tranquilizer, food as 37
trans fatty acids 115
  FDA regulations regarding 116
transplant team 14, 43
type 2 diabetes 26, 37, 43
  among children 111

U

underweight 57
USDA Food Guide Pyramid 27, 71-77

V

vacation strategy 99
Valentine's Day 106
vegetable proteins 32
vegetables 41, 103 - 104

W

walk the dog 28, 35
warning, carbs - calories 25
water 26, 126
weight 85
  rule of thumb 86
weight loss
  equipment 102
  risks 37
  strategies 97
weight-loss strategies 97
white carbs 26, 40
white rice 26
white sugar 40
whole grains 27, 39
whole wheat bun 33
whole wheat crackers 27
whole wheat flour 27
whole wheat pasta 26
whole wheat pita 34
women, teenage girls 30
women's diet books 44
wrist band 101
www.ducttapediet.com 18, 102

Y

yams 26
yo-yo effect 38